LIBRARY OF VETERINARY PRACTICE

Digestive Disease in the Dog and Cat

JAMES W. SIMPSON

SDA, BVM & S, MPhil, MRCVS
Department of Veterinary Clinical Studies

RODERICK W. ELSE

BVSc, PhD, MRCVS, MRCPath
Department of Veterinary Pathology

Both of the
Royal (Dick) School of Veterinary Studies,
Summerhall, Edinburgh

OXFORD

BLACKWELL SCIENTIFIC PUBLICATIONS

LONDON EDINBURGH BOSTON

MELBOURNE PARIS BERLIN VIENNA

© 1991 by
Blackwell Scientific Publications
Editorial Offices:
Osney Mead, Oxford OX2 0EL
25 John Street, London WC1N 2BL
23 Ainslie Place, Edinburgh EH3 6AJ
3 Cambridge Center, Cambridge
  Massachusetts 02142, USA
54 University Street, Carlton
  Victoria 3053, Australia

Other Editorial Offices:
Arnette SA
2, rue Casimir-Delavigne
75006 Paris
France

Blackwell Wissenschaft
Meinekestrasse 4
D-1000 Berlin 15
Germany

Blackwell MZV
Feldgasse 13
A-1238 Wien
Austria

First published 1991

Set by Setrite Typesetters, Hong Kong
Printed and bound in Great Britain by
The Alden Press, Oxford

DISTRIBUTORS

Marston Book Services Ltd
PO Box 87
Oxford OX2 0DT
(*Orders*: Tel: 0865−791155
        Fax: 0865−791927
        Telex: 837515)

USA
Mosby−Year Book, Inc.
11830 Westline Industrial Drive
St Louis, Missouri 63146
(*Orders*: Tel: 800 633−6699)

Canada
Mosby−Year Book, Inc.
5240 Finch Avenue East
Scarborough, Ontario
(*Orders*: Tel: 416 298−1588)

Australia
Blackwell Scientific Publications
(Australia) Pty Ltd
54 University Street
Carlton, Victoria 3053
(*Orders*: Tel: 03 347−0300)

British Library
Cataloguing in Publication Data

Simpson, James W.
  Digestive disease in the dog and cat.
  1. Dog−pet disease   2. Cat−pet disease
  I. Title   II. Else, Roderick W.
  III. Series
  636.0896

  ISBN 0−632−02931−5

Contents

Introduction

The accurate diagnosis and effective long-term therapy or control of alimentary disease in the dog and cat have often proved difficult goals to achieve. This has been largely due to a lack of comprehensive information on the specific conditions affecting the alimentary tract together with a lack of suitable practical methods of investigation. Recently, veterinary gastroenterology has advanced rapidly and a great deal of information is now available which can assist the clinician in reaching a definitive diagnosis. Such knowledge allows for more specific and effective treatment.

Some causes of alimentary disease are being elucidated through newer methods of functional investigation and as a result there are only a few cases where a firm diagnosis is difficult to attain. Even in this group, some degree of control of disease is now possible with the advent of specific drugs and management regimes.

One obstacle to the diagnosis and prognosis of some alimentary diseases has been the inaccessability of parts of the gut, such as the small intestine, for visual examination other than by surgical means. This situation has improved substantially with the development of fluoroscopy and endoscopy in tandem with dynamic function tests and the greater availability of suitable equipment for these procedures. Such techniques have obviated the need to resort to laparotomy in some cases, although the latter is still an important and useful approach, particularly in practice situations where sophisticated facilities and equipment may not be readily available.

About 20% of patients entering the consulting room are presented with some form of alimentary disorder characterized by vomiting, diarrhoea or constipation and weight loss. Vomiting and diarrhoea may be simple transient acute disorders which are related to management or dietary upset in young animals or more chronic debilitating diseases in mature and geriatric patients. The majority of these cases have a straightforward aetiology, responding to simple treatment. Other cases, however, require extensive alimentary tract investigation using sophisticated techniques in order to reach a diagnosis. Yet other cases have presenting symptoms of alimentary malfunction as a result of disease in other body organs and in this connection the differential diagnosis of gastrointestinal disease should include a consideration of the hepatobiliary and pancreatic systems, since these organs play major roles in the regulation of digestive and metabolic processes.

A proper investigation of alimentary abnormalities is initiated with a detailed history and should be coupled with a full physical examination since factors which appear to be trivial or irrelevant to the casual observer may be important diagnostic clues. Only on this basis can the clinician decide whether a simple diagnosis can be obtained or whether further investigation is required, and in which direction it should proceed.

The object of this book is to provide the general practitioner with an understanding of the range of conditions affecting the alimentary tract together with a practical approach to the investigation of diseases of this system in the dog and cat. It is *not* intended to be a comprehensive account of all alimentary diseases but rather an account of the types of condition that the authors have encountered in a practice and referral situation.

We have attempted wherever possible in our cases to correlate clinical features with biopsy and clinicopathological findings, and also with autopsy examination, where the latter is relevant in confirming clinical findings or providing information on cases of undiagnosed alimentary disease, or where the clinical diagnosis was in doubt. In addition to describing the clinical symptoms, diagnosis and therapy of a range of alimentary tract conditions, we have included a working approach to the differential diagnosis of alimentary disease, particularly vomiting and diarrhoea. Because investigation of chronic alimentary diseases continues to provide the practitioner with problems in diagnosis we have included a chapter on laboratory methods indicating how such tests may be applied in practice and how they may be interpreted. In addition, because more veterinarians are undertaking alimentary biopsy following endoscopy, as a means to securing a diagnosis, we have included information on these techniques.

Our hope is that the book will be useful in a practical way to clinicians faced with the daily business of investigation of alimentary disease in the dog and cat.

James W. Simpson
Roderick W. Else

1/Diseases of the Oral Cavity and Pharynx

Introduction

The mouth is the entry to the alimentary tract and consists of an oral cavity bordered by fleshy upper and lower lips. It connects via the pharynx to the oesophagus in close proximity and virtual continuity to the larynx and trachea. Although closely related anatomically, the maintenance of the separate integrities of these two passageways is vital.

Dogs and cats with oropharyngeal disease are usually poorly nourished and stunted. Lesions in the oral cavity are often valuable clues to the presence of disease in other parts of the body (e.g. ulceration in uraemia).

There are other closely associated structures such as salivary glands, teeth and regional head and neck lymph nodes which may be primarily or secondarily involved in oropharyngeal disease.

Anatomical considerations

The oral orifice is formed by the upper and lower lips. The free borders of these structures are often heavily pigmented in canines and have exaggerated serrations of their margins near the junctions at the angles of the mouth. The lips and cheeks are lined by stratified squamous epithelium which is reflected onto the mandible and maxilla and becomes continuous with the buccal mucosa and gingival margins. The outer hairy surface of the upper lips adjacent to the nose in cats and dogs has several large sensory tactile hairs.

The lateral margins of the oral cavity are framed by the jaw bones and teeth, with the tongue forming the floor and the hard and soft palates constituting the dorsal roof. The hard palate is covered by stratified squamous epithelium which is thrown into prominent horizontal folds. The caudal part of the soft palate is a soft mobile muscular flap-like structure which forms a nasopharyngeal closure mechanism during swallowing.

The tongue is a highly muscular fleshy structure which is anchored caudally at its root by muscles arising from the hyoid apparatus which forms a sling-like attachment. The tongue is covered by stratified squamous epithelium with modifications on the dorsal surface forming papillae. These papillae are projections covered by epithelial cells containing nerve endings (taste buds). In the cat, there are prominent horny spike-like projections present, the foliate papillae. In the dog, there are many foliate

1

papillae but in addition there are four to six prominent circumvallate papillae (raised, round and surrounded by pits) on the caudodorsal surface.

Teeth are very hard modified epithelial structures which are anchored in the upper and lower jaw bones. The dog and cat have simple or brachydont teeth. They are composed of a central soft gelatinous pulp cavity surrounded by a larger bulk of dentine (modified bone) and coated in very hard enamel (Fig. 1.1). Both species are edentulous at birth but develop a set of deciduous teeth which start erupting at between 2 and 8 weeks after birth. Between 2 (3 in cats) and 6 months of age the deciduous teeth are shed as the permanent teeth erupt; this arrangement may lead to persistent deciduous teeth alongside permanent teeth. Eruption time tends to be earlier in large breeds of dog but even in small breeds and in all cats full crown height of permanent teeth should be achieved by 10 to 12 months of age. The normal dental formulae for dogs and cats are as follows:

	Dog	Cat
Deciduous	3I 1C 3M	3I 1C 3M
	3I 1C 3M	3I 1C 2M
Permanent	3I 1C 4PM 2M	3I 1C 3PM 1M
	3I 1C 4PM 3M	3I 1C 3PM 1M

I = incisor, C = canine, PM = premolar, M = molar.

The incisor teeth in both species have single roots. In the canine upper jaw the first cheek tooth has one root, the second and third have two roots and the rest have three roots. In the lower jaw the first and last cheek teeth have one root and the rest have two. The upper fourth premolar and lower first molar teeth are known as the carnasials. In the cat, the upper jaw first and fourth cheek teeth have single roots, the second has two and the third cheek tooth (feline carnassial) has three roots. In the lower jaw all the cheek teeth have double roots.

In both the dog and cat the mandible is smaller than the maxilla at birth but under normal circumstances of differential growth this relationship alters and the mature mandibular arch is larger than the maxillary arch. However, the maxillary teeth should overlap the mandibular teeth laterally with the maxillary canine tooth caudal to the mandibular one in both the dog and cat. This arrangement provides both species with a shearing action particularly between the cheek teeth. Brachiocephalic and doliocephalic breeds of dogs will show variations.

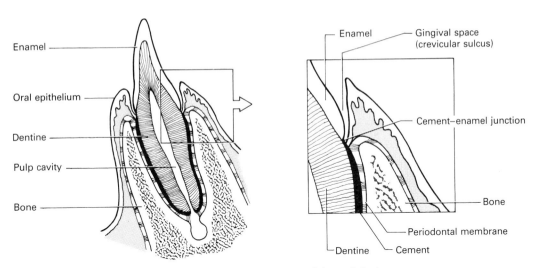

Enamel

Oral epithelium

Dentine

Pulp cavity

Bone

Enamel — Gingival space (crevicular sulcus)

Cement–enamel junction

Bone

Periodontal membrane

Dentine — Cement

Fig. 1.1 Diagram to show the arrangement of the periodonium.

The pharynx is a musculomembranous connecting passage between the oral cavity and oesophagus and also the caudal nasal passage; these regions are known as oropharynx and nasopharynx, respectively. The supporting pharyngeal muscles are striated and function in groups as constrictor or dilator muscles, and they are important in the swallowing reflex. The roof of the oropharynx is formed by the soft palate and its floor is the root of the tongue. Under normal circumstances the oropharynx is solely concerned with the passage of fluid or food except when the animal coughs or mouth breathes.

In the pharynx of the dog and cat there are areas of diffuse lymphoid tissue and solitary nodules known as the tonsils.

Physiological considerations

The functions of the oral cavity are largely controlled by muscles innervated by cranial nerves. The cheeks are innervated by the facial nerve and this activity creates facial expression in addition to altering the cheek capacity. The functions of prehension and mastication are dependent on the closing action of the masseter and temporal muscles, innervated by the mandibular branch of the trigeminal nerve and the closure action of the digastricus muscle innervated by the facial and trigeminal nerves. In both the dog and cat the jaw muscles are powerful, reflecting the carnivorous mode of feeding.

The tongue is rendered mobile by muscles attached to the hyoid and innervated by the hypoglossal nerves. Sensory nerve impulses from the tongue are conducted in the lingual chordatympanic branch of the facial nerve and glossopharyngeal nerves.

The combined efforts of jaws and tongue, together with the cheeks and hard palate serve to perform the functions of prehension and mastication of food prior to the formation of a bolus and movement of same into the oropharynx prior to swallowing.

The majority of muscles around the pharynx are constrictor in action whilst the dilator action is carried out by the stylopharyngeus muscle (attached to the stylohyoid and lateral walls of the pharynx). The vagus and glossopharyngeal nerves are motor to all the pharyngeal muscles. Sensory supply to the pharynx is via the trigeminal, glossopharyngeal and vagus nerves.

Swallowing (deglutition) is a complex mechanism by which a food bolus is transferred from the oral cavity via the pharynx and oesophagus to the stomach. It is a reflex action coordinating many muscles but divided into a voluntary first stage with an involuntary second stage mediated mainly by the glossopharyngeal, vagus and hypoglossal nerves.

In the first stage, food or liquid is forced into the pharynx as a result of a caudodorsal action of the tongue against the palate with a closed mouth. The second involuntary phase commences as the bolus enters the oropharynx. The soft palate is elevated and the oropharynx is closed by a cranial and dorsal movement of the tongue as a sequel to contraction of hyoid and pharyngeal constrictor muscles. The hyoid movement also draws the larynx forward under the root of the tongue and causes the epiglottis to close the aperture of the larynx. At the same time the oesophagus is dilated and pulled forwards to meet the food bolus. The combined effects of pharyngeal constrictor muscles and tongue movement result in passage of bolus into the oesophagus after which oesophageal contraction completes the propulsive effort. After this the soft palate, hyoid apparatus and larynx return to their normal positions and passage of air into the larynx can occur.

Diseases of the mouth and pharynx

Although the mouth is one of the most accessible parts of the alimentary tract, thorough clinical examination requires the use of sedation or anaesthesia, explaining at least in part why, except for a number of well-recognized entities, diseases of the buccal cavity have received relatively scant attention until recently.

The following is an account of the authors' experience of conditions of the canine and feline mouth and pharynx as shown in Table 1.1.

Table 1.1 Primary oral diseases

Congenital/genetic
Skeletal deformity and malocclusion
Cleft palate
Harelip
Enamel defects
Anodontia/polydontia
Anomalous tooth morphology
	Immune-mediated disease
	Autoimmune disease:
	  Pemphigus vulgaris
	  Bullous pemphigoid
	Drug sensitivity (toxic epidermal
	  necrolysis)
	Contact dermatitis
	Secondary immune complex disease
	Grey Collie syndrome

Traumatic disease Lacerations/bite wounds Fractures (bones/teeth) Foreign bodies Chemicals (caustic/toxic) Electrocution	*Neoplasia* Epulis Fibrosarcoma Squamous cell carcinoma Malignant melanoma Ameloblastoma

Infectious disease
Canine viral infections: distemper, infectious
  hepatitis, juvenile papillomatosis
Canine leptospirosis
Feline viral infections: upper respiratory
  tract disease (rhinotracheitis virus — FVR;
  calicivirus — FCV), Feline leukaemia virus
  (FeLV), Feline immunodeficiency virus (FIV),
  Feline panleukopenia virus
Mycotic stomatitis
Necrotizing ulcerative gingivitis
	Non-specific disease
	Malnutrition
	Hypervitaminosis A in cats
	Retained deciduous teeth
	Temporomandibular joint disease
	  (luxation; craniomandibular
	  osteopathy)
	Feline labial (eosinophilic) granuloma

Peridontal disease Gingivitis ($\pm$ hyperplasia) Periodontitis ($\pm$ abscessation) Feline plasmacytic–lymphocytic gingivitis	

Diseases of the lips and cheeks

Congenital and genetic defects

The commonest congenital defect of the lips is the congenital fissure or harelip. It may be midline but is usually unilateral and asymmetrically sited in the upper labium. The condition may be simple or coexist with more serious malformation of the associated maxilla and nasal septum. It is often associated with cleft palate. The defect is clinically obvious and where the nose is involved then serous nasal discharge may occur.

Surgical restructuring of simple lip lesions may be undertaken but the presence of a coexisting maxillary or palate defect complicates the situation. It is questionable whether affected animals should be allowed to breed in view of the likely hereditary implications. Some breeds of dog have coexisting exaggerated labial folds and this may lead to chronic inflammation and dermatitis (see below).

Traumatic lesions

Traumatic lip lesions in both cats and dogs are commonly the result of fighting or bite wounds. Lacerations of the lips with avulsion from their normal attachments may also occur in road traffic accidents.

In these cases the lesions are clinically obvious and require cleansing with removal of impacted grit or other foreign material, such as indriven hairs, prior to surgical restructuring. Where denudation of the mandibular symphysis occurs then difficulties in achieving skin covering may be experienced. Antibiotic coverage should be given in trauma cases. Some authorities (Harvey 1989, Sams & Harvey 1989) have reported lip necrosis as a result of burns acquired by chewing through electrical cords.

Inflammation/infectious diseases

Inflammation of the lips (chelitis) may arise from a number of causes. It may be a response to contact with abrasive or sharp mechanical objects such as tree branches or contact with irritants of chemical, animal or plant origin. Excessive labial folding in certain breeds (e.g. Cocker Spaniels) predisposes to entrapment of saliva and debris, thereby promoting inflammation. Lips frequently become affected in generalized skin diseases such as demodectic mange, pemphigus vulgaris and bullous pemphigoid.

Clinically affected animals are often presented with halitosis and a history of pawing at the mouth or rubbing the muzzle along the ground. Excessive salivation (ptyalism) may be a feature, together with brown staining of the skin. If the condition is chronic then the lips may be irregularly thickened or have multiple nodules as a result of inflamed hair follicles or small chronic abscesses on the non-glabrous surface.

In cats the so-called eosinophilic granuloma or chronic labial ulcer may form an initial lesion which is aggravated into a more generalized chelitis by licking. The initial lesion is usually on an upper lip near the midline and may be accompanied by lesions elsewhere, notably the skin of the hind limbs. Diagnosis of the condition is made by histopathological examination of lesion biopsy.

Treatment of chelitis depends on the removal of the inciting cause. Injuries to the lips should be repaired and any foreign bodies removed. Infected and hairy lesions should be cleansed and excessive hair removed.

In the case of lip fold dermatitis, resection of excess tissue and remodelling may be carried out. Antibiotic or sulphonamide preparations should be used but in our experience topical creams are of little benefit since patients tend to lick them off. Elizabethan collars may be useful in preventing self-trauma. In the case of feline eosinophilic granuloma, systematic cortico-steroids given orally are helpful (prednisolone at a dose of 0.5 mg/kg twice daily until lesions regress, then on a reducing dose over the next 2 weeks) and megestrol acetate (Ovarid; Coopers Pitman-Moore) may be used at a dosage of 2.5 mg twice weekly.

Neoplasia

Tumours affecting the lips are often found to arise from the mucosal surface and because of their position are subject to abrasion and ulceration.

In the dog the buccal surfaces of the lips are often involved in melanotic tumours and over the last decade the authors have seen an increasing number of lymphohistiocytic labial neoplasms. A wide variety of skin and connective tissue tumours may affect the outer surface of the lips; these are often benign (e.g. sebaceous adenomas, hair follicle tumours) but more aggressive tumours may also occur (mast cell tumours). Surgical excision with histopathological diagnosis should be carried out.

In the cat, the lips may become involved in squamous cell carcinoma arising in the adjacent buccal cavity. Eosinophilic granuloma may masquerade as neoplasia and biopsy should be undertaken to determine a diagnosis.

Disorders of the jaw and teeth

The term jaws refers here to the maxillary and mandibular bones delineating the buccal cavity.

Congenital defects

Genetic factors can influence the degree of normal occlusion. In some canine breeds the degree of prognathia or retrognathia can be excessive resulting in malocclusion; the Boxer and English Bulldog are prime examples. Since these features are often the result of intentional breeding programmes, appropriate breeding advice should be given to eliminate excesses of malocclusion.

Retained or persistent deciduous teeth may cause displacement of permanent teeth (Dillon 1986). This situation is not uncommon in some toy breeds of dog (Yorkshire Terriers) and leads to disinclination to eat and pain on mastication. Surgical removal of temporary supernumerary teeth should be effected.

Abnormalities of permanent teeth of genetic origin occur rather uncommonly and include abnormal morphology, ectopia or absence (anodontia)
of one or more teeth. Occasionally enamel defects occur and these have
been related to a porphyria syndrome in cats (Sams & Harvey 1989).

Trauma

The commonest type of traumatic jaw lesion is that of skeletal fracture,
usually as a result of a road traffic accident. Cats particularly suffer from
mandibular symphyseal separation or more extensive mandibular fracturing.

Affected animals are presented with a history of trauma or road traffic
accident. On examination they often have clear evidence of jaw asymmetry,
and radiography confirms the extent and sites of damage.

Treatment involving fixation with figure-of-eight wiring around the canine
teeth or more extensive pinning is usually successful in cats. Canine patients
may require more extensive orthopaedic correction using pins, plates or
wire suturing. Maxillary lesions may not require surgical intervention,
depending on the degree of compression of adjacent structures and the
degree of dental malocclusion.

Temporomandibular joint luxation is seen in dogs and cats as a result of
trauma but may occur spontaneously in some breeds of dogs (Irish Setters,
Bassett Hounds, Golden Retrievers). Radiography is essential in differentiating
a subluxation from a fracture since the clinical presentation of a painful
dropped jaw is the same in both cases. The luxation can be corrected under
general anaesthesia using a wooden or plastic rod to separate the teeth
whilst pushing the mandible in a cranial or caudal direction as required.
Where the condition is the result of joint dysplasia then mandibular condyl-
ectomy is said to be beneficial (Lantz 1985).

Trauma to teeth is usually associated with road traffic accidents; broken
teeth should be extracted under general anaesthesia taking care to remove
all root material.

Inflammation

Osteomyelitis of the jaw bones is rare although localized inflammation may
follow severe periodontal disease and infection (see below). Craniomandibular
osteopathy is characterized by bony proliferation and exostosis of the base
of the skull and mandible and is occasionally seen in young West Highland
Terriers causing dysphagia and pain on jaw opening. Radiographic examination reveals the abnormal exostosis which usually involves the temporomandibular joint. The cause of the condition is unknown and the prognosis
very guarded in view of the joint involvement.

Enamel hypoplasia is uncommonly encountered in dogs. True hypoplasia of enamel is the result of failure of enamel to form before dental eruption rather than posteruptive damage. The major cause of enamel hypoplasia is canine distemper infection. The virus damages the inner enamel-forming epithelium and when teeth erupt they have a dull chalky surface which is often pitted or grooved with dark brown staining of pitted areas. The dark areas are caused by secondary deposits of dentine. Hypoplastic enamel has also been produced in puppies by feeding pregnant bitches on diets deficient in fat-soluble vitamins but dietary induction of enamel hypoplasia does not seem to be a major problem in the authors' experience.

Dental caries is caused by the local fermentation of starches and sugar residues lodged in the centres of the tooth table. This reaction results in decalcification of enamel and dentine. It occurs in dogs but not in cats because of the absence of retaining centres of teeth in the latter species. The first upper molar teeth are usually affected (Lane 1982). The lesions do not progress to produce the pain and abscessation associated with human caries because secondary dentine fills the pulp cavity throughout life, thereby preventing infection of the cavity.

Neoplasia

Neoplasms affecting the jaw bones in both cats and dogs are usually soft tissue tumours (e.g. squamous cell carcinoma, fibrosarcoma) which have eroded and invaded bony areas adjacent to their sites of origin. Such neoplastic invasion manifests itself as pathological jaw fractures although the tumour mass may often be apparent well before this stage is reached.

Neoplasia of the dental structures is uncommon in the dog and cat. Occasionally tumours arise from the enamel organ and form an ameloblastoma usually in the mandible.

In common with other oral tumours these lesions are often well advanced by the time they are recognized by pain and bloody salivation. Lesions are often proliferative and ulcerated. Diagnosis can be achieved through biopsy and histological examination. Cytological examination may be helpful although in this particular type of tumour it is of less assistance. Therapy usually involves surgical excision or debulking. At least one report suggested that radiotherapy may be effective for this type of tumour (Langham *et al.* 1977).

Diseases of the oral cavity

The oral cavity is subject not only to primary disease but also to secondary disease i.e. systemic diseases which cause oral changes.

Congenital defects

The commonest congenital defect in the dog and cat is a midline defect of the hard palate resulting in a variably-sized connection between the buccal cavity and the nasal chambers. The soft palate is less commonly affected in our experience and cats have a lower incidence of the defect. It is generally agreed that whereas hare-lip has a definite hereditary basis, clefts of the hard palate may be the result of a complex interaction of chromosomal aberration, teratogenic influences, mechanical and traumatic effects during gestation. Purebred dogs have three times the risk of crossbred animals (Johnston 1980).

Severely affected animals are presented early with dramatic fluid discharges from the nose but more subtle defects may not be so readily apparent. Affected animals may be stunted and have other congenital defects such as cardiac anomalies. Diagnosis can be made on clinical examination, the extent of the defect being assessed with the assistance of radiographs.

Repair can be effected surgically in both species using overlapping or double-flap techniques (Harvey 1987) although success is usually greater in dogs because the tissues are more delicate in cats.

Trauma

Disruption and distortion of the oral cavity may occur as part of road traffic accident trauma where the jaws are fractured. Lacerations of cheeks and associated structures require surgical repair but buccal mucosa heals rapidly unless there is secondary infection or embedded foreign material such as hair or grit.

Foreign body lodgement in the oral cavity of dogs and cats is occasionally seen, especially in animals which are indiscriminate feeders or stick chewers. Pieces of wood, fragments of bone or pieces of plastic have been encountered in dogs; they are usually wedged between teeth or across the roof of the mouth. In cats, fish bones may become similarly lodged; other foreign bodies in this species include needles and fish hooks. A major complication of sharp foreign bodies is that they may become impaled in the gingivae or palates and work their way into the deeper tissues. In dogs sharp plant awns may produce nodular granulomatous inflammation (McKeever & Klausner 1986).

The presence of foreign bodies is usually indicated by pawing at the mouth and attempts to dislodge the object by rubbing the muzzle along the ground. Dysphagia may be accompanied by hypersalivation and retching. If the object has been present for a while then a foul odour may be detected. Foreign bodies are usually identified and removed by careful manipulation under light anaesthesia unless the patient is cooperative, when sedation alone may be sufficient. Artery forceps are particularly useful for removing bone fragments and wood splinters; deeply-embedded material requires more extensive surgical removal. The presence of embedded needles may be detected by radiography. Postoperative treatment should include antibiotic as well as antiseptic cleansing if the degree of abrasion or penetration has been severe.

Chemical agents may cause oral damage and generalized oral inflammation (stomatitis). Phenolic disinfectants or alkaline caustic agents may be involved and immediate treatment should aim to neutralize any strong alkaline effects by lavage with dilute acids such as vinegar or lemon juice. Subsequent management should consist of cleansing with mild antiseptic or sodium bicarbonate solutions. Acid damage should be treated with dilute sodium bicarbonate.

Inflammatory and infectious diseases

Generalized inflammation of the mouth (stomatitis) rarely occurs without the involvement of a similar reaction in the gums (gingivitis) and the tongue (glossitis). Stomatitis may be a relatively uncomplicated primary condition associated with chemical, thermal or mechanical irritations, or more frequently arising from the action of infectious agents. A state of secondary stomatitis may result from systemic viral infections (e.g. canine distemper, feline immunodeficiency virus) and, in the cat, nutritional deficiency. However, the commonest cause of stomatitis in mature and older dogs and cats is probably an extension of gingivitis accompanying periodontal disease.

Clinical signs of stomatitis may vary considerably depending on the causal mechanism. Chemical or mechanical irritants usually result in sudden and dramatic symptoms characterized by pain, severe ptyalism and complete dysphagia. Infections of viral origin on the other hand induce more insidious anorexia, variable thirst, halitosis and escalating pain depending on the degree of tissue damage. Complete examination usually requires sedation or light anaesthesia. Although clinical examination alone is usually sufficient to establish the presence of stomatitis, lesion swabbing and cytological examination may be helpful in indicating the nature of the reaction. In addition, in the case of the cat, a test for feline leukaemia virus (FeLV) and feline immunodeficiency virus (FIV) should be carried out where there is stomatitis or ulceration.

General therapy for stomatitis not associated with more severe systemic disease should include cleansing with sterile saline or weak sodium bicarbonate solution. Lavage with a weak antiseptic (0.2% chlorhexidine) may be helpful and use of antibiotics, fungicides or metronidazole preparations may be necessary. Recalcitrant ulceration may require cautery to initiate resolution.

Stomatitis and gingivitis may be caused by a variety of infectious agents as follows:

1 Infectious oral papillomatosis — occurs in young dogs and is characterized by the development of benign papillomas. Lesions may affect the mouth, lips, tongue and pharynx and although they are usually self-limiting and resolve within 3 months, occasionally cases are severe enough to cause dysphagia or dyspnoea. Florid lesions (Fig. 1.2) require surgical removal and electrocautery. Recurrence is not usually seen although it has been recorded in some individuals; in these cases cyclophosphamide therapy may be necessary.

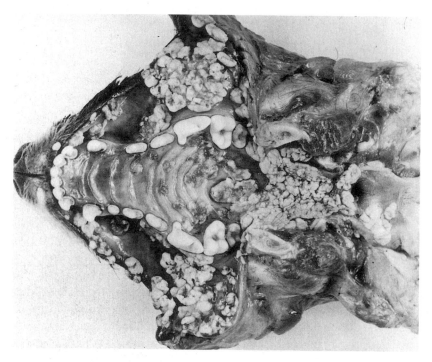

Fig. 1.2 Multiple nodular growths characteristic of severe papillomatosis in the oropharynx and on the lips of a 2-year-old crossbred dog.

2 Feline viral diseases — oral lesions are often seen in association with systemic viral infections of cats.

(a) Feline calicivirus (FCV) and FVR — cause respiratory infections but also induce ulcerative stomatitis with painful ulceration of the tongue, hard palate and fauces regions. The lesions are usually most severe in calcivirus infection and start as small vesicles on the dorsolateral margins of the tongue which then coalesce and rupture. The hard palate, lips and pharynx can become involved leading to anorexia. Feeding hard dry food exacerbates lesions. Affected cats and kittens often present primarily with respiratory disease but pyrexia and anorexia due to mouth pain continue after respiratory signs subside. Treatment of affected animals is supportive with antibiotic coverage to prevent secondary bacterial infection. High quality protein should be fed, if necessary through a pharyngostomy tube, together with parenteral fluids to correct dehydration. Vitamin B preparations are also useful.

Oral lesions are caused less frequently by feline rhinotrachietis virus but can be extensive and severe when they occur (Sams & Harvey 1989).

(b) Feline panleucopenia virus. Although the usual manifestation of panleucopenia virus infection in susceptible cats and kittens is gastro-intestinal upset, oral lesions may also be seen. These include ulcerative stomatitis and necrotic gingivitis with ulceration of hard and soft palates. Therapy should be supportive with broad spectrum antibiotic coverage to prevent secondary bacterial infection.

(c) Feline leukaemia virus and FIV. Oral lesions are not uncommon in FeLV-positive cats and these usually take the form of chronic stomatitis and gingivitis. Ulcers occur on the tongue, gingivae and in the fauces region. Presenting symptoms are those of anorexia and dysphagia in addition to other signs related more directly to FeLV infection. Treatment of oral lesions should be supportive but the overall prognosis is poor. More recently FIV has been associated with oral ulceration or stomatitis progressing to gingivitis (Pedersen *et al.* 1987). In these cases, as in the case of FeLV infection, the oral involvement is probably a reflection of

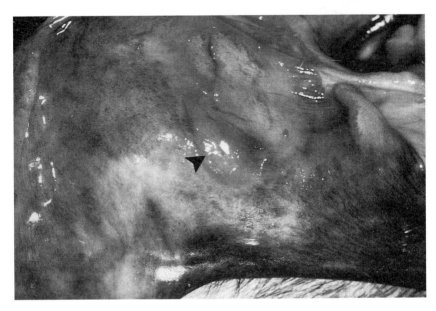

Fig. 1.3 Buccal ulceration at the angle of the jaws in an 8-month-old dog with suspected distemper.

the immune suppression inherent in the infection. Serological tests are necessary to differentiate FVR, FCV and FIV infections.

3   Canine viral infections — ulceration (Fig. 1.3) followed by a non-specific stomatitis has been associated with infectious canine hepatitis (ICH) and distemper in young dogs and susceptible unvaccinated adults which develop chronic forms of these diseases. The oral lesions are part of a generalized viral onslaught on epithelial cells, and clinical symptoms are usually attributable to damage in other parenchymatous organs. In addition to the symptoms classically associated with ICH or distemper, oral lesions lead to pain, dysphagia and anorexia. Therapy should be supportive and aimed at prevention of secondary bacterial infection.

4   Mycotic stomatitis — stomatitis resulting from fungal infection is uncommon in the dog and has not been seen by the authors in the cat. *Candida albicans* may cause a severe stomatitis in dogs, usually in immunosuppressed individuals or dogs that have received long-term or high doses of corticosteroids. The lesions are irregular ulcerations surrounded by inflammation, and yeast-like organisms can be cultured. Pseudomembranous white lesions (thrush) are less likely. Aspergillus infections may rarely spread from the nasal chambers into the oral cavity. Systemic antifungal therapy (e.g. ketaconazole) is often more effective than local application alone and patients should be carefully assessed for bacterial infections and immune suppression since fungal infection is often a complication of these diseases.

Immune-mediated diseases

Immune-mediated diseases have become increasingly important in veterinary medicine over the last decade and oral lesions may be seen in both immune deficiency disease and autoimmune disorders as part of a generalized syndrome. Immune deficiency states often lead to worsening of local oral disease such as stomatitis or periodontal disease and allow fungal infections to become established. Autoimmune diseases affecting the skin, ears and oral cavity are commonly seen in the dog and occasionally in the cat. These are bullous diseases of the skin and mucosae which result from the reaction of circulating autoantibodies to intercellular epidermal antigens.

1   Pemphigus vulgaris — this is now a well-recognized condition in the dog (Stannard *et al.* 1975, Bennett *et al.* 1980) and more recently in the cat (Scott 1984). There is no particular breed or sex distribution. Lesions affect principally the oral mucosa (Fig. 1.4), nares, lips, periorbital skin, anus, prepuce or vulva. Initially lesions form as vesicles and develop into larger intraepidermal bullae which rupture to leave well-defined ulcers. In advanced cases bullae may not be obvious, but rather extensive non-responsive ulcers may be found.

Clinical symptoms are those of dysphagia, pain and halitosis although

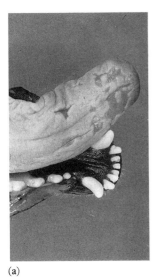

(a)

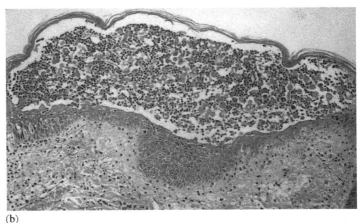

(b)

Fig. 1.4 (a) Tongue of a 3-year-old Border Collie with pemphigus vulgaris. Note extensive ulceration following bullous lesions, and (b) histopathological section of a typical bulla lesion from case (a).

affected dogs are usually presented because of the more obvious nasal and periocular skin lesions. Diagnosis depends on biopsy and histological detection of bullae and clefting within the epidermis, together with immunofluorescent detection of immunoglobulin G in the epidermis or circulating antibodies to intracellular cement (Ackerman 1985a). Treatment is dependent on high corticosteroid therapy (2 mg/kg/day prednisolone) to control lesions initially, together with antibiotics and local antiseptic dressing as adjuncts. Some cases may respond and go into remission thus allowing a tapered down dosage of corticosteroids. Others do not attain remission on corticosteroids and cyclophosphamide therapy may be contemplated (2.2 mg/kg/day initially tapering to 1 mg/kg every second day).

2   Bullous pemphigoid — this is a less common but macroscopically similar autoimmune disease with relatively greater skin involvement. The lesions in this disease are also vesicles and bullae but they develop with clefting immediately below the epidermis. Affected dogs are often presented with skin lesions which are non-responsive to simple antibiotic and low-dose corticosteroid therapy. Diagnosis depends on careful histopathological examination of biopsies and immunofluorescent demonstration of immunoglobulin G and complement (C3) at the basement membrane zone (Ackerman 1985b). The therapy for bullous pemphigoid is essentially the same as for pemphigus vulgaris, namely corticosteroids or cyclophosphamide.

3   Other immune-mediated diseases — the oral cavity is often a site of expression of known or suspected immune-mediated stomatitis. These conditions are in many cases poorly understood; they include contact dermatitis, secondary immune complex disease, toxic epidermal necrolysis caused by adverse reactions to drugs or Staphyloccocal organisms or in the case of the cat, FeLV and FIV infections. Stomatitis and gingivitis have been described

as part of the Grey Collie syndrome which is characterized by cyclic neutro-penia, thrombocytopenia, lameness and malabsorption (Cheville 1968).

Periodontal disease

Periodontal disease is perhaps the most common oral disease seen in dogs and cats and involves the periodontium, the tissues surrounding and sup-porting the teeth in their sockets (i.e. alveolar bone, periodontal membrane, cementum, gingivae, see Fig. 1.1). Periodontal disease is the major cause of tooth loss in both dogs and cats although there are some significant species differences. As far as dogs are concerned there are significant breed differ-ences in the incidence of periodontal disease, e.g. small breeds such as Miniature Poodles have a high incidence compared with German Shepherds (Harvey 1989). Local oral factors are involved in the genesis of periodontal disease but the relationship with nutrition and total body health is not fully understood. However, it is clear that a soft diet correlates positively with periodontal disease (Golden *et al.* 1982).

Under normal circumstances there is a balance between destruction and repair of the epithelial lining of the crevicular groove which maintains normal integrity of the periodontal membrane. Periodontal disease is caused essentially by the accumulation of plaque on the tooth surfaces and the severity correlates directly with the quantity of such deposit. The plaque accumulation is initiated by the deposition of an acid glycoprotein coating which is precipitated from the saliva. Oral bacteria adhere to this pellicle and produce a matrix of polysaccharide−protein complexes which incorporate other substances, such as dead epithelial cells, leukocytes, lipid, carbo-hydrate, polysaccharide−protein complexes, calcium and phosphorus.

The bacterial flora change as the plaque forms; initially there are many gram-positive cocci but as the plaque matures and thickens gram-negative cocci predominate and an increase in anaerobic, spirochaetal and motile rod-shaped bacteria occurs. The micro-organisms induce ulceration and erosion of the crevicular epithelium and this induces inflammation in the surrounding gingiva (gingivitis). At the same time plaque accumulation distorts the crevicular groove and enamel cuticle, forming a periodontal pocket. The pocket encourages accumulation of plaque and provides the environment which is supportive of growth of gram-negative anaerobic bacteria. These changes lead to destruction of the gingival tissue with recession of the gums and retraction of the periodontal membrane. Ultimately there is infection of the tooth root, destruction of alveolar bone and dental loss.

Initially plaque may be difficult to see except with plaque-disclosing dyes (e.g. erythrosin) but it undergoes mineralization as calcium salts are precipitated and deposited from saliva. The mineralized product is seen as

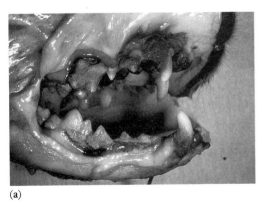
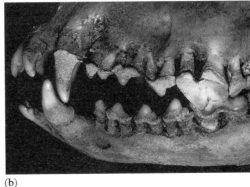

(a)   (b)

Fig. 1.5 (a) Extensive dental calculus deposition in a 13-year-old & King Charles Spaniel dog, and (b) Skull of a 15-year-old male Collie showing alveolar osteoporosis following severe long standing calculus deposition similar to Fig. 1.5(a).

an off-white, yellow or brown deposit (calculus or tartar). Large deposits (Fig. 1.5) contribute to gingival trauma and gingivitis.

Periodontal disease therefore is a progressive syndrome which starts as gingivitis and develops into advanced periodontitis with tooth loss unless treated successfully.

Gingivitis may also be triggered by systemic diseases or immune suppression and this is particularly true in cats (e.g. FeLV and other feline virus infections, Fig. 1.6). Nutritional disorders involving protein deficiency may predispose to gingivitis and hypervitaminosis A may also be implicated in cats.

Clinically the initial stages of gingivitis are marked by reddening of the gum margin adjacent to the teeth with thickening or rolling of the free gingival margin. Progressive changes produce oedema and friable gums which bleed on minimal handling or probing. With the formation of the periodontal pocket, a purulent exudate develops accompanied by accumulations of necrotic debris. Bacterial organisms cause ulceration of the canine lingual and buccal mucosae and these ulcers are painful. If the gingivitis is low grade but chronic, gingival hyperplasia may develop. This should be differentiated from the dysplastic gum hypertrophy seen in some breeds of dog (e.g. Boxers) and more rarely in cats.

Simple gingivitis is a reversible inflammatory condition. Treatment should aim to remove the causative factors of bacterial plaque and calculus with hand or ultrasonic descaling followed by dental polishing. Necrotic gingiva should be curetted away and affected areas swabbed with 0.1% chlorhexidine solution. Antibiotic therapy with a broad spectrum drug (tetracycline) may be required. Metronidazole is effective particularly where there are anaerobic and spirochaetal bacteria present. Some animals, however, do not tolerate this drug readily.

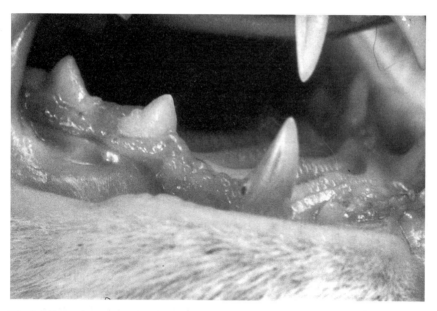

Fig. 1.6 Lower jaw of an adult cat showing extensive chronic gingivitis.

A more severe gingivitis known as acute necrotizing ulcerative gingivitis
has been described in the dog (Harvey 1989). The condition is thought to
be in part the result of infection by *Fusibacterium fusiformis* and a spirochaete
(*Borrelia* spp.). The authors have not seen this condition in either the dog
or the cat.

A lymphocytic plasmacytic gingivitis has been reported in cats. Clinically
affected cats have dysphagia, halitosis and weight loss. Pain is a feature.
Lesions are proliferative and ulcerative gingivitis develops with extension to
involve soft palate, palatopharyngeal region and oropharynx. There may be
raw nodular lesions at the fauces which crack and ulcerate when the mouth
is opened. Histopathologically there is hyperplastic ulcerated mucosa with
heavy infiltrations of plasma cells with lymphocytes, polymorphs and histiocytes in attendance. Serum proteins are elevated due to increased gamma-
globulin (Johnessee & Hurvitz 1983). It has been suggested that the
condition may be immune-mediated or related to calcivirus infection. The
prognosis for affected cats is generally poor although metronidazole, prednisolone and megestrol acetate have variably successful suppressive effects
on the inflammatory response.

Periodontitis is often the sequel to gingivitis and is the result of extension of
inflammation into the periodontal ligament, tooth and alveolar bone
(Fig. 1.5). It is thought that the increasing content of gram-negative bacteria in
plaque cause higher levels of endotoxins and together with high levels of
bacterial hyaluronidase these agents breach the epithelial integrity of the
dental sulcus. Interaction of the endotoxins with host antibodies results in

antibody—antigen complexes and these in turn lead to enhanced inflammation involving the alveolar bone. The involvement of bone invariably leads to tooth loss, either as a generalized horizontal loss or more focal single tooth deletions. Some dogs may exhibit gum recession following initial inflammation and the exposure of the cemento—enamel junction hastens the dental loss. Other dogs, however, may have gingival hyperplasia in the face of bone loss. Cheek and lingual contact ulceration is common in dogs with periodontal disease but this is not the case in cats.

Cats suffer severely with progression of periodontitis and are severely anorexic. Gingival recession is common with marked tooth loss as a result of external tooth root resorption where the inflammation at the cemento—enamel junction leads to collapse of the tooth crown with retention of the roots. These roots may become chronically inflamed or cystic and very painful with periodontal abscessation.

Treatment should aim to remove degenerate teeth and any retained roots. Curettage of necrotic debris and gingivectomy may be necessary; the latter is designed to eliminate the gingival sulcus in an attempt to facilitate future plaque control. Remaining teeth should be thoroughly descaled and the oral cavity cleansed with antiseptic such as chlorhexidine. Antibiotic or metronidazole therapy may be necessary in addition.

Periodontal abscesses may accompany periodontitis or may occur as a sequel to foreign body penetration. They may be sited as a swelling in the gingiva or adjacent to tooth roots in alveolar bone. In the dog the carnassial abscess is associated with maxillary fourth premolar or mandibular first molar tooth. The former (malar abscess) produces a swelling below the orbit on the affected side of the skull and may lead to a discharging sinus on the dorsum of the nose. These lesions are best dealt with by dental extraction, thereby allowing the abscess to drain with appropriate antibiotic cover if deemed necessary.

Secondary stomatitis

It is important to remember that some systemic diseases cause marked oral lesions which may lead to initial presentation of a patient or give the clinician important clues as to the nature of the systemic disease.

The most important disease in this category is generalized uraemia resulting from renal failure. The clinical oral symptoms which accompany uraemia in the dog and cat are principally ulceration of the cheeks and tongue with necrosis of the tip or edges of the tongue. The exact mechanism of ulceration and necrosis is unknown but the lesions are probably a direct reflection of high levels of circulating urea and breakdown of urea in localized sites such as the mouth. A more severe complication in long-standing canine cases is the decalcification and fibrosis of the jaws (rubber jaw) as a consequence of secondary hyperparathyroidism.

In the authors' experience however this is not a common condition nowadays.

Treatment of uraemia is largely supportive and difficult where there is severe renal disease and many cases are in end-stage renal disease if they present with advanced mouth lesions.

Dogs and cats with diabetes mellitus may develop unresponsive stomatitis which progresses to periodontitis. The exact nature of this relationship is not known but the oral lesions may be associated with decreases in the flow rate and the composition of saliva as is suspected in man (Marder *et al.* 1975). Treatment of ulceration in diabetic patients is often difficult because of poor tissue healing but correction of the necrotic gums and teeth should be attempted as described above.

Reticuloendothelial diseases are invariably accompanied by bleeding disorders and these are often seen as buccal haemorrhaging of the petechial type. Thrombocytopenias particularly may initially be detected by owners as multiple small haemorrhages of gums and palate. Similarly, poisoning by anticoagulant rodenticides such as warfarin may manifest as buccal petechiation before more serious symptoms develop.

Oral neoplasia

Oral neoplasia is important in the dog and cat particularly of the older age group. It is not uncommon for extensive tumour growth to affect the pharynx as well as the buccal cavity and some tumours may invade surrounding tissues or alternatively spread from adjacent sites (especially the nasal chambers) into the mouth.

CANINE TUMOURS

Some studies have indicated that primary oral neoplasia comprises the fourth most common site of malignancy in dogs (Dorn *et al.* 1968). There are undoubtedly age and breed susceptibilities and different types of tumour have different patterns of biological behaviour (Todoroff & Brodey 1979). The latter observation has implication for prognosis and therapeutic considerations.

In general terms the first abnormality observed by an owner is excessive salivation which is blood-tinged if the tumour is ulcerated. Many large lesions result in dysphagia, pain and halitosis accompanying necrosis and dental decay. Rapidly invasive tumour growth by malignant lesions may result in spontaneous fractures of the jaw. Some dogs are initially presented with an owner's complaint of a neck lesion; on examination these lesions are regional lymph nodes with metastatic tumour deposits from a primary oropharyngeal malignancy (e.g. squamous cell carcinoma).

Where oral neoplasia is suspected it is mandatory to carry out a full visual examination under sedation or general anaesthesia. Radiography may be of assistance is assessing degrees of bone involvement and if malignancy is likely then chest or regional tissue radiographs are helpful in assessment.

Lesions are usually clearly identifiable as neoplastic and if exposed are often traumatized with ulceration or necrosis with adherence of food debris. Some inflammatory lesions may however masquerade as neoplasms. Pathological diagnosis is essential for prognosis and instituting appropriate therapy. The type of diagnostic assessment of choice is usually excision biopsy since this procedure provides complete information for diagnosis and should remove the lesion, thereby providing a major step in therapy. Where this is not feasible then cytological examination of the exfoliated cells may be helpful. This can be achieved by making touch impression smears of the lesions or scraping the lesion with a spatula or blunt blade to collect cells (Else 1986). Several neoplastic conditions affect the canine oropharynx.

Papilloma. This condition used to be common, particularly in puppies, but within the last two decades has become rare in our experience. The lesions can range from single or multiple smooth nodules to multiple confluent, rough, white verrucose lesions on the lips, cheeks, tongue and less commonly, hard palate and pharynx. The benign tumours are caused by a papovavirus infection and spontaneously undergo necrosis after 6 to 8 weeks. If large or extensive they may cause dysphagia and pain and require surgery.

Epulis. These lesions are benign gingival neoplasms of fibromatous type and said to be the most frequently seen oral neoplasm in the dog (Dubielzig *et al.* 1979). They may occur as solitary fibromatous and ossifying lesions which are often discovered incidentally during dentistry procedures and appear to be relatively inocuous with no association with calculus or gingivitis/ periodontal disease. They may have metaplastic bone spicules present but are often pedunculated and are easily resected. However if metaplastic bone is left behind at surgery the lesions tend to recur.

A more serious form of lesion is the condition of multiple bilateral epulides sometimes known as bilateral gingival hyperplasia (Fig. 1.7). In this situation there is thickening of gum tissue around all teeth and particularly in the upper jaw. There is said to be familial incidence of this condition in the Boxer breed but it does not seem to be associated with calculus deposition or periodontal disease. In other breeds (West Highland Terrier, Labrador) in our experience however, calculus does appear to be associated. The epulides of this type are histologically similar to the simple type. The main problem associated with these lesions is the fact that they interfere with mastication. Complete surgical removal is often impractical but debulking and palliative surgery can be helpful.

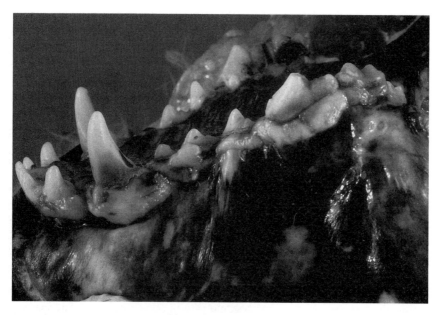

Fig. 1.7 Multiple fleshy gum enlargements characteristic of gingival hyperplasia in a 7-year-old Labrador dog. The upper gums were similarly affected.

Squamous cell carcinoma. This is one of the most common malignant tumours of the oropharynx in the dog. In our series the tonsils used to be the most common site affected but more recently gums and lips have been the more usual sites. Affected dogs usually present with pain on handling the mouth, halitosis and blood-tinged salivation over periods of 1 to 3 months. Male dogs seem to be more often affected than females. Lesions affect the gums of the anterior lower jaw and posterior upper jaw and less commonly the lips (Fig. 1.8). The tumours are white or pink, firm or fleshy swellings and are usually unicentric. These tumours are slow to metastasize and favour local deep invasion into mandibular or maxillary bone. This poses a problem of adequate surgical removal and these cases may require varying levels of radical maxillectomy or mandibulectomy (White *et al.* 1985) to affect complete removal. Radiation therapy may also be desirable but may not be practical.

Melanotic tumours. Melanotic tumours are equally distributed between the gums and non-gingival sites. In our experience lesions are commonest in the upper jaw at the molar regions and in the canine or premolar region in the lower jaw (Fig. 1.9). Tumours can also affect lips, tongue or cheek. There does not seem to be any greater incidence of melanotic tumours in dark

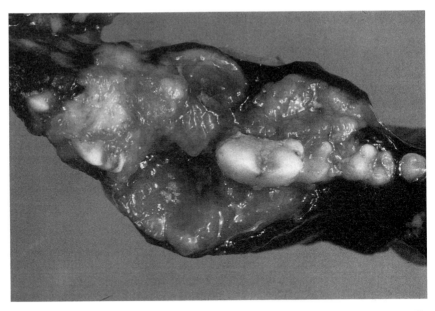

Fig. 1.8(a) Squamous cell carcinoma affecting the mandible of a 12-year-old Standard Poodle dog.

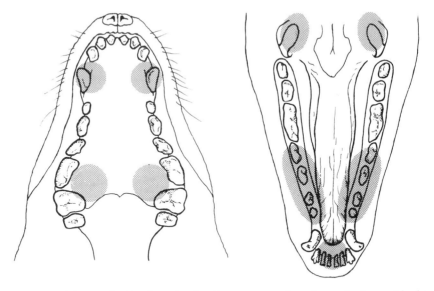

Fig. 1.8(b) Diagram showing the major sites for squamous cell carcinoma development in the canine mouth.

skinned dogs but the risk of developing melanoma increases with age. Male dogs are affected more often than females.

Macroscopically amelanotic melanomas and tumours with little pigment histologically are locally aggressive and highly malignant but at the same

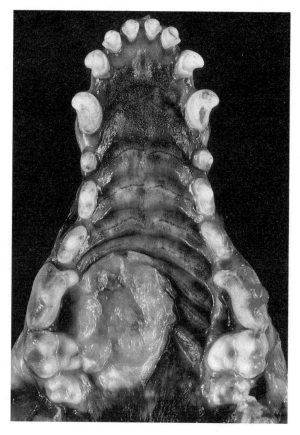

Fig. 1.9(a) Malignant melanotic tumour affecting the palate in an 8-year-old female Retriever.

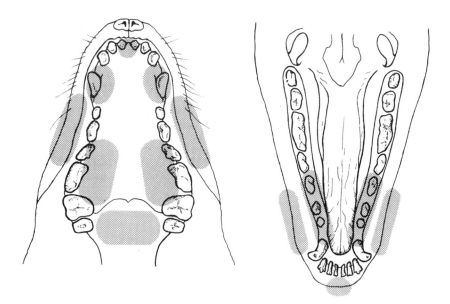

Fig. 1.9(b) Diagram showing the major sites for oral melanotic tumours.

time heavily pigmented tumours can also be highly invasive (Borthwick *et al.* 1982). Metastasis to regional lymph nodes is rapid with lung metastasis heading the list of widespread organ involvement usually as a result of lymphohaematogenous involvement. Melanomas, particularly the amelanotic type, tend to be invasive and surgical removal is difficult if tumour growth is advanced. Cryosurgery has been found to be merely palliative and surgical resection with chemotherapy is probably the treatment of choice (Gorman 1986).

Fibrosarcoma. This tumour is said to be more common in larger breeds (Todoroff & Brodey 1979) but our evidence does not confirm this. Gum tissue is usually the site of these tumours especially the molar region of the maxilla and hard palate. The tongue and sublingual mucosa may also be sites for development.

These tumours are non-pigmented but have a rougher more fibrous texture than carcinomas. Small lesions grow rapidly and like squamous cell carcinomas infiltrate underlying soft and bony tissue. Although spread to other sites is possible, the majority tend to recur locally after surgery unless radical excision procedures (with radiotherapy) are performed. Previous dental extraction or diseased teeth may be associated with the sites of tumour formation (Borthwick *et al.* 1982).

Other tumours. Tumours arising from the enamel organ of the tooth or other parts of the odontogenic apparatus occur very uncommonly. Tumours such

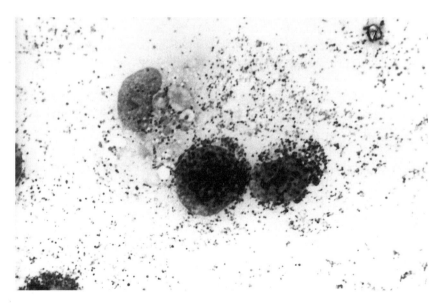

Fig. 1.10 Touch impression preparation of mast cell from an oral lesion in a 10-year-old Irish Setter dog.

as ameloblastomas may cause space-occupying lesions in the mandible or maxilla in relatively young dogs; they are biologically benign.

Mast cell tumours may arise from the oral subepithelial tissue and form lip nodules but more often they are extensions of cutaneous facial lesions. Cytological examination is helpful in diagnosis. Touch impressions stained with Romanovsky stains show characteristic metachromatic cytoplasmic granules (Fig. 1.10). Excision biopsy is usually effective but it is worth remembering that the individual tumour may be one expression of a more generalized mastocytosis with a more serious prognosis as a consequence.

Lymphoid buccal tumours were considered uncommon (Brodey 1960) but the present authors are becoming accustomed to seeing labial lesions with the histological characteristics of malignant lymphohistiocytic tumours or lymphosarcomas. Although some of these cases are solitary buccal lesions, recurrence is not uncommon and a significantly high proportion develop generalized multicentric lymphosarcoma of body lymph nodes.

FELINE TUMOURS

Cats may potentially develop the same range of oral tumours as dogs although lesions equivalent to epulides in dogs are uncommon and melanomas are much less common (Stebbins *et al.* 1989). Almost all oral masses seen in cats are either periodontal disease, gingival hyperplasia, labial granulomas or malignant tumours. Of the latter the most common are squamous cell carcinoma and fibrosarcoma.

The clinical symptoms are similar to those in the dog with anorexia, dysphagia, halitosis and blood-tinged salivation prominent features.

Squamous cell carcinomas usually affect the tongue itself or the sub-lingual area caudal to the frenulum, resulting in swelling and immobility of the tongue. The upper or lower gums may also be sites of tumour growth. Many of the tongue lesions present difficult surgical problems by the time of presentation since degrees of growth are considerable and surgical resection is not compatible with retention of functional activity. Palliative debulking merely gives temporary relief since recurrence is rapid. Radiation and chemotherapy are not effective. Many gingival tumours lead to rapid invasion of mandibular or maxillary bone and metastasis to local lymph nodes and lungs may occur simultaneously with bony invasion. If lesions are still localized however, mandibulectomy may give good results (Harvey 1986).

Fibrosarcomas are also associated with destructive growth locally but no site predilection is apparent. Although of low metastatic potential, extensive local infiltration usually means that complete surgical removal may be difficult and probably requires varying degrees of jaw resection to stand any chance of success.

Diseases of the tongue

The tongue is frequently involved in the diseases which affect the buccal cavity and other oral structures.

Congenital abnormalities of the tongue alone are uncommon and even if puppies or kittens have marked malformations such as cleft palate, the tongue is often normal. A condition known as bird tongue has been described in puppies. It is characterized by abnormal narrowing with distortion and impairment in swallowing. The defect is thought to be associated with a simple recessive gene (Hutt & De Lahunta 1971).

The majority of diseases of the tongue are acquired and the most common groups are traumatic and inflammatory disease (glossitis), the latter often occurring as part of a stomatitis syndrome.

Tongue injuries result from bite wounds or licking sharp objects and rough surfaces. Other injuries include chemical or electrical burning and more rarely snaring of the tongue with nylon fishing line or cotton.

Clinical signs are usually obvious with blood-tinged salivation and pawing at the mouth. Damage to the tongue is self-evident. Treatment includes control of bleeding, suturing of lacerations and possible amputation of part of the tongue if necessary (dogs manage fairly well with the anterior third of the tongue missing). Snares and embedded foreign bodies should be removed under general anaesthesia with subsequent broad spectrum antibiotic support.

Glossitis is perhaps the most common lesion of the tongue, particularly in cats, where ulcerative glossitis associated with herpesvirus (FVR) and calicivirus (FCV) can be a chronic intractable problem. The main problem in these cats is to maintain adequate nutrition and hydration in the face of severe pain and resultant dysphagia. Pharyngostomy intubation may be necessary to get affected cats over the acute phase of the condition.

Severe lingual ulceration in dogs often accompanies acute and chronic renal failure and pancreatitis but the pathogenesis remains uncertain. Affected dogs are anorexic, depressed, have halitosis and hypersalivate. The tongue may become necrotic at the free borders (Fig. 1.11) with sloughing as an end result. Many dogs can withstand loss of lingual tissue in this way if the basic systemic disease is corrected and if parenteral antibiotic and antifungal agents are given.

Cats with labial (eosinophilic) granulomas may have lingual or sublingual involvement.

Squamous cell carcinomas may involve the feline tongue, either at the root or invading from a primary gingival site. Such tumours may be suitable candidates for radio or thermal therapy (Thompson 1986) where suitable facilities are available. Tumours of the canine tongue are rare (Beck et al. 1986).

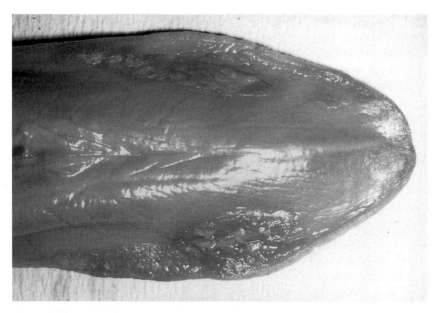

Fig. 1.11 Ventral surface of the tongue of a 13-year-old Labrador with renal failure: there are necrotic foci along the free borders of the tongue.

Diseases of the pharynx

There is a close anatomical relationship between the oral cavity and the pharynx which results in many diseases being oropharyngeal in nature rather than involving one compartment alone.

Congenital defects of the pharynx are rarely identified; any malformations are usually part of a severe defect which has more obvious manifestations in the oral cavity. Some toy breeds of dog (Yorkshire Terriers) have elongated soft palates which can cause difficulties in deglutition although the more common problem encountered is one of interference with airflow into the larynx. In cases of prolonged soft palate, surgical amputation may be attempted but enthusiasm for such procedures should be tempered with the knowledge that resultant postsurgical scarring and stricture can be undesirable side effects.

Although primary inflammatory disease of the pharynx, pharyngitis, is not common, the condition may often accompany stomatitis, rhinitis or more widespread systematic disease, e.g. in dogs with distemper and in feline leukaemia infection.

Acute pharyngitis is usually accompanied clinically by dysphagia, gagging and production of frothy saliva. Pyrexia and coughing may be noted and where there is submandibular oedema, dyspnoea may be an added complication. More chronic pharyngitis may develop with a non-productive cough and anorexia as presenting signs. Examination reveals foamy mucus in the oropharynx with hyperaemia of the mucosa and possibly ulceration and enlarged reddened tonsils in the dog. Ulceration and mucosal hyperaemia are features in the cat.

Very often the pharyngitis is of bacterial origin and in these cases response to suitable antibiotic therapy is usually dramatic. Where there is extensive inflammation and ulceration, as is often the case in cats, low doses of corticosteroids may be beneficial but they should be covered with adequate antibiotic therapy. Severely affected cats should be given supportive fluid therapy if required and pharyngostomy tube feeding may be necessary.

Foreign bodies are often problematic in the pharyngeal region, particularly in the cat. Solid non-perforating foreign bodies are seldom a problem in dogs although smooth rounded objects (e.g. small balls, chunks of meat) may become wedged in the pharynx with serious results. Perforating objects such as needles, bone spicules or hard plastic fragments may lodge in tonsillar crypts at the pillars of the oropharynx or caudolateral pharynx. In these sites the objects usually provoke an inflammatory reaction which is characterized by painful coughing, retching and dysphagia. External palpation of the pharyngeal region may elicit pain and usually provides evidence of uni- or bilateral swelling.

Bloody salivation is often seen, and affected animals require carefully induced general anaesthesia and examination to locate the seat of the reaction. Radiography is a major aid to diagnosis particularly if the penetrating body has migrated dorsally towards the temporal region or caudolaterally into the neck. Where foreign bodies are not radio-opaque diagnosis can be difficult.

Penetrating foreign bodies frequently present clinically as painful, asymmetrically-positioned retropharyngeal abscesses in the pharyngeal region or lateral upper neck. Affected animals may be pyrexic and usually anorexic. In cats it is important to differentiate relatively superficial bite abscesses from deeper-seated retropharyngeal abscesses. Radiography will demonstrate any radiodense foreign body which should be surgically removed and the accompanying abscess drained. Where foreign bodies are not demonstrable the region should be explored surgically with care and again any abscess cavities drained. Broad spectrum antibiotic should be provided until healing is complete.

The tonsils form a ring of lymphoid tissue at the oropharynx. In the dog, the organs are larger with more protrusion from their crypts; in the cat the tonsils are not so obvious with the bulk of the tissue lying laterally below the oropharyngeal mucosa. The most common condition of the tonsils is inflammation, with dogs apparently more commonly affected than cats. Tonsillar neoplasia occurs in dogs less commonly nowadays in our

Table 1.2 Differentiation of tonsillitis and tonsillar neoplasia

Feature	Tonsillitis	Squamous cell carcinoma	Lymphosarcoma
Clinical signs	Cough, retching, dysphagia ± pyrexia	Dysphagia, dyspnoea, anorexia, weight loss, pain, mass in neck	Dysphagia, anorexia, depression, weight loss
Age	Young to adult	Old animals	Middle-aged to old animals
Blood picture	Leukocytosis or leukopenia	Normal?	Leukocytosis or leukaemia
Radiography (chest)	Normal	± Lung metastasis	± Neoplasia thymic or bronchial nodes
Tonsillar size	Both uniformly enlarged	Unilateral, nodular or ulcerated plaque	Bilateral diffuse mass
Tonsillar colour	Red ± focal abscesses	White/grey ± ulceration	Pink
Tonsillar consistency	Friable	Firm/hard	Firm
Regional lymph nodes	Bilateral enlargement ± pain	Unilateral, nodular, non-painful	Usually bilateral, uniformly enlarged
Other body lymph nodes	Probably not involved (?general infection)	Unlikely	Many other nodes ± other organs

experience but it is important to differentiate between tonsillitis and neo-plastic involvement (Table 1.2).

In young dogs and to a lesser extent kittens, the tonsillar lymphoid tissue is normally prominent and often undergoes benign hyperplasia presumably as a response to a low-grade bacterial stimulation from the environment and part of the maturation process.

More clinically significant tonsillitis may be a primary condition arising from bacterial infections (e.g. Streptococcal, Staphylococcal, coliform, *Proteus* spp.) and this seems to be more common in young small breed dogs. Affected dogs retch and cough and may produce mucus; they are often depressed and anorexic. On examination the tonsils may be enlarged (Fig. 1.12) but size may be misleading. Bright red colouration with petechiation and/or focal white abscesses are clear indicators of tonsillitis. It is worth remembering that tonsillitis may be one manifestation of a more generalized systemic inflammatory or infectious disease, or may be secondary to vomiting or respiratory disease (e.g. kennel cough). Therefore in making a diagnosis the clinician should eliminate other organ involvement.

Acute primary tonsillitis of bacterial origin usually responds to antibiotic therapy but it may be necessary to give lengthy courses of these drugs to extinguish any bacterial infection fully. Chronic or recurrent tonsillitis, where affected tonsils become sufficiently enlarged to cause mechanical interference with swallowing or respiration, may warrant tonsillectomy.

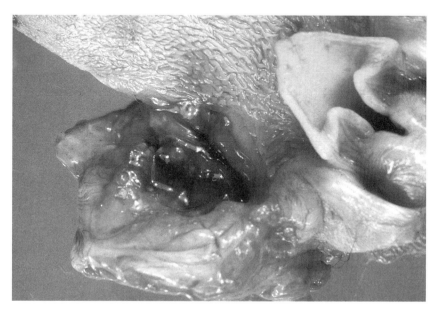

Fig. 1.12 Enlarged reddened tonsil with hyperaemia of the crypt characteristic of acute tonsillitis in a 4-year-old Border Collie dog.

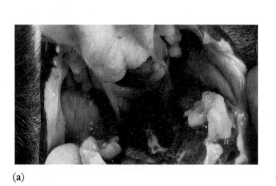

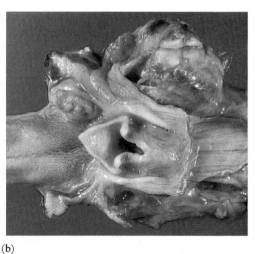

(a)   (b)

Fig. 1.13 (a) Opened mouth of a dog showing an irregularly enlarged tonsil on one side of the pharynx, and (b) the oropharynx and adjacent retropharyngeal lymph node of a dog with tonsillar squamous cell carcinoma. The node is enlarged by metastatic neoplasia.

Tonsillar neoplasia may masquerade as chronic tonsillitis in older dogs and cats. The most common tonsillar neoplasm is squamous cell carcinoma (Fig. 1.13). Lymphosarcoma also occurs in middle aged and older cats and dogs.

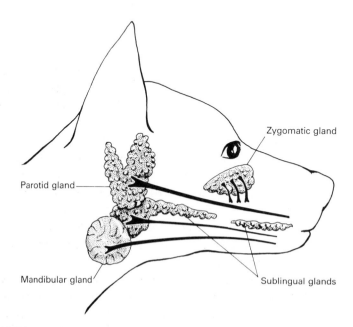

Fig. 1.14 Diagram showing anatomical location of salivary glands and ducts in the dog.

Clinical symptoms of tonsillar neoplasia are often those of chronic oral lesions with anorexia and dysphagia the major reasons for presentation by owners. Weight-loss is an additional feature and dogs with tonsillar carcinomas may present with unilateral upper cervical swellings which are retropharyngeal lymph nodes affected by metastatic disease. Owners of affected dogs sometimes note that there has been a loss of voice. On examination tonsillar carcinomas are often unilateral firm ulcerated masses whilst lymphosarcomas tend to be bilateral symmetrical with more diffuse involvement. Lesions should be biopsied or surgically removed for histopathological assessment. Complete surgical excision is often not possible and many cases have regional lymph node involvement or more distant metastasis (lungs) by the time of initial presentation. Prognosis is invariably grave for tonsillar carcinoma; chemotherapy adjuncts to surgery are ineffective although some reports have suggested that localized irradiation therapy may increase survival time (MacMillan *et al.* 1982) Lymphosarcoma of the tonsils is similarly unrewarding to treat because of its locally diffuse nature and the fact that the tonsil lesion is often one manifestation of a multicentric distribution.

Disease of the salivary glands

The salivary glands are associated anatomically with oral structures and are physiologically part of the alimentary system. The glands are not all in close association with the buccal cavity but they all drain into the mouth.

Anatomical and physiological aspects

In both species there are four major pairs of salivary glands — the parotid, mandibular, zygomatic and sublingual (Fig. 1.14). The parotid gland is an irregularly triangular pale pink organ situated in the retromandibular fossa. Dorsally it locates below the ear canal and ventrally extends to the wing of the atlas vertebra at the caudal angle of the mandible. It comprises lobules of serous glandular acini held together by fibrous connective tissue resulting in a finely nodular organ. Medial to the gland are the facial nerve, maxillary artery and vein and the parotid lymph node. The gland is drained by the prominent parotid duct which drains into the mouth by a papilla on the mucosa of the cheek at the level of the upper carnassial tooth. Innervation for secretory activity is via the glossopharyngeal nerve and auriculotemporal branch of the trigeminal nerve.

The mandibular gland is a large but well-circumscribed, slightly flattened ovoid organ lying caudoventrally to the parotid gland beneath the maxillary vein. It has a strong fibrous capsule and is distinct from the parotid gland with a firm well-defined lobulated structure. The gland is drained by a mandibular duct which runs along the floor of the mouth and opens on the lateral surface of the sublingual frenulum. The gland secretion is mixed, serous and mucous.

The sublingual gland is a loose connected series of lobules with caudal and cranial concentrations situated between the mylohyoideus muscle and lateral surface of the tongue. The caudal part is closely associated with the mandibular gland. There is a sublingual duct draining this area which either joins the mandibular duct or opens close to it on the sublingual frenulum. The cranial part is polystomatic, opening directly on a fold of mucosa at the floor of the mouth via numerous small ducts. The sublingual gland secretion is also mixed in nature.

The zygomatic gland is another mixed type salivary gland which is a well-circumscribed irregularly ovoid gland situated ventrocaudally to the orbit and medial to the zygomatic arch and masseter muscles. Multiple ducts (the cranial one is largest) open onto the buccal mucosa lateral to the last upper molar tooth. Small buccal glands are presented irregularly in the cheeks.

Canine and feline saliva has no appreciable enzyme activity and the saliva serves mainly to lubricate food boluses although in dogs lubrication of the buccal mucosa and tongue is important in facilitating heat loss.

Diseases of the salivary glands

Primary salivary gland disease is uncommon in both dog and cat. It is generally agreed that the most common conditions seen in both species are cystic or sialocoele abnormalities (Table 1.3).

Sialadenitis

Salivary gland inflammation is an uncommon condition as a primary clinical entity although low grade non-specific inflammation may be part of a systemic infectious disease (e.g. distemper). More specifically infections may arise from haematogenous infections or ascending infections from oral trauma (foreign bodies). The glands most affected are the parotid or zygomatic. Clinical signs usually include swelling and pain in the affected region especially when the mouth is opened. Abscessation may be evident and retrobulbar abscessation is often the result of zygomatic sialadenitis.

Autoimmune sialadenitis has been reported in about 20% of dogs with keratoconjunctivitis sicca. A condition of salivary gland necrosis has been described in Jack Russell Terriers (Kelly et al. 1979) but in the past decade the present authors have not seen this condition in some 1600 canine necropsies.

Early treatment with parenteral antibiotics is usually effective in low-

Table 1.3 Pharyngeal and salivary gland diseases

Pharyngeal diseases	
Congenital defects	Elongated soft palate ± malformation
	Parapharyngeal cysts
Pharyngitis	Specific viral, e.g. FCV, FVR, FeLV/FIV
	Non-specific bacterial, e.g. Staphylococcal, coliform, *Pasteurella* spp.
	Mechanical irritation, e.g. foreign bodies (wood, awns); chemicals
Retropharyngeal abscess	Non-specific bacterial
	Related to foreign bodies
Tonsillitis	Juvenile lymphoid hyperplasia
	Infectious, general or local bacterial or viral
	Secondary to chronic respiratory disease or regurgitation syndromes (e.g. persistent aortic arch)
Neoplasia	Squamous cell carcinoma ⎫
	Lymphosarcoma ⎬ usually tonsillar
	Benign polyps (rare) ⎭
Salivary glands	
Sialadenitis	Usually non-specific; sterile or bacterial/ viral
Sialocoele (salivary mucocoele) (+ ranula)	More common in dogs
Neoplasia	Usually adenocarcinoma, uncommon in cats

grade infections but abscessation may be incised at the most superficial ventrolateral point to ensure drainage. Zygomatic gland abscesses should be drained via an incision through the oral mucosa just behind the last upper molar. Longstanding lesions should be irrigated with antiseptic solutions and the patient given broad spectrum antibiotic post surgery.

Sialocoele (salivary mucocoele)

This is the most common salivary abnormality in the dog; it occurs much less commonly in cats.

A salivary mucocoele is an abnormal collection of salivary gland secretion (often mucus) in a non-epithelial-lined swelling. The swellings are usually sited where salivary secretion from damaged gland seeps into connective tissue and takes the line of least resistance along fascial planes. The most frequent sites are sublingual tissues and the intermandibular or cranial cervical areas and the pharynx may become involved. The swelling may be unilateral or bilateral if sited in the neck. The sublingual lesions are often unilateral fluctuating smooth submucosal swellings and are known as ranulas (Karbe & Nielson 1966).

The cause of the lesions is unknown. There is some evidence that trauma from foreign bodies may involve salivary glands and it is considered most likely that leakage direct from gland tissue or via ruptured ducts is the initiating cause (Spreull & Head 1967) rather than obstruction to duct drainage. Studies in cats (Harrison & Garrett 1972) however have shown that experimental ligation of the sublingual duct produces sialocoele and therefore ductal obstruction or stricture may in fact play a role.

Clinically sialocoeles tend to develop gradually although enlargement may be dramatic. Lesions in the lingual region tend to produce swellings which interfere in normal prehension and deglutition, and eventually interfere with normal positioning of the tongue. Neck lesions can present as unilateral or bilateral firm cystic swellings; they rarely cause dysphagia or dyspnoea and because of this affected dogs or cats may not be presented until swellings are very large.

Diagnosis is made on the basis of the site, nature and consistency of the swelling. Aspiration biopsy is important in confirming the diagnosis; aspirated fluid is clear, blood tinged or brown, turbid or mucous. Sometimes small nodules resembling calculi are found free in the swelling. These are small folds of inflammatory lining of the cyst which slough into the cavity. In cases where the exact extent of the lesion cannot be ascertained contrast radiography may be helpful in delineating the cyst.

Treatment of sialocoeles by aspiration alone usually only brings temporary relief since the cysts frequently reform. Surgical drainage and removal of affected salivary gland tissue is the treatment of choice although dissection and removal of cervical lesions can be a lengthy and delicate procedure. It has been suggested that ranulas may be treated by a marsupilization procedure involving creation of a fistula between the cyst and buccal cavity but removal of mandibular and sublingual gland tissue on the affected side is probably more satisfactory and recurrence is not a problem.

Neoplasia

Neoplasms of salivary glands of the dog and cat are uncommon. They are usually locally invasive adenocarcinomas which develop fairly slowly. They frequently affect the mandibular and parotid glands; neoplasia in the zygomatic gland results in fairly dramatic exophthalmos following retrobulbar invasion. Metastasis to regional lymph nodes and lungs also occurs.

Clinically affected animals are presented with unilateral masses which have developed fairly slowly. Pain and dysphagia tend to be manifest only when the tumours are large. Thoracic radiographs should be obtained to check for metastatic disease if salivary neoplasia is suspected.

Surgical removal with histopathological examination is the treatment of choice although total extirpation may be difficult because of the diffuse nature of the glands and in the case of the parotid gland, the adjacent vascular and nervous structures.

References

Ackerman L.J. (1985a) Canine and feline pemphigus and pemphigoid. Part I; Pemphigus. *Compendium on Continuing Education for the Practicing Veterinarian*, 7; 89−97.

Ackerman L.J. (1985b) Canine and feline pemphigus and pemphigoid. Part II; Pemphigoid. *Compendium on Continuing Education for the Practicing Veterinarian*, 7; 281−286.

Beck E.R., Withrow S.J., McChesney A.E., Richardson R.C. & Henderson R.A. (1986) Canine tongue tumours: A retrospective review of 57 cases. *Journal of American Animal Hospital Association*, 22; 525−532.

Bennet D., Lauder I.M., Kirkham D. & McQueen A. (1980) Bullous autoimmune disease in the dog 1; Clinical and pathological assessment. *Veterinary Record*, 106; 497−503.

Borthwick R., Else R.W. & Head K.W. (1982) Neoplasia and allied conditions of the canine oropharynx. In: *The Veterinary Annual*, G.S.C. Grunsell, F.W.G. Hill & M.E. Raw (eds). Scientechnica, Bristol, 248−269.

Brodey R.S. (1960) A clinical and pathologic study of 130 neoplasms of the mouth and pharynx in the dog. *American Journal of Veterinary Research*, 21; 787−812.

Dillon A.R. (1986) The oral cavity, In: *Canine and Feline Gastroenterology*. B.D. Jones & W.B. Liska (eds), W.B. Saunders, Philadelphia, 1−53.

Cheville N.F. (1968) The Gray Collie syndrome. *Journal of American Veterinary Medical Association*, 152; 620−630.

Dorn C.R., Taylor D.O.N., Schneider R., Hibbard H.N. & Klanber M.R. (1968) Survey of animal neoplasms in Alameda and Contra Costa Counties, California II: Cancer morbidity in dogs and cats from Alameda County. *Journal of the National Cancer Institute*, 40; 307−318.

Dubielzig R.R., Goldschmidt M.H. & Brodey R.S. (1979) The nomenclature of periodontal epulides in dogs. *Veterinary Pathology*, 16; 209−214.

Else R.W. (1986) Biopsy-principles and specimen management. *In Practice*, 8; 112−116.

Golden A.L., Stoller N. & Harvey C.E. (1982) A survey of oral health in small animals. *Journal of American Animal Hospital Association*, 18; 891−899.

Gorman N.T. (1986) *Oncology, Contemporary Issues in Small Animal Practice*, 6, Churchill Livingstone, New York.

Harrison J.D. & Garrett J.R. (1972) Mucocoele formation in cats by glandular duct ligation. *Archives Oral Biology*, 17; 1403−1414.

Harvey C.E. (1986) Oral surgery; Radical resection of maxillary and mandibular lesions. *Veterinary Clinics of North America*, 16; 983−993.

Harvey C.E. (1987) Palate defects in dogs and cats. *Compendium on Continuing Education for the Practicing Veterinarian*, 9; 402−420.

Harvey C.E. (1989) Oral, dental, pharyngeal and salivary gland disorders. In; *Textbook of Veterinary Internal Medicine*. S.J. Ettinger (ed.), W.B. Saunders, Philadelphia, 1203−1254.

Hutt F.B. & De Lahunta A. (1971) A lethal glossopharyngeal defect in the dog. *Journal of Heredity*, 62; 291−293.

Johnessee J.S. & Hurvitz A.I. (1983) Feline plasma cell gingivitis. *Journal of American Animal Hospital Association*, 19; 179−181.

Johnston, M.C. (1980) Animal models for craniofacial disorders: a critique. *Progress in Clinical Biological Research*, 46; 33−38.

Karbe E. & Nielson S.W. (1966) Canine ranulas, salivary mucocoeles and bronchial cysts. *Journal of Small Animal Practice*, 7; 625−630.

Kelly, D.F., Lucke, V.M., Denny, H.R. & Lane J.G. Histology of salivary gland infarction in the dog. *Veterinary Pathology*, **16**; 438−443.

Lane J.G. (1982) *ENT and Oral Surgery of the Dog and Cat*, P.S.G. Wright, Bristol.

Langham R.F., Mostosky U.V. & Schirmer R.G. (1977) X-ray therapy of selected odontogenic neoplasms in the dog. *Journal of American Veterinary Medical Association*, **170**; 820−822.

Lantz G.C. (1985) Tempero-mandibular ankylosis; surgical correction of three cases. *Journal of Amercian Animal Hospital Association*, **21**; 173−177.

McKeever P.J. & Klausner J.S. (1986) Plant awn, candidal, nocardial and necrotizing ulcerative stomatitis in the dog. *Journal of American Animal Hospital Association*, **22**; 17−24.

MacMillan R., Withrow S.J. & Gillette E.L. (1982) Surgery and regional irradiation for treatment of canine tonsillar squamous cell carcinoma: retrospective review of eight cases. *Journal of American Animal Hospital Association*, **18**; 311−314.

Marder M.Z., Abelson D.C. & Mandel I.D. (1975) Salivary alterations in diabetes mellitus. *Journal of Periodontal disease*, **46**; 567−569.

Pedersen N.C., Ho E.W., Brown M.L. & Yamamoto J.K. (1987) Isolation of a T lymphotrophic virus from domestic cats with an immunodeficiency-like syndrome. *Science*, **235**; 790−793.

Sams D.L. & Harvey C.E. (1989) Oral and dental diseases. In; *Cat Diseases and Clinical Management*, R.G. Sherding (ed.), Churchill Livingstone, New York, 875−906.

Scott D.W. (1984) Feline dermatology 1972−1982: introspective retrospections, *Journal of American Animal Hospital Association*, **20**; 537−564.

Spreull J.S.A. & Head K.W. (1967) Cervical salivary cysts in the dog. *Journal of Small Animal Practice*, **8**; 17−35.

Stannard A.A., Gribble D.H. & Baker B.B (1975) A mucocutaneous disease in the dog resembling pemphigus vulgaris in man. *Journal of American Veterinary Medical Association*, **166**; 575−582.

Stebbins K.C., Mrose C.C. & Goldschmidt M.H. (1989) Feline oral neoplasia: A ten year survey, *Veterinary Pathology*, **26**; 121−128.

Thompson J.M. (1986) Advances in the use of hyperthermia in oncology. In: *Contemporary Issues in Small Animal Practice*. 6. N.T. Gorman (ed.), Churchill Livingstone, New York, 89−119.

Todoroff R.J. & Brodey R.S. (1979) Oral pharyngeal neoplasia in the dog: a retrospective study of 361 cases, *Journal of American Veterinary Medical Association*, **175**; 567−571.

White R.A.S., Gorman N.T., Watkins J.B. & Brearley M.J. (1985) The surgical management of bone involved oral tumours in the dog. *Journal of Small Animal Practice*. **26**; 693−708.

2/Conditions of the Oesophagus

Oesophageal anatomy

The oesophagus starts as the cricopharyngeal sphincter in the caudal pharynx, initially lying dorsal to the trachea, moves to the left in the mid-cervical region then dorsal to the trachea at the thoracic inlet. In the thorax it lies dorsal and to the right of the aortic arch. It continues ventral to the aorta and enters the oesophageal hiatus of the diaphragm ending at the cardia where a physiological distal sphincter is formed, which guards entry to the stomach.

The oesophagus has four layers; the mucosa, submucosa, muscle and serosa. The mucosa lies in longitudinal folds of stratified squamous epithelial cells with ducts from the submucosal glands opening on the mucosal surface which secrete mucus. In the cat, the mucosal surface at the distal oesophagus has a scale-like surface and the muscularis mucosae run the entire length of the oesophagus unlike that in the dog which is only found in the distal oesophagus.

The submucosa contains blood vessels, nerves and many elastic fibres which create the longitudinal mucosal folds observed when the oesophagus is empty. Mucus secreting glands are found in this layer throughout the length of the oesophagus in dogs but only in the proximal oesophagus in cats.

The muscle layer differs in the dog and cat. In the dog the muscle layers lie obliquely round the oesophagus although they form an inner circular layer at the distal end. The muscle layer is entirely composed of striated muscle with only a very small area of smooth muscle at the distal end of the oesophagus. In the cat, striated muscle is found in the proximal oesophagus and this changes to smooth muscle in the thorax. The serosa is a thin sheet of fascia which is contiguous with the pleura.

Oesophageal physiology

The function of the oesophagus is to transfer food and fluids from the oral cavity to the stomach. Swallowing is controlled via a group of sensory and motor neurones originating from the cranial nerves. Sensory input is derived from the fifth, ninth and tenth cranial nerves and motor function from the fifth, seventh, ninth, tenth, eleventh and twelfth cranial nerves. Initiation of swallowing is voluntary but is completed by involuntary reflexes. The involuntary reflexes are controlled centrally through sensory neurones in the pharynx and oesophagus which travel to the swallowing centre in the medulla. The swallowing centre sends inhibitory messages to the respiratory centre, also in the medulla, to stop breathing while food is being swallowed.

Following prehension of food, muscles of the pharynx and the base of the tongue push a bolus to the caudal pharynx under voluntary control, sensory fibres in the pharynx respond to this bolus by inducing contraction of pharyngeal muscles with relaxation of the cricopharyngeal muscle allowing the bolus to enter the oesophagus. Presence of the bolus in the oesophagus initiates a primary peristaltic wave which travels down the oesophagus carrying the bolus and secondary peristaltic waves follow, ensuring the bolus reaches the distal oesophagus where sensory neurones detect the bolus and relax the physiological sphincter to allow passage into the stomach. In the cat it is thought that the longitudinal muscles actually contract, shortening the length of the oesophagus and speeding the transit of the food bolus (Leib 1986). Regurgitation of food from the stomach is normally prevented by the distal physiological sphincter and distention of the fundus making a flap-like valve at the cardia.

Both congenital and acquired conditions of the oesophagus have been documented. These conditions will be discussed in the remaining part of this chapter (Table 2.1).

Dysphagia

Dysphagia means difficulty in swallowing but is non-specific giving no indication as to cause. There are many causes of dysphagia which can be divided into: (1) functional disorders, associated with motor disorders of the swallowing process; and (2) mechanical disorders due to local anatomical defects preventing swallowing. Lesions of the tongue, hyoid, soft and hard palate, jaw, pharyngeal muscle, cheeks and cranial oesophageal sphincter may be involved. Collection of a thorough history and conduction of a

Table 2.1 Conditions of the oesophagus

Condition	Congenital	Acquired
Cricopharyngeal achalasia	+	+
Megaoesophagus	+	+
Vascular ring anomaly	+	−
Oesophageal foreign body	−	+
Oesophageal neoplasia	−	+
Peri-oesophageal mass	−	+
Oesophagitis	−	+
Oesophageal diverticulum	+	+
Disorders of gastro-oesophageal junction	+	+

Table 2.2 Differentiation of dysphagia based on location of barium entrapment following barium swallow

Region	Oral	Pharyngeal	Cricopharyngeal	Oesophageal
Oropharynx	+	+/−	+/−	−
Nasopharynx	−	+	+/−	+/−
Pharynx	−	+	+	+/−
Larynx/trachea	−	+	+	+/−
Oesophagus	−	+/−	−	++

detailed physical examination will often allow a distinction to be made between the presence of a systemic and local lesion. Dysphagia may be further divided by symptomatology into oral, pharyngeal and oesophageal dysphagias (Table 2.2).

Oral dysphagias involve difficulties in prehension of food and bolus formation at the base of the tongue. The tongue is essential for lapping fluids and moving solids along its midline to the base where a bolus forms and is projected into the pharynx. Lateral deviation of food indicates a problem and is identified by collection of food in the buccal folds. Oral swallowing is voluntary and involves the fifth, seventh and twelfth cranial nerves. Frequently animals modify their behaviour to cope with oral dysphagias. They chew food excessively, throw their head about or hold their head up to get food into the pharynx. As pharyngeal swallowing is intact this adaptive behaviour is effective in overcoming the problem. There is no retching, no aspiration pneumonia and no food regurgitated down the nasal passages in oral dysphagia. Food accumulation in the buccal folds, food falling out of the mouth or crusting round the muzzle suggest oral dysphagia.

Pharyngeal dysphagia occurs when involuntary swallowing is not initiated by presence of a food bolus at the base of the tongue. Either there is a failure in pharyngeal muscle contraction, failure of the pharyngeal openings to close (nasal, laryngeal and oral), or failure of the cranial oesophageal sphincter to open. Attempts at swallowing are accompanied by gagging and retching with food returning to the mouth or inhaled or passing down the nose. Occasionally retention of food in the pharynx occurs which may be regurgitated hours later. Weight loss occurs in such cases because adaptive behaviour will not correct the problem and no food enters the oesophagus (Watrous 1983).

Cricopharyngeal achalasia

This is an uncommon condition of the dog which has not been recorded to date in the cat. Cricopharyngeal achalasia may be due to failure of the muscle to relax, asynchronous relaxation or permanent opening of the muscle (chalasia) (Pearson 1970, Watrous 1983). It may occur as a congenital condition or may be seen at any age. The exact cause of dysphagia may be due to hypertrophy, atrophy or fibrosis of the muscle. Any interference with neurological supply to the muscle will also cause this condition (Shelton 1982). With incoordination some food may pass into the oesophagus, while with achalasia food never enters the oesophagus. Food is retained in the pharynx inducing choking and retching.

Clinical diagnosis

Cricopharyngeal achalasia normally affects dogs less than 1 year-old, often being observed at weaning when solid food is introduced (Shelton 1982). There is difficulty in swallowing both solids and liquids and there is failure to gain adequate weight. Retching and gagging are principal signs together with regurgitation of food and more commonly fluids down the nostrils or into the trachea. This frequently results in aspiration pneumonia and upper respiratory tract infection with coughing, sneezing, nasal discharge, pyrexia and dyspnoea (Pearson 1970).

Diagnosis can be difficult because of the different types of swallowing problem which may be present and because single X-ray plates do not provide adequate diagnostic information. The only satisfactory method of diagnosing the condition is by using barium-coated food and fluoroscopy to monitor swallowing (Table 2.3). In this way the actual site of the swallowing defect can usually be determined and in particular a differentiation between pharyngeal and cricopharyngeal dysfunction can often be made (Table 2.2).

Treatment

This depends on the underlying cause of the dysphagia. If cricopharyngeal achalasia is diagnosed, then treatment involves surgical section of the muscle permitting the bolus of food to enter the oesophagus following contraction of the pharyngeal muscles.

If the cause of the swallowing defect is oral or pharyngeal in origin then section of the cricopharyngeal muscle should not be carried out as this may

Table 2.3 Diagnostic aids for investigation of oesophageal disease

Observation	Dysphagias
Plain radiographs	Foreign bodies, neoplasms
Barium studies	Megaoesophagus, strictures
Fluoroscopy	Motility disorders
Endoscopy	Foreign bodies, neoplasms, strictures, oesophagitis

make the condition worse. The underlying cause for cranial nerve dysfunction must be found and corrected (Suter & Watrous 1980).

Feeding management should involve the use of small frequent meals which are soft or liquid in consistency. This is unlikely to be of value alone or in the long-term management of the condition.

Megaoesophagus

Megaoesophagus is a condition where the oesophagus becomes dilated in association with a loss of motor function. The aetiology of the condition is not known although it can be congenital or observed secondary to other disease states. It is not caused by increased lower sphincter tone as occurs in man, termed oesophageal achalasia, but is due to failure of the physiological sphincter to dilate.

Primary megaoesophagus appears to be related to a deficit in the sensory neurones supplying the oesophagus or in neurones supplying or within the swallowing centre itself. As there is no sensory input, there is no detection of sensation if a bolus of food is presented. Thus peristalsis is not initiated and the distal sphincter does not dilate, so the food is retained in the oesophagus (Zawie 1987). Any abnormality along the pathway which controls reflex peristalsis in the oesophagus associated with the passage of a bolus of food will lead to retention in the oesophagus. The condition can also be described as being due to an asynchronous motor function of the oesophagus and distal oesophageal sphincter. In addition it is thought that the condition seen in very young dogs is due to immaturity of oesophageal tissue which may improve with the passage of time. In the adult form the problem appears to be irreversible due to an acquired defect in neurological control of the oesophagus.

Secondary causes of megaoesophagus may occur associated with myasthenia gravis (Palmer & Barker 1974), polymyositis, systemic lupus erythematosis (Krum et al. 1977), hypoadrenocorticism (Feldman & Tyrrell 1977, Zawie 1987) or lead poisoning (Shelton 1982). In cats secondary megaoesophagus is seen as part of the typical clinical picture observed in cases of feline dysautonomia (Key–Gaskell) syndrome. Myasthenia gravis has also been reported in the cat with associated megaoesophagus (Mason 1976). A form of megaoesophagus in cats associated with pyloric obstruction has been observed which improves following pyloromyotomy (Zawie 1987).

The aspiration pneumonia which is commonly observed in this condition is thought to be due to failure of the respiratory centre in the medulla to inhibit breathing during swallowing.

Megaoesophagus is reportedly more common in the Great Dane, Irish Setter and German Shepherd dog (Harvey et al. 1974). It is said to be inherited as a simple autosomal recessive gene in the Miniature Schnauzer and Fox Terrier (Cox *et al.* 1980) and has been shown to be heritable as a recessive non-sex-linked disease in the cat (Clifford *et al.* 1971). The condition is more common in females (Harvey *et al.* 1974) and is generally less common in cats than in dogs.

Clinical diagnosis

The classical features of megaoesophagus are thin, depressed dogs which regurgitate undigested food and fluids. Regurgitation may be intermittent initially and in some cases there is no regurgitation observed by the owner, only signs associated with aspiration pneumonia.

The regurgitation of food some 12 h after feeding has been observed and in these cases there is a smaller amount of undigested food often in a sausage shape and coated in mucus. Food is more likely to be regurgitated soon after feeding when the patient is exercised, excited or stressed. The regurgitated food should contain no bile and have a high pH indicating it has not been in the stomach. Many owners will report the dog or cat to be vomiting when in fact it is passive regurgitation which is occurring. Gagging is sometimes reported by the owner and this appears to be due to passive regurgitation into the pharynx where it induces choking. Frequently the patient will consume the regurgitated food immediately and this may be repeated on several occasions.

Aspiration pneumonia is a common complication and leads to symptoms such as dyspnoea, coughing, lethargy and pyrexia. Occasionally there is upper respiratory infection with mucopurulent nasal discharge. It is the respiratory infection which accounts for the greatest mortality in this condition. Appetite is usually intact and described initially as ravenous but often declines especially when aspiration pneumonia develops or the oesophagus becomes dilated and impacted which ensures further loss of muscle tone.

A careful history and a full physical examination will ensure there is no evidence for secondary causes of megaoesophagus. Assuming there is no systemic involvement then the following procedures may be used to confirm idiopathic megaoesophagus.

Diagnosis is achieved following radiography. Plain X-rays will normally reveal a dilated thoracic oesophagus and frequently an air-filled stomach. A barium swallow using solid food coated in barium sulphate is a useful method of confirming retention within the oesophagus (Fig. 2.1). It is usually the entire thoracic oesophagus which is dilated, the oesophagus having greater ability to dilate in the thorax than in the cervical region, although dilation of the cervical oesophagus may occur especially in cats. Fluoroscopy will assist in confirming there is a failure of peristalsis and that there is no other form of oesophageal disease present. It is rare for the food

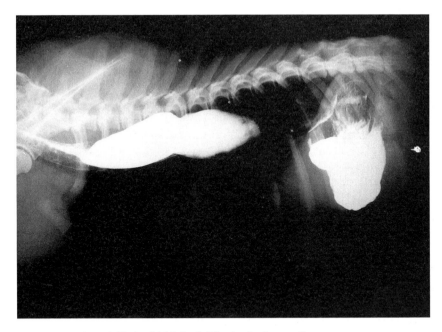

Fig. 2.1 Oesophageal dilation highlighted following barium swallow.

to actually reach the stomach and the distal oesophagus may appear to cone down at the diaphragm before entering the stomach. This is due to normal distal sphincter function.

Treatment

The prognosis is poor in the majority of cases with many dogs continuing to lose weight associated with aspiration pneumonia. Death from aspiration pneumonia is common. Euthanasia is also commonly carried out because medical management fails and these two situations account for over 70% of cases. Care is needed in the case of very young animals which have congenital megaoesophagus as their oesophageal tissue continues to mature for several months after birth and spontaneous recovery can occur. In addition a transient form of the condition with complete recovery has been documented in young adult dogs (Cox *et al.* 1880, Hendricks 1984).

Treatment falls into two possible categories; medical and surgical. The use of a modified Heller's myotomy has been advocated where the oesophageal muscle and that of the gastric cardia is sectioned to allow food to enter the stomach more readily. However there is still no peristaltic contractions present so food does not reach the stomach following surgery without accompanying medical management. For this reason it is rarely employed and medical treatment alone is more commonly adopted (Sokolovsky 1972).

In fact it has been suggested that mortality is greater in surgically-treated cases (Harvey *et al.* 1974).

Feeding the patient from an elevated level is advocated. This position should be maintained for up to 30 min post-feeding to assist the entry of food into the stomach. Cats can be carried on the owners shoulder to assist the passage of food into the stomach. Liquid foods are more readily accepted than solid foods. Feeding the patient several small meals daily may also assist in the management. Variation on this basic method may be required with individuals and owners should be encouraged to experiment with the dietary regime to find the most effective method for their pet. Medical management of puppies is definitely worthwhile as some spontaneously improve by 6 to 12 months of age.

Tracheal wash with subsequent culture and sensitivity is recommended to determine the bacteria associated with the aspiration pneumonia. A suitable antibiotic should be used and maintained for at least 3 weeks or until the symptoms of respiratory disease subside. Earlier presentations have better prospects as treatment can be started before the nerve plexus in the muscularis degenerate further because of stasis.

Vascular ring anomaly

This condition comprises a group of congenital malformations of the aorta and sometimes root of great vessels. It results in obstruction of the oesophagus by external mechanical pressure and induces regurgitation of food. Various congenital vascular anomalies can occur, the most frequent being the persistent right aortic arch (Zawie 1987) where the oesophagus is trapped between an abnormal right aorta and a patent ductus arteriosus. Rarer forms include a double aortic arch and abnormalities of the brachiocephalic and subclavian arteries (Woods *et al.* 1978).

Normally the aorta, pulmonary artery and ligamentum arteriosum lie to the left of the oesophagus causing no obstruction to the passage of food. Occasionally the right fourth aortic arch persists instead of the left fourth aortic arch and this results in the aorta lying on the right of the oesophagus and the base of the heart. The pulmonary artery lies ventral and to the left and the ligamentum arteriosum on the left and dorsal to the oesophagus (see Fig. 2.2). This completes the vascular ring and leads to obstruction of the oesophagus at the level of the heart base. The trachea is frequently included in the vascular ring but it is rare for respiratory obstruction to be a feature of the condition (Lawson & Pirie 1966).

If the obstruction remains untreated for some time then fibrosis and stricture formation of the oesophagus occur or permanent dilation due to degeneration of the myenteric plexus so that following surgical correction, regurgitation may persist (Clifford *et al.* 1971).

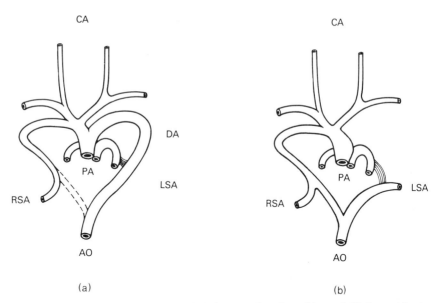

Fig. 2.2 Diagrammatic representation of (a) the normal aortic position and (b) the position in persistent right aortic arch. CA = carotid artery, PA = pulmonary artery, DA = ductus arteriosus, LSA = left subclavian artery, RSA = right subclavian artery, AO = aorta.

Vascular ring anomaly is seen in puppies and rarely in the kitten (Uzuka & Nakama 1988). It is said to occur more commonly in German Shepherd, Irish Setter and Boston Terrier dogs. In the authors' experience the condition can occur in any breed and there appears to be no obvious sex predisposition.

Clinical diagnosis

The condition is observed soon after weaning when solid food is introduced (Jessop 1960). Regurgitation of undigested food occurs 1 or 2 h after feeding (Pearson 1970). If the dilation proximal to the vascular ring is large then there may be a delay in regurgitation of food for several hours following feeding. A bulge may be observed at the thoracic inlet following feeding and prior to regurgitation due to dilation of the oesophagus with food. Fluids may be taken without regurgitation as the obstruction is often incomplete. Affected animals are often weaker and smaller than littermates due to malnutrition and complicating pneumonia. Aspiration pneumonia is common and the signs include dyspnoea, coughing, lethargy and pyrexia. Cardiac or vascular dysfunction may also occur in this condition.

The clinical signs of vascular ring anomaly are very similar to those observed in megaoesophagus. Radiographs, barium studies and fluoroscopy are the most useful procedures for detecting this condition. Dilation of the oesophagus proximal to the base of the heart is observed in vascular ring

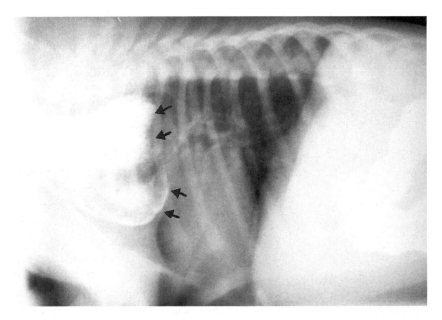

Fig. 2.3 Vascular ring anomaly highlighted following barium swallow.

anomaly (Clifford & Malek 1969). The oesophagus is not dilated between the heart and the diaphragm (see Fig. 2.3). If liquid barium is administered then some may reach the stomach because the obstruction is incomplete although the bulk of the barium will remain in the dilated oesophagus. However barium mixed with food is always retained in the proximal oesophagus. In addition, radiographic examination will frequently reveal changes to the lungs consistent with aspiration pneumonia.

Treatment

The prognosis must be guarded because a thoracotomy is required to correct the vascular defect in an animal which is a poor risk, being weak, malnourished and with aspiration pneumonia. An additional risk follows successful surgery where there may be permanent stenosis of the oesophagus or failure of oesophageal peristalsis. A reduction in the number of myenteric ganglion cells in the mid-oesophagus has also been recorded following the development of vascular ring anomaly (Clifford *et al.* 1971). If surgery is carried out early before fibrosis and stricture formation occurs, the prognosis is likely to be favourable.

It is recommended to treat any aspiration pneumonia and to drain the oesophageal dilation of accumulated food and fluid prior to surgery. Thoracotomy via the left fourth intercostal space will expose the vascular ring, and once identified the obstructing vessel, which is normally the ligamentum arteriosum, is ligated and sectioned. Once the obstruction has been relieved it is necessary to check there is no stricture of the oesophagus and that peristalsis is still present. This is best achieved through follow-up radiographs and barium studies. Oesophagoplasty has been carried out in order to free such stricture of the oesophagus (Funkquist 1970).

Oesophageal foreign body

Although the oesophagus has a remarkable ability to dilate, foreign body obstruction is common in dogs, although less common in cats (Pearson 1966). Dogs have a general tendency to scavenge and cats frequently hunt, and it is these activities which can lead to foreign body obstruction. The most common foreign body observed in dogs is a vertebral bone although it is possible for many different objects to obstruct the oesophagus. In cats, fish and chicken bones are the commonest foreign bodies found, although needles with thread attached are also observed. The sites where the oesophagus is narrowest and where obstruction is likely to occur include the proximal and distal sphincters, thoracic inlet and base of the heart (Ryan & Greene 1975). The base of the heart appears to be the commonest site for foreign body obstruction in the authors' experience. The condition can occur in any breed although the Poodle and Terriers seem to be more commonly involved (Ryan & Greene 1975).

Clinical diagnosis

Often there is a history of eating household scraps especially vertebral bones. The typical clinical signs of the condition include acute onset of regurgitation of food shortly after eating, salivation and frequent swallowing movements with attempts to retch. In most cases the appetite remains good in the early stages although food is regurgitated and the patient often salivates and appears bright and active. As the condition advances the situation changes. The patient becomes anorexic, depressed and regurgitation is reduced as are repeated swallowing efforts.

Complications are common and include perforation of the oesophagus leading to mediastinal infection, pleurisy with exudative pleural effusion. If this occurs then marked depression, pyrexia, dyspnoea and dehydration rapidly occur. The mortality rate increases sharply when these complications occur.

If the obstruction is incomplete, fluids, and occasionally food may reach the stomach. Under these circumstances the condition may remain undiagnosed and persist until oesophageal perforation occurs.

The history and clinical signs are typical but confirmation of the obstruction and its location are essential. The careful passage of a stomach tube will

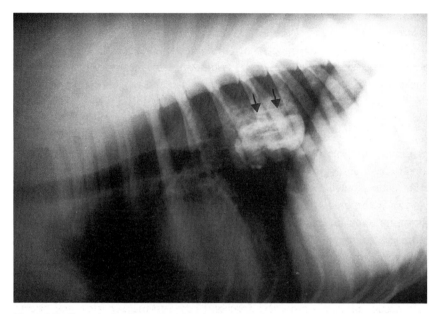

Fig. 2.4 Radiograph showing radio-dense foreign body in the oesophagus.

reveal if an obstruction is present and its location. Plain radiographs are also useful in diagnosing and locating the obstruction (Fig. 2.4). Barium studies should not be performed as there may be a perforation of the oesophagus leading to barium passage into the mediastinum and thorax. The radiographs will also assist in determining if pleurisy or aspiration pneumonia has occurred.

Endoscopy is a very valuable method of diagnosis, allowing a careful examination of the foreign body and any tissue damage that has occurred. This will aid the clinician in deciding the best method of removing the foreign body. Endoscopy will also allow evaluation of the oesophagus following removal of the foreign body to determine if laceration or perforation has occurred, indicating the need for surgical intervention.

Treatment

The prognosis in the early stages of foreign body obstruction is good especially if there is no laceration or perforation of the oesophagus. The longer the foreign body has been in place the more likely tissue necrosis and eventual perforation will occur. Where pleurisy has developed the prognosis must be very guarded. Following removal of the foreign body, common complications include stricture formation, perforation and diverticulum formation.

The removal of the foreign body can be achieved by one of several methods: (1) removal *per os* using an endoscope and grasping forceps,

(2) pushing the foreign body into the stomach; and (3) removal via thoracotomy.

The use of a rigid or flexible endoscope with grasping forceps introduced *per os* is the commonest method of visualization and removal of the foreign body (Ryan & Greene 1975). Occasionally this is not possible especially if the foreign body lies near the distal end of the oesophagus. In these cases the foreign body may be pushed into the stomach and allowed to dissolve in gastric acid or may be removed via laparotomy which is a less hazardous procedure than thoracotomy. If it is left in the stomach then careful monitoring is required using radiography. In each case it is important to use an endoscope to examine the extent of tissue damage following removal of the foreign body, as soft tissue damage may require further treatment. Where perforation or serious laceration has occurred thoracotomy may still be required.

Thoracotomy is hazardous because; (1) infection may lead to poor wound healing, (2) the foreign body often lodges at a site where there are major blood vessels surrounding the oesophagus; and (3) there may be extensive soft tissue damage round the foreign body making suturing and repair difficult.

Following removal of the foreign body conservative medical treatment should include small liquid meals, use of antacids to prevent acid damage should any gastric reflux occur, and the use of antibiotic to guard against secondary infection. The latter is essential if pleurisy has occurred following perforation. In this case it is advisable to carry out culture and sensitivity testing prior to selecting an antibiotic.

Oesophageal neoplasia

Tumours of the oesophagus are rare in the dog. Primary tumours may include squamous cell carcinoma, fibrosarcoma, osteosarcoma, leiomyoma (Ridgeway & Suter 1979). Although *Spirocera lupi* is found in Africa, Asia, southern Europe and America but not in the UK, it may be observed causing tumour formation in imported dogs. Secondary tumours include bronchiogenic, gastric, thyroid and mammary carcinomas. Oesophageal tumours in cats are very rare but when present are likely to be squamous cell carcinomas (Fernandes *et al.* 1987). Neoplasia of the oesophagus is seen more frequently in the middle to old age group.

Clinical diagnosis

Signs are those associated with a slowly developing obstruction of the oesophagus with eventual dilation proximal to the obstruction. This results in a slow insidious onset of regurgitation of food following feeding, but not fluids, and persistent salivation in the early stages. Eventually total obstruction leads to regurgitation of both food and fluids and this change in the clinical picture may take several months to develop. Weight loss is a feature as the condition advances and the tumour may be seen as a swelling in some cases where the cervical oesophagus is involved. If the tumour is secondary then signs associated with the primary tumour are also expected. Snoring and dysphagia are other signs which have also been reported (Lawson & Pirie 1966). Occasionally there may be pain on movement or palpation of the neck.

Plain radiographs may reveal a soft tissue mass in the oesophagus and barium studies will assist in determining the exact site of the obstruction. Endoscopy will confirm that a tumour is present by allowing visualization of the mass and collection of biopsy samples. Biopsy of any mass is essential if an accurate prognosis is to be given. The condition is clinically similar and must be differentiated from oesophageal dilation, foreign body obstruction, vascular ring anomaly and perioesophageal obstructing mass.

Treatment

Surgical removal of a diagnosed tumour may be possible but often by the time clinical signs of regurgitation are established the tumour has advanced beyond surgery. Equally many of the tumours are malignant and will have spread to other tissues or the tumour itself may have origins in other tissues. The prognosis must therefore be very guarded.

Perioesophageal masses

Rather than a tumour directly affecting the oesophagus there may be a change in tissue closely associated with the oesophagus leading to compression and interference with oesophageal function. Vascular ring anomaly, heart base, thymic or thyroid tumours, retropharyngeal or bronchial lymph node enlargement and paraoesophageal abscesses are examples of such masses.

When the thymus is involved, obstruction of the oesophagus occurs at or just proximal to the thoracic inlet with dilation of the cervical oesophagus, often seen as a bulge in the neck following feeding (Gruffydd-Jones et al. 1979, Fig. 2.5). Although fluids may initially be retained, regurgitation shortly after feeding together with salivation and repeated swallowing may be observed. In addition anorexia, depression, weight loss and respiratory signs may be detected, such as dyspnoea and coughing. There may be hydrothorax and associated symptoms in advanced cases due to thymic interference with vascular function.

Diagnosis is based on radiography and barium studies which highlight

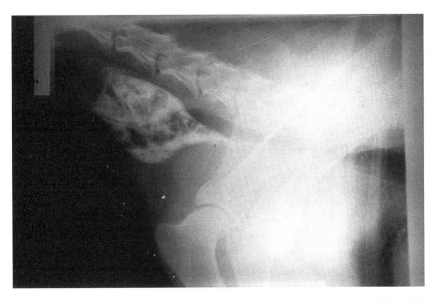

Fig. 2.5 Radiograph showing perioesophageal mass in the cervical oesophagus highlighted by food mixed with barium sulphate.

the site of obstruction. If a thoracic effusion is present then thoracocentesis and cytological examination of the fluid are very useful.

Where there is pulmonary disease the bronchial lymph nodes may become enlarged, although they are unlikely to compress the oesophagus. Heart-base tumours may be large enough to cause oesophageal obstruction (Zawie 1987).

Treatment in many cases is unlikely to be successful because of the extensive invasion of tissue which has occurred by the time clinical symptoms are observed. However exploratory surgery and careful dissection of the mass, followed by antibiotic if infective, is the only method of treatment likely to be effective.

Oesophagitis

The ingestion of strong acids or alkalis or very hot food can cause oesophagitis. In the cat calcivirus infection can cause oesophagitis. Oesophageal papillomatosis associated with oesophagitis has been reported in the cat (Wilkinson 1970). More commonly reflux of gastric secretion into the oesophagus is known to cause irritation and inflammation, referred to as reflux oesophagitis.

Reflux oesophagitis may be observed following general anaesthesia as the premedication and anaesthetic agents used tend to relax the distal oesophageal sphincter and reduce oesophageal peristalsis. Gastric acid at very low pH then enters the oesophagus together with pepsinogen which is activated by the acid; both cause considerable inflammation and tissue damage (Pearson *et al.* 1978). This inflammation leads to further relaxation of the sphincter and so allows the entry of more acid to the oesophagus and thereby establishes a vicious cycle (August 1983). Other initiating causes may occur at surgery, e.g. tilting the patient so the head is lower than the abdomen, increasing intra-abdominal pressure.

The actual contact time of acid on oesophageal mucosa is also important. Gastric juice only needs to be in contact with the oesophagus for some 20 min to induce damage to the mucosa and underlying tissues, resulting in inflammation and ulceration. Stricture of the oesophagus due to healing by fibrous tissue is a common sequel, especially if the condition is allowed to advance without treatment.

Clinical diagnosis

The history may include knowledge of injurious types of food ingested or access to dangerous chemicals or recent surgery. The predominant clinical signs are dysphagia, regurgitation and pain on eating. Other symptoms include lethargy, mild pyrexia, salivation, coughing and retching.

Plain radiographs are of little value, while barium studies especially where fluoroscopy is employed are of great value in detecting reflux oeso-phagitis (Fig. 2.6). A definitive diagnosis is obtained from endoscopy where the tissues can be examined for signs of inflammation and ulceration. Biopsy samples should be collected in order to confirm the diagnosis, rule out neoplasia and assess the extent of the changes.

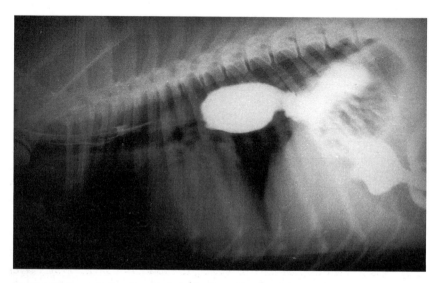

Fig. 2.6 Radiograph showing oesophageal reflux of barium from the stomach.

Treatment

Where acid or alkali is known to have been ingested, emesis should not be induced but the chemical should be neutralized. Corrosive chemicals should be neutralized using egg white. It goes without saying that further ingestion of the chemical should also be prevented. In addition antacids particularly those with local anaestheic (Mucaine; Wyeth Laboratories) 5 to 10 ml qid will relieve the pain of inflammation and treatment to reduce the level of acid as described below will also be beneficial.

With regard to reflux oesophagitis the objective is to break the vicious cycle by reducing the amount of available gastric acid for reflux into the oesophagus. Reduction of gastric acid is achieved through use of H_2 blocking agents such as cimetidine (Tagamet; SmithKline Beecham Pharmaceuticals) 4 mg/kg tid. In addition restoration of normal oesophageal motility and lower sphincter tone can be achieved following administration of meta-clopramide (Emequell; SmithKline Beecham Pharmaceuticals) 0.5 to 1 mg/kg bid. bethanechol (Myotonine; Glenwood Laboratories) 2.5 to 10 mg every 8 h may be used in place of metaclopramide to restore oesophageal tone, but this drug only works effectively on the smooth muscle of the oesophagus which forms only a small component of the canine oesophagus (Dodds *et al.* 1976).

The dog or cat should be given several small meals each day rather than one large meal. The case should be reviewed at frequent intervals and if there is any indication of stricture formation then prednisolone at 1 mg/kg/day in divided doses may reduce healing by fibrous tissue. Local anaesthetic agents incorporated in antacid suspensions may also be used to reduce the pain. Drugs in this group include mucaine (Wyeth Laboratories) 5 to 10 ml qid depending on the size of dog.

Resection of the portion of oesophagus involved has been suggested but is not practical. The prognosis should always be guarded especially in advanced cases where deep tissue change has occurred with subsequent risk of stricture formation.

Oesophageal diverticulum

This is a rare condition of dogs and cats which may be either congenital or acquired. When it does occur it is most likely to be located either at the thoracic inlet or between the heart and the diaphragm. Congenital forms occur most often at the thoracic inlet while the acquired forms occur as a consequence of some other oesophageal disease. Conditions such as foreign bodies, vascular ring anomaly, stricture formation and tumours may lead to diverticulum formation cranial to the obstruction. The foreign body itself may weaken the oesophageal wall leading to breakdown of the muscle layer and diverticulum formation. Such acquired diverticula occur most frequently in the thoracic oesophagus and may be lined by only connective tissue and epithelial cells.

Once formed the diverticulum may become impacted with food, become inflammed and infected or may rupture emptying contents into the mediastinum.

Clinical diagnosis

Clinical signs observed in most cases include pain on eating, regurgitation of food and secondary infection with pyrexia. Occasionally the lesion may be so painful that animals are reluctant to move and may be anorexic.

Diagnosis is based on radiographic evidence from plain films and following a barium swallow. Endoscopy may be used to detect a diverticulum or the extent of the mucosal changes associated with the condition.

Treatment

When the congenital form is diagnosed, treatment usually orientates around frequent small meals of homogenized food. When the acquired form is present this usually requires thoracotomy and correction of the oesophageal defect.

Disorders of the gastro-oesophageal junction

Gastro-oesophageal intussusception and sliding hiatus hernia have been recorded in the dog. The causes of these conditions are not known but dysfunction of the lower oesophageal sphincter, widening of the gastro-oesophageal hiatus 'patulous cardia' and congenital defects in the diaphragm have all been suggested (Gaskell *et al.* 1974). The authors have experience of a case where marked increase in thoracic negative pressure associated with laryngeal stridor caused increased intrathoracic pressure and herniation (Burnie *et al.* 1989). Either a portion of the stomach herniates into the thorax and returns to the abdomen or a portion of stomach slides into the oesophagus associated with oesophageal peristalsis or breathing. There is an association with reflux oesophagitis and the condition appears more common in young dogs although the case observed by the authors was in an 11 year-old crossbred dog.

Clinical diagnosis

The most common clinical sign is regurgitation of food shortly after eating together with fluids which may be blood tinged (coffee grounds) due to ulceration caused by gastric acid. Salivation, weight loss and hunger have

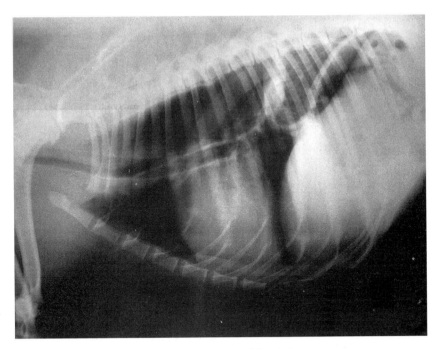

Fig. 2.7 Plain radiograph showing gastro-oesophageal herniation.

been described. Associated respiratory signs include inspiratory effort and stridor with use of thoracic muscles to aid breathing.

Plain radiographs are often of little value while barium studies may help but are best interpreted with the aid of fluoroscopy. In this way the gastro-oesophageal junction can be closely observed for herniation (Fig. 2.7). Endoscopic examination of the oesophagus usually reveals inflammation and ulceration of the distal oesophagus.

Treatment

Fundopexy and gastropexy or repair of the oesophageal hiatus have been described and associated with some success. Where inspiratory stridor is the cause correction of the laryngeal obstruction results in cessation of the stridor and gastro-oesophageal herniation. Cimetidine (Tagamet; Smith-Kline Beecham Pharmaceuticals) at 4 mg/kg tid may be used to treat any associated oesophagitis together with the other drugs described for that condition.

References

August J.R. (1983) Gastrointestinal disorders of the cat. *Veterinary Clinics of North America,* **13**; 585–597.

Burnie A.G., Simpson J.W. & Corcoran B.M. (1989) Gastro-oesophageal reflux and hiatus hernia associated with laryngeal paralysis in a dog. *Journal of Small Animal Practice*, **30**; 414–416.

Clifford D.H. & Malek R. (1969) Diseases of the canine oesophagus due to prenatal influences. *American Journal of Digestive Diseases*, **14**; 578–602.

Clifford D.H., Soifer F.K., Wilson C.F., Waddell E.D. & Guilloud G.L. (1971) Congenital achalasia of the oesophagus in four cats of common ancestory. *Journal of American Veterinary Medical Association*, **158**; 1554–1560.

Cox V.S., Wallace L.J., Anderson V.E. & Rushmere, R.A. (1980) Hereditary oesophageal dysfunction in the Miniature Schnauzer dog. *American Journal of Veterinary Research* **41**; 326–330.

Dodds W.J., Hogan W.J. & Miller W. (1976) Reflux oesophagitis. *American Journal of Digestive Diseases*, **21**; 49–67.

Feldman E.C. & Tyrrell J.B. (1977) Hypoadrenocorticism. *Veterinary Clinics of North America*, **7**; 555–570.

Fernandes F.H., Hawe R.S. & Loeb W.F. (1987) Primary squamous cell carcinoma of the oesophagus in a cat. *Companion Animal Practice*. **1**; 16–22.

Funkquist B. (1970) Oesophagealplasty as a supporting measure in the operation for oesophageal constriction following vascular malformation. *Journal of Small Animal Practice*, **11**; 421–427.

Gaskell C.O., Gibb C. & Pearson H. (1974). Sliding hiatus hernia with reflux oesophagitis in two dogs. *Journal of Small Animal Practice*, **15**; 503–509.

Gruffydd-Jones T.J., Gaskell C.J. & Gibb C. (1979). Clinical and radiographical features of anterior mediastinal lymphosarcoma in the cat: A review of 30 cases. *Veterinary Record*, **104**; 304–307.

Harvey C.E., O'Brien J.A., Durie V.R., Miller D.J. & Veenema R. (1974). Megaoesophagus in the dog: A clinical survey of 79 cases. *Journal of American Veterinary Medical Association*, **165**; 443–446.

Hendricks J.L. (1984). Transient oesophageal dysfunction mimicking megaoesophagus in three dogs. *Journal of American Veterinary Medical Association*, **185**; 90–92.

Jessop L. (1960) Persistent right aortic arch in the cat causing oesophageal stenosis. *Veterinary Record*, **72**; 46–47.

Krum S.H., Cardinet G.H., Anderson B.C. & Holliday T.A. (1977) Polymyositis and poly-arthritis associated with SLE in a dog. *Journal of American Veterinary Medical Association*, **170**; 61–66.

Lawson D.D. & Pirie H.M. (1966). Conditions of the canine oesophagus: II vascular rings, achalasia, tumours and perioesophageal lesions. *Journal of Small Animal Practice*, **7**; 117–127.

Leib M.S. (1986) Megaoesophagus in the dog. In: *Current Veterinary Therapy IX*, R.W. Kirk (ed.), W.B. Saunders, Philadelphia, 848–852.

Mason K.V. (1976). A case of myasthenia gravis in a cat. *Journal of Small Animal Practice*, **17**; 467–472.

Palmer A.C. & Barker J. (1974). Myasthenia gravis in the dog. *Veterinary Record*, **95**; 452–454.

Pearson H. (1966). Symposium on conditions of the canine oesophagus. I Foreign bodies in the oesophagus. *Journal of Small Animal Practice*, **7**; 107–116.

Pearson H. (1970). The differential diagnosis of persistent vomiting in the young dog. *Journal of Small Animal Practice*, **11**; 403–415.

Pearson H., Darke P.G.G., Gibb C., Kelly D.F. & Orr C.M. (1978). Reflux oesophagitis and stricture formation after anaesthesia: A review of seven cases in dogs and cats. *Journal of Small Animal Practice*, **19**; 507–519.

Ridgeway R.L. & Suter P.F. (1979) Clinical and radiographic signs in primary and metastatic oesophageal neoplasms of the dog. *Journal of American Veterinary Medical Association*, **174**; 700–707.

Ryan W.W. & Greene R.W. (1975). The conservative management of oesophageal foreign bodies and their complications: A review of 66 cases in dogs and cats. *Journal of American*

Animal Hospital Association, **11**; 243–249.

Shelton G.D. (1982). Swallowing disorders in the dog. *Compendium on Continuing Education for the Practicing Veterinarian*, 7; 607–611.

Sokolovsky V. (1972). Achalasia and paralysis of the canine oesophagus. *Journal of American Veterinary Medical Association*, **64**; 943–955.

Suter P.F. & Watrous B.J. (1980). Oropharyngeal dysphagia in the dog: A cinefluorographic analysis of experimentally induced and spontaneously occurring swallowing disorders. *Veterinary Radiography*, **21**; 24–39.

Uzuka Y. & Nakama S. (1988). Persistent right aortic arch in a cat. *Companion Animal Practice*, **2**; 14–16.

Watrous B. (1983). Oesophageal disease. In: *Textbook of Veterinary Internal Medicine*, S.J. Ettinger (ed.), W.B. Saunders, Philadelphia. 1191–1233.

Wilkinson G.T. (1970). Chronic papillomatous oesophagitis in a young cat. *Veterinary Record*, **87**; 355–356.

Woods C.B., Rawlings L., Barber D. & Walker M. (1978). Oesophageal deviation in four English Bulldogs. *Journal of American Veterinary Medical Association*, **172**; 934–939.

Zawie D.A. (1987). Medical diseases of the oesophagus. *Compendium on Continuing Education for the Practicing Veterinarian*, **9**; 1146–1152.

3/Conditions of the Stomach

Gastric anatomy

The stomach is a direct continuation of the oesophagus lying caudal to the liver and deep under the costal arch. The fundus of the stomach lies on the left side of the abdomen while the pylorus lies to the right, continuing as the duodenum. The stomach is semi-lunar in shape with a convex greater-curvature and concave lesser-curvature, the latter being divided by a fold called the angular incisure. The cardiac zone is small and continuous with the oesophagus while the fundus forms the largest zone linked to the pylorus by the body. The pyloric zone is divided into the pyloric antrum which leads to the pyloric canal with its associated pyloric sphincter (Fig. 3.1).

The stomach wall has four layers; from the outside inwards, the serosa, muscle, submucosa and mucosa. The serosa is a transparent sheet of meso-thelial cells attached to the underlying muscle by loose connective tissue. The muscle layer comprises of three layers of smooth muscle, the outer

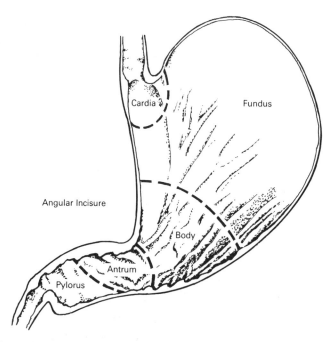

Fig. 3.1 Anatomical divisions of the stomach.

longitudinal muscle fibres are continuous with those of the oesophagus and duodenum and merge with the external oblique fibres at the greater- and lesser-curvature. The inner circular muscle fibres line all zones except for the fundus, and the fibres become especially thinkened at the pylorus where they form a true anatomical sphincter. Some internal oblique fibres exist, and fan out from the cardiac zone and form the weak cardiac sphincter. The submucosa contains elastic fibres and other connective tissue, blood vessels, nerves and lymphoid tissue (Miller *et al*. 1964). Mast cells are commonly found in the mucosa and submucosa (Aures *et al*. 1968).

The mucosa is thrown into folds called rugae formed by the muscularis mucosae. The surface mucosa is covered in mucus-secreting columnar epithelial cells which extend into numerous invaginations forming the gastric pits. The proliferative zone for epithelial renewal lies at the isthmus of the gastric pits from where cells migrate onto the mucosal surface. Epithelial cell turnover occurs every 3 days (Eastwood 1977).

Each zone in the stomach contains specific types of glandular cells. In the cardiac zone epithelial cells secrete mucus. In the fundus and body regions the parietal cells found in the mid-region of the gastric pits secrete hydrochloric acid while chief cells found near the base of the pits secrete pepsinogen which digests protein. Renewal of parietal and chief cells occurs from sites deep in the pits at the much slower rate, of approximately 25 days (Eastwood 1977). Argentaffin cells are found in the gastric pits of the fundus region secreting serotonin and the antrum where gastrin is produced from G cells (Grube & Forssmann 1979). These cells are part of the (amine precursor uptake and decarboxylation (APUD) cells). The lamina propria of the mucosa contains connective tissue and the muscularis mucosae.

Gastric physiology

The stomach has three main functions: (1) it acts as a reservoir for ingested food without any increase in intragastric pressure, (2) it mixes food with hydrochloric acid and pepsin to start the digestive process; and (3) it controls the flow of ingesta into the intestine.

Food reservoir

When food is ingested, relaxation of the stomach allows filling to occur without increases in intragastric pressure. The capacity of the stomach is very variable and ranges between 0.5 and 8 litre depending on the size of the dog or cat (Miller *et al*. 1964). The ability of the stomach to relax is centrally mediated so with each swallowing process there is relaxation of the fundus and body of the stomach. This is reinforced by a local reflex where distention of the stomach itself further induces relaxation.

Digestion

Initial digestion occurs by addition of hydrochloric acid and pepsin from the fundus and body of the stomach, and following thorough mixing of the contents in the pyloric antrum there is slow release of chyme into the duodenum. Gastrin is produced by the G cells in the mucosa of the pyloric antrum and duodenum. In order for the parietal cells to produce hydrochloric acid it is necessary for receptor sites on these cells to be occupied by one or more of acetylcholine, histamine and gastrin (Moreland 1988). Blocking one of these receptors seriously reduces the amount of hydrochloric acid produced by the cells. Natural inhibition of gastrin occurs by negative feedback mechanism from high acid levels in chyme reaching the antrum. Gastrin not only stimulates hydrochloric acid production, it also causes hypertrophy of the fundal mucosa, increases antral motility and increases the tone of the gastro-oesophageal sphincter. Gastrin is normally catabolized by cells in the kidney or liver among other tissues (Breitschwerdt et al. 1986). Hydrogen ion is produced from the breakdown of carbonic acid to bicarbonate and hydrogen ions, involving the enzyme carbonic anhydrase. Production of large amounts of hydrogen ion is an energy-dependent process involving active transport at membrane levels.

Vagal fibres are stimulated by the sight, smell and taste of food, resulting in the release of gastrin and consequently hydrochloric acid and pepsinogen (Walsh et al. 1972). Distention of the stomach together with the presence of digested protein also stimulates gastric secretion. Finally the presence of amino acids and peptides in the duodenum leads to increased gastric secretion via gastrin and histamine release. Histamine output occurs mainly during the early phase of gastrin secretion.

Pepsinogen, the inactive precursor of pepsin, is produced by the chief cells found in the fundus of the stomach. Control of secretion is determined by the same mechanisms as those controlling acid production. Pepsinogen is converted to pepsin in the lumen of the stomach by the presence of hydrochloric acid. If the pH of gastric juice rises, pepsin is rapidly inactivated and this happens naturally when gastric chyme enters the duodenum where bicarbonate neutralizes the gastric acid and thus pepsin.

Mucus is composed of glycoproteins, protein and carbohydrate. It coats the gastric mucosa and protects it from acid and mechanical damage and also functions as a lubricant. Mucus secretion is stimulated by irritation of the mucosa and also by acetylcholine action. Mucus contains pepsin inhibitors and some buffering capacity against hydrochloric acid.

Gastric mucosal barrier

The gastric mucosal barrier is designed as a defence mechanism to protect the stomach from irritant ingested food, hydrochloric acid and excessive pepsin activity. It consists of two parts: a layer of mucus covering the gastric mucosa; and secondly columnar epithelial cells lining the surface of the mucosa. Although the mucus has some buffering capacity and can inactivate pepsin, its role in barrier formation is minor. The major component of the barrier is provided by the epithelial cells and more specifically the lipoprotein layer on their apical surface. Damage to this barrier leads to disruption of the epithelial cells and breakdown of tight junctions between the cells. Such damage may follow use of various drugs, e.g. aspirin, phenylbutazone, interferences with gastric blood flow leading to ischaemia, reflux of bile or pancreatic enzymes into the stomach and the possible involvement of autoimmune mechanisms (Twedt & Magne 1986). Damage to the barrier allows acid and pepsin to inflame the mucosa and underlying tissues with disruption of mast cells releasing histamine which stimulates further acid production and thus further damage (Fig. 3.2).

Emptying

The fundus acts as a hopper and controls emptying of liquids while the antrum acts as a mixing chamber grinding solid foods. The pyloric sphincter has little control over emptying of liquids but may influence the particle size of solids emptied into the duodenum. In addition it prevents reflux

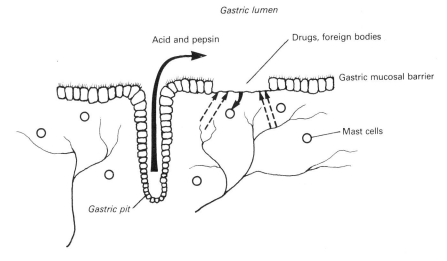

Fig. 3.2 Mechanism of gastric ulceration.

of duodenal contents into the stomach (Hall *et al.* 1988, Stemper & Cooke 1976).

The stomach has an inbuilt electrical pacemaker located in the greater-curvature which produces five slow waves per minute which spread over the stomach and may initiate muscle contraction (Weber & Kohatsu 1970). Contractions only occur if the slow wave triggers a spike potential and this does not always occur, as hormones and neural control mechanisms influence the initiation of spike potentials. Three types of gastric motility are recognized. The first, digestive motility, occurs after ingestion of a meal when there are slow continuous antral mixing contractions. Interdigestive motility occurs when the stomach is empty, and involves high amplitude contractions which cleanse the stomach, emptying any stomach contents into the duodenum. Lastly are the intermediate contractions which are a transition between the above types of motility (Itoh *et al.* 1977).

The stomach empties liquids faster than solids and carbohydrates faster than fats. Solids are retained for further antral mixing until they are reduced in size to 2 mm, suspended in liquid and then emptied into the duodenum. When large undigestible plastic spheres were fed as an experiment they remained in the stomach (Hinder & Kelly 1977). The greater the nutrient density of the diet, the slower the stomach empties (Hunt & Stubbs 1975). Gastric emptying is controlled by other factors such as the presence of chyme of low pH, or chyme containing fats and products of protein digestion in the duodenum, all of which reduce gastric emptying (Cooke 1975, Hunt & Stubbs 1975).

Acute gastritis

True vomiting may be due to acute or chronic gastritis for which there are many causes (Table 3.1). It is also important to remember that true vomiting may be due to non-gastric causes (see Chapter 4). Apparent vomiting, or in reality regurgitation, may be associated with oesophageal disease and this should be carefully differentiated (see Chapter 4).

Acute gastritis occurs where sudden and significant inflammation of the mucosa occurs, often involving some dietary indiscretion. In particular the history may suggest access to spoiled foods, foreign bodies, grass, bones and chemicals, e.g. detergents, antifreeze, which abrade and inflame the mucosa. Although infectious agents may cause acute gastritis they rarely do so exclusively, so enteritis or other systemic symptoms would be expected. The mucosal damage created allows acid and pepsin to diffuse back onto the mucosal surface leading to inflammation, cellular infiltration and ulceration where the condition is severe or chronic. Mast cell disruption releases histamine which induces further acid production and so potentiates the damage. Afferent nerves are stimulated leading to vomiting through the

Table 3.1 Conditions of the stomach

Acute gastritis
Chronic gastritis
  Idiopathic
  Atrophic
  Hypertrophic
  Eosinophilic
Gastric ulceration
Gastric neoplasia
Gastric foreign body
Gastric motility disorders
Pyloric stenosis
Gastric dilation/torsion

vomiting centre, and distention of inflamed stomach by further food or liquid intake acts as a powerful stimulus to vomiting (Burrows 1986).

Clinical diagnosis

Acute sudden onset of vomiting is initially associated with food or liquids but as anorexia develops so vomiting may occur at any time. Weakness, depression, dehydration, collapse and occasionally fever may be detected, although a reduced temperature once collapsed is more common. It is important to differentiate acute gastritis from gastric or intestinal obstruction, intussusception, acute pancreatitis, acute hepatitis, poisoning and specific infections.

A diagnosis is usually based on history and clinical findings. If symptomatic treatment fails, then it is usual to instigate an investigation. Such an investigation might include radiography and barium studies and blood chemistry if a secondary non-gastric cause of vomiting is suspected.

Treatment

Total gastric rest for at least 24 h prevents gastric distention and so reduces the frequency of vomiting. Gastric rest also inhibits acid and pepsin production which would further inflame the mucosa. Administration of kaolin or bismuth oral preparations when vomiting stops, acts as protectants. Antiemetics such as metaclopramide (Emequell; SmithKline Beecham Pharmaceuticals) 0.5 to 1.0 mg/kg every 8 h may be given as long as there is no evidence of obstruction. Rehydrate with intravenous Hartmans solution or isotonic dextrose saline. Once vomiting has stopped for at least 24 h start oral electrolyte solution (Lectade; SmithKline Beecham Pharmaceuticals) as an oral rehydrant instead of water, and if vomiting does not recur feeding bland easily-digested food in small amounts should be initiated.

Chronic gastritis

Chronic gastritis may be described as a condition where there is chronic vomiting of variable frequency and character. It clinically describes any patient with chronic vomiting for which there is no diagnosis. Pathologists generally describe chronic gastritis by the changes observed on histopathology. Unfortunately it is possible to have histopathological changes but no clinical signs and clinical signs but no pathological changes. Any definition therefore has to be confined to those conditions where there are clinical signs and positive histopathology. Two forms occur: ulcerative and non-ulcerative. The non-ulcerative conditions may be further divided into idiopathic, atrophic, hypertrophic and eosinophilic gastritis. Ulcerative gastritis is associated with advanced forms of the above or other more serious conditions such as neoplasia. Non-ulcerative idiopathic gastritis is the type most commonly observed clinically, but the cause is rarely determined (Burrows 1986).

The aetiology of chronic gastritis is complex and varied and will be discussed in more detail when describing the specific conditions in the following sections. However it includes dietary factors, interference with microcirculation leading to mucosal ischaemia, excess hydrochloric acid production, reflux of bile and enzyme into stomach, autoimmune disease and release of gastric antigen following physical damage (Twedt & Magne 1986).

Idiopathic gastritis

Idiopathic gastritis is a reversible condition which occurs following repeated exposure to a specific agent. It may be an early phase of a more serious form of gastritis when ulceration may develop and before changes have become irreversible.

The dog is often in good physical condition, with the exception of intermittent vomiting. There are rarely any changes in blood picture or radiographs, and endoscopy reveals very little, except that on histopathological examination of biopsy tissue, there is infiltration of the mucosa by plasma cells and lymphocytes with some degree of fibrosis in the lamina propria (Burrows 1986).

Treatment may require correction of dehydration but this is only likely in advanced cases. The use of metaclopramide (Emequell; SmithKline Beecham Pharmaceuticals) 0.5 to 1.0 mg/kg every 8 h is frequently helpful and dietary correction or modification using a low fat diet may also be beneficial. Any underlying cause should always be sought, although this is rarely found.

Atrophic gastritis

Introduction

A rare condition of older dogs in which there is atrophy of the gastric mucosa and loss of secretory power which is thought to be immune-mediated (Burrows 1986). There is a reduction in the thickness of the mucosa, and histopathologically in the size and depth of gastric pits. Parietal cells are replaced by mucus-secreting cells and there is cellular infiltration similar to that observed in idiopathic gastritis. Although the cause has not been determined, it may be the end-stage of idiopathic gastritis occurring over many months. A model has been produced where a dog was experimentally immunized with its own gastric juice resulting in changes similar to those produced in naturally occurring disease, indicating a possible autoimmune aetiology (Twedt & Magne 1986).

In this condition there is a reduction in the volume of hydrochloric acid produced and this can lead to small intestinal bacterial overgrowth, malabsorption and chronic diarrhoea. Plasma gastrin is elevated in affected dogs because the normal negative feedback mechanism is inhibited by low gastric acid levels.

Clinical diagnosis

Chronic intermittent vomiting is the feature of this condition often occurring over several months. The vomitus may contain mucus, bile or food and there is rarely a direct association with feeding. Eructation and anorexia may also occur and occasionally there is evidence of abdominal pain, manifest by the dog assuming a praying position. Chronic diarrhoea and weight loss have occurred when bacterial overgrowth develops.

The clinical signs are non-specific and radiographs rarely provide additional diagnostic information. To obtain a diagnosis, endoscopy and biopsy of the gastric mucosa is required. Macroscopically there may be flattened rugal folds. The mucosa may bleed easily when touched by the endoscope and submucosal blood vessels may be easily observed. Microscopically there is loss of glandular tissue, plasma cell infiltration of the lamina propria and varying amounts of fibrosis.

Treatment

Prognosis is generally good in the majority of cases but treatment may be required for life. A meat and not a cereal-based diet should be fed and ideally a hypoallergen diet should be offered in frequent small meals each day. Azathioprine (Imuran; Calmic Medicals Division) has been suggested where autoimmune disease is suspected. Corticosteroids although anti-inflammatory, stimulate parietal cells to produce hydrochloric acid. However prednisolone may be of value when given at 1 mg/kg daily for 1 week to reduce the immune response (Burrows 1986). Antibiotic in the form of tylosin at 20 mg/kg bid (Tylan; Elanco Products) may be required to control bacterial overgrowth and chronic diarrhoea.

Hypertrophic gastritis

This is a condition characterized by gross thickening of the gastric mucosa occurring as a diffuse or focal form involving the fundus, body or pylorus of the stomach (Clark 1985). It appears to be similar to a condition seen in man termed 'Menetrier's Disease' (Burrows 1986). The condition has been described in the cat (Dennis *et al.* 1987) as well as the dog (Van der Gaag *et al.* 1976). The focal form often involves the antrum and pylorus causing outflow obstruction or may appear like a polyp. In the diffuse form the majority of the mucosa is involved with macroscopic thickening of the mucosa and large rugal folds (Fig. 3.3 and Plate 1). This is due histologically to glandular hyperplasia and cystic dilation of mucus glands with cellular infiltration of plasma cells and lymphocytes. Metaplastic changes lead to a loss of differentiation between the parietal and chief cells. Occasionally there is ulceration and hypertrophy of the muscle layer as well as the mucosa.

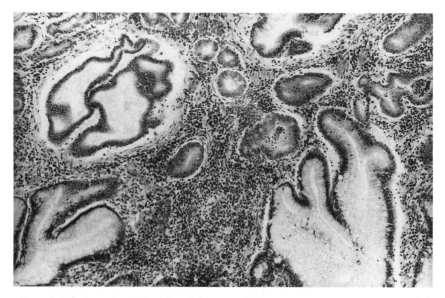

Fig. 3.3 Microscopic appearance observed in hypertrophic gastritis.

The aetiology is not known but may include autoimmune disease, genetic predisposition in Boxers and Basenjis, hormonal influence especially through excessive levels of acetylcholine, gastrin or histamine which have a trophic effect on the mucosa (Twedt & Magne 1986). It may also occur where there is renal disease with failure to metabolize gastrin leading to hyperacidity and gastric mucosal hypertrophy. Parasitic conditions may also be implicated, and one case in a Siamese cat reported the presence of *Ullalonus tricuspis* in the stomach (Dennis *et al.* 1987). Pyloric stenosis may coexist with hypertrophy gastritis and is especially seen in small breeds, nervous dogs, behaviour-associated cases and with neuroendocrine disease (Twedt & Magne 1986).

Clinical diagnosis

Chronic vomiting usually occurring over several months is a feature in diffuse cases and the vomitus varies considerably from large volumes of fluid at low pH, to haematemesis where ulceration is present. If there is outflow obstruction vomiting may be described as projectile, associated with feeding and usually containing food. Anorexia, abdominal pain, diarrhoea and weight loss do occur (Sikes *et al.* 1986).

In the diffuse form, barium studies may reveal prominent rugal patterns while in the focal form these changes may be confined to the antrum and pylorus. Delayed gastric emptying is a feature when the focal pyloric form is present, together with narrowing of the antrum. Endoscopy is more helpful and reveals enlarged rugae, while biopsy confirms the diagnosis.

Treatment

Treatment must be supportive as there is no cure and thus the prognosis must be guarded. Renal and liver disease and gastrin-producing tumours should be considered. Surgical intervention is required when the focal form causes pyloric stenosis by carrying out pyloric resection (Dennis *et al.* 1987, Twedt & Magne 1986) or pyloroplasty (Sikes *et al.* 1986). In the diffuse form frequent small meals using hypoallergen diets together with cimetidine (Tagamet; SmithKline Beecham) 5 to 10 mg/kg every 8 h or ranetidine (Zantac; Glaxo Laboratories) 0.5 mg/kg every 12 h will effect control in many cases.

Eosinophilic gastritis

This is a rare condition in which there is eosinophilic infiltration and diffuse fibrosis of all layers of the stomach wall. Occasionally there is focal granuloma formation which may resemble gastric neoplasia. The cause is not known but it has been suggested that immunological mediation involving allergens or parasites may be involved (Twedt & Magne 1986). In particular *Toxocara canis* has been implicated (Hayden & Van Kruiningen 1973). An eosinophilic lymphadenitis and vasculitis may be seen.

Clinical diagnosis

The history may reveal chronic intermittent vomiting over a long period of time. There may be an association with dietary changes or increased levels of parasitism. Vomitus may contain blood and may or may not be associated with feeding. Signs of ascites and subcutaneous oedema may also develop in advanced cases, where hypoproteinaemia has occurred through protein loss across the gastric mucosa.

Routine haematology often reveals a persistent circulating eosinophilia and some degree of hypoproteinaemia. Barium studies may reveal filling defects, narrowing or thickening of the mucosa. The mucosa may bleed easily and ulceration has also been observed on endoscopy. The diagnosis is confirmed by histopathology of biopsy tissue which shows eosinophil infiltrates in mucosa, submucosa and muscle layers. The infiltration may be diffuse or focal and vasculitis often with thrombosis occurs.

Hayden & Fleischmann (1977) described a scirrhous eosinophilic gastritis of three female dogs between the ages of 3 and 5 years, where there was weight loss, lethargy and recurrent vomiting with peripheral eosinophilia. These dogs had a palpably thickened stomach and sometimes pendulous abdomen.

Treatment

The use of a hypoallergen diets frequently results in a fall in the circulating eosinophil count without need for other treatment. Any evidence of endoparasites such as *Toxocara canis* should also be treated using a suitable anthelmintic. In addition prednisone at 0.5 mg/kg daily for 2 weeks, tailing off to alternate day therapy should be provided. However in some cases longer-term therapy, in the order of several weeks is required.

Gastric foreign bodies

A wide range of foreign bodies have been found in the stomachs of dogs. They range from stones and balls to spoons, razor blades and fish hooks. On the other hand cats are fastidious eaters and foreign bodies are rare in this species. The exception is the fur or hairball which does occur but is grossly overdiagnosed. This occurs following excessive self-grooming especially in long haired breeds of cat.

Very often foreign bodies are detected by accident as they are asymptomatic unless they cause valve-like obstructions in the pylorus. However they can also account for acute episodes of vomiting. If the objects are sharp or abrasive then physical damage to the mucosa occurs and leads to chronic gastritis which gives more persistent symptoms. Earth or sand are good examples of abrasive foreign material ingested by puppies. In the authors' experience depraved appetite and polydipsia in dogs with gastric foreign bodies may be seen.

Clinical diagnosis

There may be no clinical signs at all, or there may be episodes of acute vomiting with periods of complete remission. This occurs when the foreign body obstructs the pylorus and then moves back into the fundus relieving the obstruction. Occasionally vomiting occurs with blood present but this is not typical. Vomiting may or may not occur associated with feeding. The foreign body may in rare cases cause perforation of the stomach with resultant peritonitis. If this occurs the signs change to include marked abdominal pain and guarding on palpation. There will be pyrexia together with depression and dehydration. An exudative ascites may be detected on paracentesis of the abdomen.

Diagnosis of foreign bodies is usually simple following X-ray of the abdomen to reveal a radiodense mass in the stomach (Fig. 3.4). Occasionally

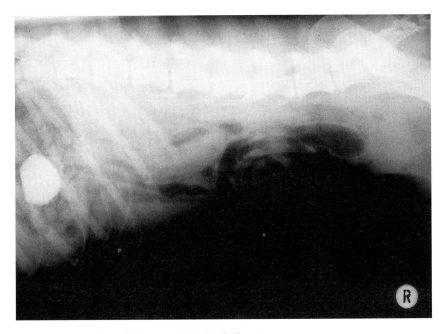

Fig. 3.4 Plain radiograph of a gastric foreign body.

however the object will be radiolucent and barium studies will be required to make a diagnosis. Evidence of peritonitis may be detected from radiographs as may ascites, giving a ground glass appearance to the abdomen and a lack of contrast (Fig. 3.5).

Treatment

Foreign bodies are usually successfully removed following laparotomy and gastrotomy. Where perforation has occurred and peritonitis has developed it is essential to obtain ascitic fluid for culture and sensitivity, followed by high doses of a suitable antibiotic. Once the patient has been rehydrated and the infection brought under control laparotomy should be carried out to repair the defect and remove the foreign body.

Gastric ulceration

Ulcers are uncommon in the dog. They are usually 'peptic' which means they develop in the presence of acid and pepsin, and are most commonly located in the body, antrum, pylorus or proximal duodenum. Normally the stomach can resist damage through protection from the gastric mucosal barrier. Anything which damages this barrier will lead to inflammation and ulceration. Acute lesions are often manifest as multiple superficial erosions,

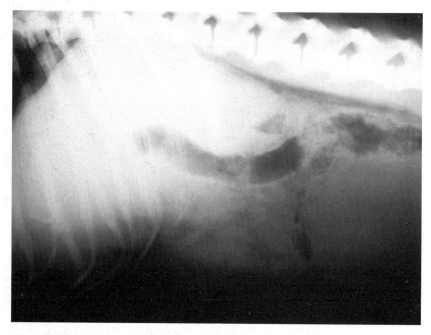

Fig. 3.5 Plain radiograph showing evidence of peritonitis.

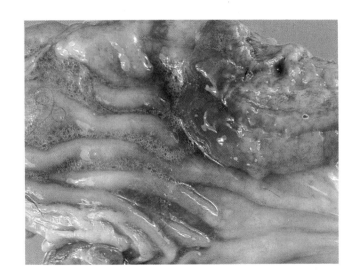

Plate 1 Macroscopic appearance of hypertrophic gastritis.

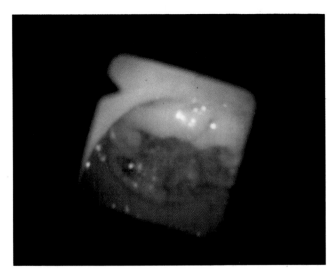

Plate 2 Endoscopic view of a gastric ulcer.

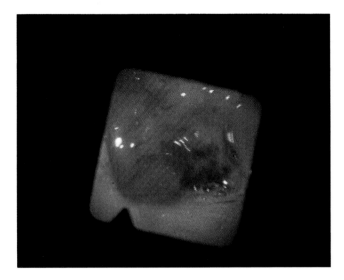

Plate 3 Endoscopic view of a gastric tumour.

while chronic lesions are single circumscribed deep ulcers with raised margins. Location, morphology and clinical manifestations vary with underlying pathogenesis. All the agents which cause acute and chronic gastritis together with anything which increases gastric acid production, changes the acid–base balance or effects the nutritional status can cause ulceration. The aetiology is large and complex and may be described as follows:

1 Drugs — such as aspirin, flunixin and phenylbutazone. They act by interfering directly with the mucosal barrier and not by increased acid production. Corticosteroids also cause ulceration by decreasing mucosal cell turnover, reducing mucus production both of which lead to loss of protection of the mucosa. In addition they increase gastrin levels, which stimulate acid production.

2 Shock, hypotension, trauma, central nervous system disease and severe illness. These are stress ulcers which occur as multiple small superficial erosions mainly in the body of the stomach.

3 Bile reflux. Bile acids are ulcerogenic and work together with factors inducing gastric ischaemia, excess acid and pepsin secretions to damage the gastric mucosal barrier. The prevalence of bile acid reflux is not clear but may be quite common.

4 Neuroendocrine. Stress causes release of cortisol and catecholamines which are thought to be ulcerogenic. If this occurs in conjunction with increased sympathetic drive causing vasoconstriction and thus mucosal ischaemia there is a real probability of ulcer formation.

5 Neurological disease. Dogs with spinal cord lesions undergoing surgery and receiving corticosteroids may develop haemorrhagic gastritis or deep ulceration of gastric mucosa often with high mortality. The spinal cord lesions are thought to lead to altered sympathetic/parasympathetic balance and stress ulceration. Vagal stimulation leads to vasodilation, increases acid and enzyme secretion. In addition to these changes animals with cord lesions often receive corticosteroids and this compounds the ulcerogenic effect.

6 Metabolic disease. In renal disease elevated blood urea and urea products occur. These toxins may damage, among many tissues, the gastric mucosa. Renal disease also delays excretion of gastrin and this continues to stimulate acid production. Ulcers may also occur in liver disease although the cause is not known but may be associated with catabolism of gastrin or other toxins. Murray *et al.* (1972) described 22 dogs with gastric ulcers, of which 16 had concurrent liver disease.

7 Hyperacidity. There are many conditions which increase acid production and hence increase risk of gastric ulceration. Increased vagal stimulation and elevated gastrin or histamine levels will have this effect. These peptic ulcers tend to be confined to the antrum and proximal duodenum. Increased gastrin comes from gastrin secreting tumours found in either the stomach or

pancreas. The condition is similar to Zollinger–Ellison syndrome observed in man and dogs (Breitschwerdt *et al.* 1986). Secondary increases in gastrin levels occur when gastrin is retained in renal disease. Further parietal cells are stimulated to produce more acid by elevated histamine levels. Such levels originate from systemic mastocytomas or mast cell tumours in the liver (Twedt 1983).

8   Ulceration can be associated with the presence of gastric neoplasia where the tumour involves the mucosa and there is a breakdown of the gastric mucosal barrier. For this reason it is essential to biopsy any dog or cat with gastric ulceration to determine if neoplasia is present.

Clinical diagnosis

Vomiting with the presence of blood usually indicates ulceration. Blood may be present in small amounts, as large clots or occur as 'coffee grounds' if retained in the stomach for some time prior to vomition. A microcytic anaemia may be observed in chronic ulceration as may dark tarry faeces if blood passes through the pylorus and intestinal tract. Nausea, variable appetite, weight loss, polydipsia and gastric pain, manifest by assuming the praying position, may all occur (Murray *et al.* 1972). Some dogs exhibit marked salivation particularly in advanced cases, while other dogs show no clinical signs at all (Twedt 1983).

Contrast studies may reveal filling defects or barium retention. Endoscopy is the best confirmatory method of diagnosis. Chronic ulcers show little inflammation but appear as craters with raised peripheries and may bleed easily. Stress ulcers appear as small punctate submucosal haemorrhages scattered over the stomach surface. Biopsy via exploratory laparotomy or endoscopy (Plate 2) is essential as ulcers may be associated with malignant neoplasia. Plasma gastrin levels should be checked, the normal fasted range for the dog being 20 to 70 pg/ml. Results should be interpreted carefully as gastrin levels may be increased in renal or hepatic disease, gastric retention and gastritis (Twedt 1983).

Treatment

The prognosis depends on the underlying cause and also whether the most frequent complication, namely perforation and peritonitis has occurred (Murray *et al.* 1972). An underlying cause should be determined and further mucosal damage prevented. If no obvious cause is found then the symptoms should be treated, thus improving the mucosal environment. The diet should be changed to a low fat diet fed as frequent small meals. In addition metaclopramide (Emequell; SmithKline Beecham) at 0.5 to 1.0 mg/kg every 8 h may be used to reduce vomiting. Oral antacids may be

Table 3.2 Antacids available to control the production or effects of gastric acid

Non-systemic antacids	Aluminium hydroxide, calcium carbonate Magnesium hydroxide: Mucaine Aludrox
Systemic antacids	H_2 blockers: Tagamet Zantec

used to neutralize the acid and to inactivate the pepsin (Table 3.2). Non-systemic antacids must be given frequently as infrequent use often leads to rebound hyperacidity. This occurs because of the failure in the negative feedback reflex where low pH reduces gastrin and hence acid production. The maximum frequency of dosing should be every 2h. At this dose rate there are risks of sodium overload, alkalosis and diarrhoea from magnesium salts. Aluminium hydroxide may lead to phosphate deficiency. Gastric acidity may also be reduced using systemic H_2 blockers which block the histamine receptor on the parietal cell. These drugs are useful in idiopathic ulceration, gastritis, mast cell tumour, gastrinomas and in uraemia. Cimetidine (Tagamet; SmithKline Beecham) at 5 mg/kg tid has been shown to be effective with no apparent toxicity. Anticholinergic drugs reduce vagal stimulation of acid production, and allow smooth muscle relaxation, but also reduce gastric emptying. This causes distention of the stomach which in turn stimulates acid production. Carbenoxolone (Winthrop) is a drug which protects gastric/duodenal mucosa by promoting mucus production and prolonging the life of epithelial cells. Sucralfate is a new drug given orally to coat and seal gastric ulcers, effectively 'bandaging' the ulcer. This prevents any further inflammation from acid or pepsin activity. It is a human preparation and as yet there is no suitable data for veterinary use.

Gastric haemorrhage may be treated with oral iced water and noradrenaline 8 mg/500 ml by stomach tube. Any absorbed noradrenaline is removed by passage through the liver. The lavage should be left in the stomach for 5 to 30 min, then removed to assess for further bleeding. Surgical resection of ulcers may be required especially in cases where tumour is involved.

Gastric neoplasia

Gastric neoplasia is rare in dogs and cats compared with man. The types of tumour detected in small animals include polyps, adenomas, leiomyomas, adenocarcinomas and lymphosarcomas. The most frequent tumour in dogs is the adenocarcinoma and the most frequent site is the antrum or pylorus of the stomach. Lymphosarcoma is the commonest feline tumour although this is not frequently seen. Tumours frequently ulcerate so symptomatology may be similar to that observed with gastric ulceration, and endoscopically they appear very similar so histopathology of surgical biopsy is essential to differentiate which is present. Tumours have been observed more frequently in Rough Collies, Irish Setter and Terrier breeds, the mean age being 10 years and possibly more common in males than females (Sullivan *et al.* 1987).

Clinical diagnosis

Classically there is a history of chronic vomiting, polydipsia and weight loss. The signs may appear over a short period of time or may develop more slowly over many months. The vomitus may be gastric juice and saliva or may contain food. There is no strong correlation between eating and vomiting but it certainly occurs in some individuals. Vomitus may also contain fresh or changed blood (coffee grounds) but this is not pathognomonic of gastric tumours. The animals frequently salivate and become anorexic and depressed in the latter stages of the condition.

A diagnosis cannot be made from clinical findings alone but usually requires confirmation from radiography, endoscopy or exploratory laparotomy. Tumours are most frequently found in the pyloric antrum or along the lesser curvature to the cardia. Plain X-rays usually fail to reveal the

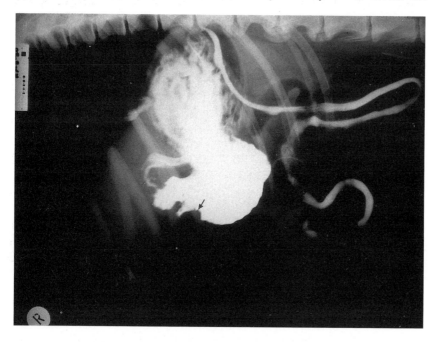

Fig. 3.6 Barium radiograph of a gastric filling defect (arrowed).

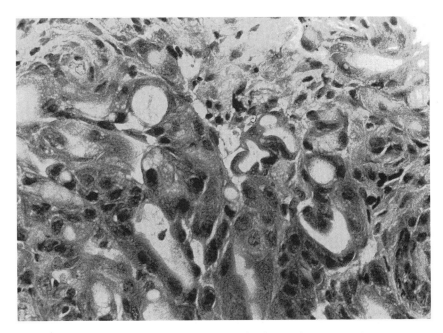

Fig. 3.7 Histological appearance of biopsy of gastric adenocarcinoma.

tumour but may show roughening of the surface or narrowing of the pyloric lumen. Contrast studies may reveal filling defects and delayed gastric emptying but these changes are not a common feature (Fig. 3.6). Endoscopy and biopsy is required to obtain a definitive diagnosis (Fig. 3.7 and Plate 3). Usually there are macroscopic changes present including ulceration, hypertrophy of the mucosa or outflow obstruction. Multiple ulcers are more frequently observed in lymphosarcoma while single large ulcers occur more frequently with adenocarcinomas. The periphery of the lesion should be biopsied and more than one sample must be collected. Adenocarcinoma frequently invades and produces a scirrhous or fibrosing reaction which results in an inflexible area of the gastric wall with distended lymphatics and early neoplastic peritonitis with adhesions. Changes may not be picked up by endoscopy and biopsy sampling if the mucosa is not involved. In such cases where no mucosal changes can be readily observed, it would be important to consider exploratory laparotomy. Although endoscopy may miss some forms of tumour, laparotomy will always allow a diagnosis to be made. However it is a very invasive technique to be employed routinely whenever a gastric condition is suspected (Sullivan *et al.* 1987).

Treatment

The prognosis must be very guarded. Surgical resection may be successful when the tumour is confined to a small area of the stomach. However the tumour is often well-established, locally spreading and may have metastasized by the time a diagnosis is obtained, necessitating euthanasia. Chemotherapy combined with surgery may be a possibility in the future but is rarely considered at the present time.

Gastric motility disorders

There are three types of normal gastric motility. The digestive, intermediate and interdigestive patterns (Itoh *et al.* 1977, Twedt 1983). When any of these motility patterns become disturbed the animal is described as having a gastric motility disorder. Such motility disorders may include situations where there is chronic vomiting of undigested food many hours after eating, gastric atony, reflux of bile into the stomach, reflux oesophagitis and even gastric dilation/torsion.

Motility disorders may occur secondarily to underlying gastric pathology. Gastric atony and retention may be associated with gastric ulceration, neoplasia or pyloric stenosis. Other conditions such as pylorospasm, bilious vomiting and reflux oesophagitis may be primary motility disorders. Stress, excitement and flight or fight reactions can account for physiological gastric atony, but primary disorders of organized gastric motility do seem to occur (Table 3.3).

Diagnosis of primary motility disorders is made on the grounds that no evidence of other gastric disease can be found following an extensive investigation. There are very few methods of diagnosing motility disorders, although our recognition of the normal physiology of gastric motility is much improved. Blood chemistry, routine radiographs, barium studies and endoscopy are of little value. The only effective method of diagnosis is through the use of fluoroscopy and observing gastric motility.

Gastric emptying time is governed by the ingesta present and not on time itself. There is hormonal and neural control as well as that of the ingesta. Liquids empty faster than solids and carbohydrates faster than fats or protein. Retention of non-digestible substances such as hair or grass may

Table 3.3 Gastric motility disorders

Primary	Pylorospasm
	Bilious vomiting syndrome
	Reflux oesophagitis
	Gastric dilation/torsion
Secondary	Fight or flight reactions
	Chronic gastritis
	Gastric ulceration/neoplasia
	Pyloric stenosis
	Gastric foreign bodies

be due to failure of 'housekeeper' contractions or 'interdigestive' contractions to occur.

Reflux gastritis

This has also been termed bilious vomiting syndrome (Burrows 1986). Reflux of bile and enzymes from the duodenum into the stomach is thought to be a normal event in fasted dogs. However if there is excess bile secretion, defective pyloric function, or reduced gastric motility, then bile is exposed to the gastric mucosa for long periods. Its detergent action damages the gastric mucosal barrier. This allows hydrochloric acid and pepsin to act on the mucosa causing further inflammation and, in severe cases, erosion and ulceration. Although the true cause is not known, it is most likely to occur where there is a failure of housekeeper contractions during periods of fasting and rest, allowing bile to pool and damage the gastric mucosal barrier.

Clinical diagnosis

Chronic vomiting of bile-stained fluid after a prolonged fast and when the animal is resting, usually occurs as an early morning event in dogs fed once daily in the afternoon. Those affected are described as having 'bad days' with total return to normal the following day. Owners describe the dog as restless early in the morning and if not fed quickly they will vomit a bile-stained fluid and remain anorexic for the remainder of the day. They rarely vomit throughout the day. Anorexia, depression, diarrhoea and borborygmi have also been reported by some owners.

Plain and contrast radiographs are of little value. Endoscopy reveals bile pooling in the stomach and biopsy confirms mild gastritis in most cases. The pylorus may be patent when examined endoscopically but this is variable. A diagnosis is made on the grounds of finding no other cause for the vomiting such as gastric or intestinal disease, in a dog exhibiting a typical history which is unresponsive to treatment.

Treatment

If an underlying cause has been found, this should be treated. The prognosis is usually good but the condition can only be controlled at present, as there is no cure, so treatment may be required for life. Dogs should be fed three times daily, by giving an early morning meal, the main meal in the afternoon and a late-night meal. Cimetidine (Tagamet; SmithKline Beecham) 4 mg/kg bid may be helpful but metaclopramide (Emequell; SmithKline

Beecham) 0.5 mg/kg given in the early morning and late at night is very effective in most cases (Minami & McCallum 1984).

Pylorospasm

It is not clear whether this is a true clinical entity as documented cases are rare in the veterinary literature. The antrum and pylorus should act together as a single unit and peristalsis of the antrum rather than pyloric closure controls emptying (Prove & Ehrlein 1982). In pylorospasm it is therefore likely that abnormal motility or peristalsis is the cause rather than true spasm of the pyloric sphincter. In the studies of Prove & Ehrlein (1982) there is outflow obstruction with radiographic evidence of retention and failure of barium to enter the duodenum. Confirmation of the diagnosis may be possible by carrying out barium studies after the administration of 0.5 mg/kg metaclopramide (Emequell; SmithKline Beecham) which causes relaxation of the pyloric sphincter. If there is no relief of gastric retention then pyloric stenosis is the most likely cause.

Pyloric stenosis

The condition may be due to abnormal pyloric motor function, or from congenital or acquired stenosis of the pylorus. Focal hypertrophic gastritis also causes outflow obstruction.

Congenital cases are seen most in brachiocephalic dogs and Siamese cats (Pearson et al. 1974). Symptoms occur at an early age associated with commencement of solid feeding and are progressive. The acquired form has no breed or sex predisposition and occurs in mid and old aged animals.

Aetiology is not known but may be due to high levels of gastrin which stimulates smooth muscle hypertrophy causing hypertrophy of the circular fibres. When food is retained by outlet obstruction this causes distention of the stomach which leads to release of gastrin. Gastrin, in addition to effects on smooth muscle, also causes release of hydrochloric acid and pepsin which can induce ulceration often observed in pyloric stenosis.

Abnormal pyloric motor function develops because of a reduction in the nerves of the myenteric plexus in the pyloric antrum so there is antral dilation and muscle hypertrophy together with nerve degeneration in the pylorus.

Clinical diagnosis

Gastric retention results in vomiting food hours after eating. Vomiting is often projectile, occurring abruptly without warning or without salivation or retching preceding the act of vomiting. Vomiting may occur at varying periods from minutes to hours after eating and frequently contains undigested or partially digested food. Bile is never found in the vomitus while saliva and gastric secretion may be observed. Young animals with the congenital form are otherwise healthy, except for vomiting, and failure to gain weight. Vomiting starts just after weaning and is progressive. There may be dehydration, anorexia and abdominal distention.

Normally the stomach will empty in 4−6h. A tentative diagnosis is made where there is a delay in gastric emptying. Vomiting of undigested food when the stomach should be empty is another diagnostic sign.

The gastric emptying time is that time required for the stomach to start emptying *not* the time for complete emptying. It should be less than 30 min in normal dogs and is often nearer 5 to 10 min. Barium retained for 12 to 24 h is abnormal. However it is a crude method of estimating gastric function. Drugs, stress and excitement will all influence the rate of emptying, together with the actual composition of the barium itself. It may be possible for liquid barium to pass through the pylorus without difficulty while barium mixed with food is retained in pyloric stenosis.

There may be failure of the pyloric canal to fill with barium, and the so-called 'pyloric beak' at the entry to the canal may be seen. Fluoroscopy is useful in assessing motility. Usually there is a loss of antral contractions, but initially there may be hypermotility then hypomotility in pyloric stenosis.

Endoscopy is of little value although it will detect hypertrophic gastritis, ulceration or tumour if they are involved in the aetiology. Exploratory laparotomy is an important diagnostic procedure where outflow obstruction is likely. It will also allow immediate surgical correction to be carried out at the same time.

Treatment

A knowledge of foods which empty fastest will allow good dietary management. For example low fat and high carbohydrate liquid diets are most effective. They should be given as frequent small meals.

Where pylorospasm is thought to be present drugs such as atropine, propanthelene bromide are useful as are parasympathomimetics such as bethanechol. Metaclopramide (Emequell; SmithKline Beecham) at 0.5 mg to 1 mg/kg orally 3/4 h before food is the most effective drug. It restores gastric tone and contractions and also relaxes the pyloric sphincter so improving gastric emptying.

Pyloric stenosis generally requires surgical correction. Either pyloromyotomy or pyloroplasty should be carried out depending on the extent of the changes observed. The muscle should always be biopsied in case there is a lesion such as a tumour present. The operation is good for improving the emptying of liquids and to some extent solids. Generally the prognosis is good in uncomplicated cases where there is no serious underlying cause. The prognosis is more guarded where tumour or destructive lesion is detected.

Gastric dilation and torsion

This condition preferentially affects the large deep-chested breeds of dog such as Bassett Hounds, German Shepherd dogs, St. Bernard, Irish Setters, Great Danes and Dobermans but Dachshunds may also be affected. There may be a predilection for young male dogs, but torsion has been observed in dogs from 2 to 10 years of age.

The cause is not known but predisposing factors include; breed, use of dry cereal-based diets, overeating or drinking, stress, exercise and aerophagia (Table 3.4). Cereal-based diets fed as one large meal per day result in larger and heavier stomachs than those found in dogs fed tinned meat and biscuit. This predisposes the dog to gastric dilation and torsion (Van Kruiningen *et al.* 1987). It is also possible that disordered gastric motility may be involved. Torsions most often occur to the left or clockwise effectively sealing off the oesophagus and pylorus (Burrows 1986). In our experience the mortality rate can exceed 68%.

Normally the pylorus is held in position on the right of the abdomen by the hepatoduodenal ligament, bile duct and lesser omentum. It can be forced to the left but returns to its original position when released. In dogs predisposed to dilation/torsion this does not occur, because there is a greater mobility of the stomach. A study of dogs with gastric dilation has shown that the stomach position may vary from the normally accepted position to that observed in gastric torsion. In some cases the stomach had rotated about 180 degrees, and returned to its normal position again. Instability of the stomach may be very important in the pathogenesis of torsion (Frendin *et al.* 1988). Therefore to create torsion there must be a gastric dilation present and increased gastric mobility. If the latter is absent then dilation is more likely to occur without torsion. Displacement of the stomach can occur if there is gastric retention and delayed gastric emptying.

Table 3.4 Predisposing causes for gastric torsion

Breed
Diet
Overeating
Stress, excitement
Gastric stasis
Aerophagia
Motility disorder
Lax gastric ligaments

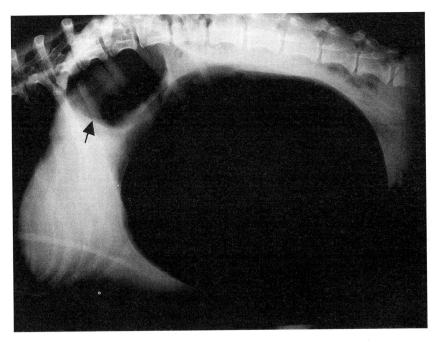

Fig. 3.8 Lateral radiograph showing the displaced pylorus in a dog with a gastric torsion.

Traction on the ligament attachments of the stomach in deep-chested dogs causes the stomach to become pendulous and so predisposed to torsion.

Aerophagia may also occur in the dog and again may lead to gastric dilation and predisposition to torsion. Gas analysis has been carried out in clinical cases and revealed the presence of a gas mixture similar to air with no evidence of methane thus ruling out possibilities of fermentation (Caywood *et al.* 1977).

Pathophysiology. When the stomach becomes dilated gastric ischaemia and circulatory shock occur. Distention of the stomach causes pressure occlusion of the vena cava and portal vein. Gastric ischaemia occurs when distention of the stomach wall is great enough to occlude the intramural arterioles. Necrosis and sloughing of the mucosa occur as a result of such ischaemia exacerbated by the action of gastric acid. If torsion has been present for some time then the muscle layer becomes necrotic and perforation is likely leading to peritonitis. Shock is frequently the cause of death, so this condition requires urgent treatment in order to save life (Table 3.5).

Baroreceptors respond to shock and hypotension by increasing sympathetic drive leading to tachycardia, vasoconstriction and splenic contraction. Right atrial receptors detect poor filling and respond by increasing anti-

Table 3.5 Pathophysiology of gastric torsion

Dilation of the stomach	Compresses blood vessels
	Compresses vena cava/portal vein
	Ischaemia of tissues
Displaced stomach	Occludes arterial supply to organ
Prolonged ischaemia	Necrosis of tissue (= perforation)
Renin	Angiotensin activation and vasoconstriction
Capillary damage	Vascular sludging
Reversible shock	Rapidly develops into irreversible shock

diuretic hormone (ADH) output, a potent vasoconstrictor. Renin from underperfused kidneys stimulates angiotensin which again leads to vasoconstriction. As shock continues multiple organ failure together with disseminated intravascular coagulation occurs, leading to death.

Clinical diagnosis

The history and symptoms are usually classical and cannot be readily confused with other conditions. There is a sudden dramatic abdominal enlargement with tympany. Initially there may be attempts at vomiting with salivation and marked restlessness. However the dog will rapidly become shocked and collapse. Occasionally there is no such history but a sudden tympany and collapse.

Diagnosis is based on the history and the presenting signs which are pathognomonic of this condition. It is however necessary to determine if dilation or torsion is present. Further diagnostic information can be obtained from radiography of the abdomen. However the dog is often critically ill and such procedures should be reduced to the minimum necessary in order to obtain a diagnosis. To this end the right lateral recumbent view will reveal a gas-filled pylorus dorsal to a gas-filled fundus in gastric torsion but not in gastric dilation (Fig. 3.8, Hathcock 1984). Evidence of haemorrhage in the gastric lavage may indicate gastric wall necrosis and risk of imminent rupture.

Treatment

It is essential that treatment is carried out promptly as these cases constitute true veterinary emergencies. There are three steps in the treatment which are carried out in the following chronological order; decompression, treatment of shock and finally surgery.

Decompression. This is the first and most important part of therapy as it improves the circulation and reduces shock and ischaemia. Passage of a stomach tube is the easiest method of decompression and can usually be carried out without sedation. If a small enough stomach tube is used, even when torsion is present, it should pass into the stomach. If the tube will not enter the stomach then gastrocentesis is an essential alternative. Prepare a site behind the costal arch and insert a large bore needle through the abdominal wall and into the stomach. Having partially decompressed the stomach, a stomach tube should be passed to allow air and fluid to be removed. Solids should be removed using a warm water lavage. If after gastrocentesis a stomach tube cannot be passed then exploratory laparotomy must be carried out immediately.

Shock. Intravenous lactated ringer solution should be administered immediately at 90 ml/kg/30 min, then the rate adjusted according to the animal's requirements (Leib & Martin 1987). If the PCV falls to less than 20% whole blood may be needed. Prednisolone at 10 mg/kg or dexamethasone at 4 mg/kg should be administered in conjunction with broad spectrum antibiotics such as ampicillin and gentamycin, trimethoprin and sulphonamides, or intravenous penicillins. Intravenous bicarbonate will be needed but the requirement is difficult to assess unless blood gas analysis is available.

Surgery. Surgery should be performed as soon as possible after decompression. Barbiturates should not be used for induction; gaseous anaesthesia should be induced using a face mask. The stomach and spleen should be repositioned by standing on the right and pulling up the pylorus and moving it over to the right while pushing the fundus down and to the left. Resection may be required if tissue is not viable. The best site to evaluate the condition of the stomach is the greater-curvature. Once the spleen is repositioned it should contract down, a splenectomy should only be performed if blood vessels are damaged.

If the tissues are viable then the stomach should be stabilized. Gastropexy is carried out by exposing the serosa and muscle layer at the antrum and suturing this at the twelfth rib on the right costal arch (Leib & Martin 1987).

References

Aures D., Hakansan R., Owman C.L. & Sporrons B. (1968) Cellular stores of histamines and monoamines in the dog stomach. *Life Sciences*, 7; 1147–1153.

Breitschwerdt E.J., Turk J.R., Turnwald G.H., Davenport D.J., Hedlund C.S. & Carakostas M.C. (1986) Hypergastrinaemia in canine gastrointestinal disease. *Journal of American Animal Hospital Association*, 22; 585–592.

Burrows C.F. (1986) Diseases of the canine stomach. In: *The Veterinary Annual*, C.S.G. Grunsell, F.W.G. Hill & M.E. Raw (eds), Scientechnica, Bristol, 270–282.

Caywood D., Teague H.D., Jackson D.A., Levitt M.D. & Bond J.H. (1977) Gastric gas analysis in canine gastric distention-volvulus. *Journal of American Animal Hospital Association*, 13; 459–462.

Clark W.A. (1985) Canine gastric hyperplasia. In: *The Veterinary Annual*. C.S.G. Grunsell, F.W.G. Hill & M.E. Raw (eds), Scientechnica, Bristol, 245–247.

Cooke A.R. (1975) Control of gastric emptying and motility. *Gastroenterology*, 68; 804–816.

Dennis R., Herrtage M.E., Jefferies A.R., Matic S.E. & White R.A.S. (1987) A case of hyperplastic gastropathy in a cat. *Journal of Small Animal Practice*, 28; 491–504.

Eastwood G.L. (1977) Gastrointestinal epithelial renewal. *Gastroenterology*, 72; 962–975.

Frendin J., Funkquist B. & Stavenborn M. (1988) Gastric displacement in dogs without signs of acute dilation. *Journal of Small Animal Practice*, 29; 775–779.

Grube D. & Forssmann W.G. (1979) Morphology and function of the enteroendocrine cells. *Hormone and Metabolism Research*, 11; 581–606.

Hall J.A., Burrows C.F. & Twedt D.C. (1988) Gastric motility in dogs. Part I. Normal gastric function. *Compendium on Continuing Education for the Practicing Veterinarian*, 10; 1282–1293.

Hathcock J.T. (1984) Radiographic view of choice for the diagnosis of gastric volvulus: The right lateral recumbent view. *Journal of American Animal Hospital Association*, 20; 967–969.

Hayden D.W. & Van Kruiningen H.J. (1973) Eosinophilic gastroenteritis in the German shepherd dog and its relationship to VLM's. *Journal of American Veterinary Medical Association*, 162; 379–384.

Hayden D.W. & Fleischmann, R.W. (1977) Scirrhous eosinophilic gastritis in dogs with gastric arteritis. *Veterinary Pathology*, 14; 441–444.

Hinder R.A. & Kelly K.A. (1977) Canine gastric emptying of solids and liquids. *American Journal of Physiology*, 233; E335–E340.

Hunt J.N. & Stubbs D.F. (1975) The volume and energy content of meals as determinants of gastric emptying. *Journal of Physiology*, 245; 209–225.

Itoh Z., Aizawa I., Takeuchi S. & Takayanagi R. (1977) Diurnal changes in gastric motor activity in conscious dogs. *American Journal of Digestive Diseases*, 22; 117–124.

Leib M.S. & Martin R.A. (1987) Therapy of gastric dilation-volvulus in dogs. *Compendium on Continuing Education for the Practicing Veterinarian*, 9; 1155–1163.

Miller M.E., Christensen G.C. & Evans H.E. (1964) The digestive system and abdomen. In: *Anatomy of the Dog*, W.B. Saunders, Philadelphia, 645–712.

Minami H. & McCallum R.W. (1984) The physiology and pathophysiology of gastric emptying in humans. *Gastroenterology*, 86; 1592–1610.

Moreland K.J. (1988) Ulcer disease of the upper gastrointestinal tract in small animals: Pathophysiology, diagnosis and management. *Compendium on Continuing Education for the Practicing Veterinarian*, 10; 1265–1279.

Murray M., McKeating F.J., Baker C.J. & Lauder I.M. (1972) Primary gastric neoplasia in the dog: A clinico-pathological study. *Veterinary Record*, 91; 474–479.

Pearson H., Gaskell C.J., Gibb C. & Waterman A. (1974) Pyloric and oesophageal dysfunction in the cat. *Journal of Small Animal Practice*, 15; 487–501.

Prove J. & Ehrlein H.J. (1982) Motor function of gastric antrum and pylorus for evacuation of low and high viscosity meals in dogs. *Gut*, 23; 150–156.

Sikes R.I., Bichard S., Patnaik A. & Bradley R. (1986) Chronic hypertrophic pyloric gastropathy: A review of 16 cases. *Journal of American Animal Hospital Association*, 22; 99–104.

Stemper T.J. & Cooke A.R. (1976) Effect of fixed pyloric opening on gastric emptying in the cat and dog. *American Journal of Physiology*, 230; 813–817.

Sullivan M., Lee R., Fisher E.W., Nash A.S. & McCandlish I.A.P. (1987) A study of 31 cases of gastric carcinoma in dogs. *Veterinary Record*, 120; 79–83.

Twedt D.C. (1983) Disorders of gastric retention. In: *Current Veterinary Therapy VIII*. R.W. Kirk (ed.), W.B. Saunders, Philadelphia, 761–770.

Twedt D.C. & Magne M.L. (1986) Chronic gastritis. In: *Current Veterinary Therapy IX*. R.W. Kirk (ed.), W.B. Saunders, Philadelphia, 852–856.

Van der Gaag I., Happe R.P. & Wolve Kamp W.Th.C. (1976) A Boxer dog with chronic hypertrophic gastritis resembling Menetrier's disease in man, *Veterinary Pathology*, **13**; 172–173.

Van Kruiningen H.J., Wotan L.D., Stake P.E. & Lord P.F. (1987) The influence of diet and feeding frequency on gastric function in the dog. *Journal of American Animal Hospital Association*, **23**; 145–153.

Walsh J.H., Csendes A. & Grossman M.I. (1972) Effects of truncal vagotomy on gastrin release and Heidenheim pouch acid secretion in response to feeding in dogs. *Gastroenterology*, **63**; 593–599.

Weber J. & Kohatsu M.D. (1970) Pacemaker localisation and electrical conduction patterns in the canine stomach. *Gastroenterology*, **59**; 717–726.

4/Investigation of Vomiting

Introduction

Although vomiting is frequently described as a diagnosis, this is inaccurate; it is merely a symptom of some specific condition. Many cases of vomiting especially in dogs follow the ingestion of contaminated or unsuitable foods, resulting in gastritis which rapidly responds to symptomatic treatment. However vomiting has a very large differential diagnosis and many cases will not respond to this regime, and will require full investigation.

The vomiting centre lies in the medulla oblongata and may be directly stimulated via the vagus nerve or may also be stimulated from input via the vestibular apparatus, cerebrum or the chemoreceptor trigger zone (CTZ) (Fig. 4.1). The dog has a well-developed vomiting centre and higher centres of the brain may stimulate this centre whenever environmental changes occur, such as excitement, fear and emotion. The vagus nerve may be stimulated by inflammatory conditions in the thorax and abdomen. Cardiac, hepatic, renal and pancreatic disease together with conditions of the oeso-phagus, stomach and intestine may result in vomiting through this type of mechanism. Inflammation of the vestibular apparatus which occurs in otitis interna and motion sickness often result in vomiting mediated through the vomiting centre. The final important input to the vomiting centre is through the chemoreceptor trigger zone which accounts for vomiting associated with many toxaemic states such as uraemia, pyometra, hepatoencephalo-

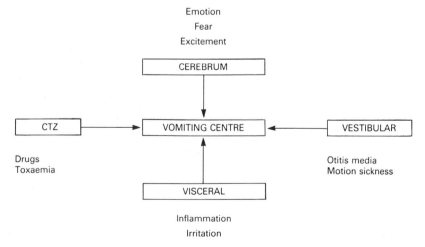

Fig. 4.1 Methods by which vomiting may be induced.

pathy and ketoacidosis. It is also stimulated by the action of certain drugs such as digoxin and apomorphine.

Although vomiting may be due to disorders of the digestive tract, there are a significant number of non-gastric conditions which may also cause vomiting (Table 4.1). It is because of the large group of non-gastric conditions that the clinician must be careful in making a diagnosis of gastritis, when presented with a vomiting patient. The only way in which a diagnosis can be made is by following some form of investigation into the primary complaint. In many cases, all that is required in the form of investigation, is the collection of a detailed history and performance of a thorough physical examination of the patient. This clinical examination is of great value to the clinician, if the correct diagnosis is to be reached and the treatment to be successful. The clinical examination will allow several very important questions to be answered:

1 Is the patient actually vomiting?
2 Is the vomiting due to primary digestive tract dysfunction or due to some other body system dysfunction?
3 What further investigation is required to reach a definitive diagnosis?

By answering these questions a systemic problem should not be missed and the spectrum of differential diagnosis significantly narrowed. In order that the full diagnostic potential of the clinical examination is appreciated, it is important to consider in detail the actual method of carrying out the clinical examination.

History

It is always tempting to ask questions about the presenting complaint and to ignore the other body systems. However, whenever a patient is presented with vomiting it is important to assess all the body systems for the reasons given above. For example, a dog may be presented with vomiting, dehydration and polydipsia. Further questioning may reveal a recent oestrus, vaginal discharge and history of pseudo-pregnancy or use of progestogens; all of which may point to a reproductive disorder such as pyometra. The physical examination should be used to substantiate the findings obtained

Table 4.1 Non-gastric causes of vomiting in small animals

Brain tumour	Uraemia	Enteritis	Distemper
Brain trauma	Ketoacidosis	Colitis	Leptospirosis
Motion sickness	Addisons disease	Obstructions	Hepatitis
Otitis media	Drugs (digoxin)	Constipation	Cardiac disease
Meningitis	Toxaemias		Pancreatitis
			Peritonitis

from the history, and may allow a diagnosis to be made, or will provide a firm foundation from which to conduct a further investigation.

When questioning the owner about the function of the digestive tract, there are specific questions which will yield valuable clues as to the likely origin of the vomiting. In particular questions regarding the behaviour of the vomiting patient (Table 4.2) and the character of the vomitus itself will provide valuable information (Table 4.3).

Retching, regurgitation, vomiting

At this point it may be helpful to consider one other important feature of the vomiting patient. It is not unknown to have a primary complaint of 'vomiting' when in fact the animal is retching and gagging which occasionally

Table 4.2 Symptoms associated with vomiting determined from the history

Association with feeding
  Present: oesophageal disease, gastritis
  Absent: systemic disease, small intestine obstruction

Appetite
  Intact: oesophageal disease, chronic gastritis
  Poor: dysphagia, systemic disease, gastric neoplasia

Persistent vomiting
  Acute gastritis, obstructions, systemic disease

Intermittent vomiting
  Chronic gastritis, gastric neoplasia
  Intestinal disease

Weight-loss
  Degree of loss reflects severity of condition

Timing of vomition
  Immediately after food: oesophageal disease
  Hours after food: gastric retention conditions
  Early morning only: bilious vomiting syndrome

Age of patient
  Congenital versus acquired conditions

Salivation
  Oral conditions, oesophageal disease and gastric diseases

Scavenging
  Common in dogs leading to gastritis

Other symptoms
  Consider systemic disease states

Associated diarrhoea
  Gastroenteritis more common than gastritis

Table 4.3 Characteristics of the vomitus

Coffee grounds
    Gastric origin, ulceration, neoplasia, gastritis

Fresh blood
    More common in oral, pharyngeal and oesophageal
    conditions, and occasionally gastric lesions

Food
    Oesophageal disease, gastric retention, motility disorders

Bile
    Bilious vomiting syndrome, persistent vomiting,
    intestinal obstruction

Faecal
    Lower intestinal obstruction (rare)

Unproductive
    Persistent vomiting, impaction of stomach

terminates with vomiting, due to the presence of upper respiratory tract infection. Dogs with kennel cough may vomit occasionally but frequently cough and retch.

Equally, animals with oesophageal disease passively regurgitate the food which has been trapped in the oesophagus. There is no active process of vomiting in this situation. Regurgitation also tends to occur shortly after eating and the vomitus has a high pH compared with vomitus of gastric origin. There is often evidence of aspiration pneumonia in oesophageal disease and occasionally dogs will be presented exhibiting signs of pneumonia rather than regurgitation or vomiting.

True vomiting on the other hand is an active process and involves marked muscle activity. The animal will initially appear restless and anxious. It will then hold a deep breath on a closed glottis, arch its neck, contract the abdominal muscles against a fixed diaphragm and compress the gastric contents into the oesophagus and out of the mouth with some force.

The clinician should attempt to differentiate between retching, regurgitation and vomiting. The differential diagnosis can be greatly reduced (Table 4.4) and this in turn reduces the need for an extensive investigation which in some cases may become totally unnecessary.

Vomiting characteristics

It is useful to determine if there is any association with feeding. If the owner describes the dog as being hungry and eager to eat, but when it does so, the food is promptly 'vomited' within a short time, this suggests oesophageal disease. It may also indicate gastric disease such as gastritis, gastric

Table 4.4 Conditions associated with retching, regurgitation and vomiting

Retching	Regurgitation	True vomiting
Pharyngitis	Oesophageal foreign	Primary gastric disease
Laryngitis	body	Systemic disease
Tracheitis	Oesophageal neoplasia	Toxaemias
Pharyngeal neoplasia	Oesophageal dilation	Drug reaction
Pharyngeal foreign	Oesophageal stricture	Intestinal obstruction
body	Reflux oesophagitis	Vagal vomiting
Cricopharyngeal	Hiatus hernia	
achalasia	Vascular ring anomaly	

foreign body or pyloric stenosis. When there is no association with feeding and the animal vomits even when the stomach is empty then advanced gastric disease, obstruction, neoplasia or systemic disease is likely to be involved. Where the appetite is intact it is less likely that the animal is systemically ill, and the problem is more often of local origin. Persistent vomiting, even when the stomach is empty suggests either acute gastritis or systemic involvement such as a toxaemia, while intermittent vomiting, especially in an animal which is bright and eating, suggests chronic gastritis or perhaps gastric ulceration or neoplasia. If weight loss is present, then the degree of such loss may reflect the severity of the problem, no matter where it originates.

Animals which vomit shortly after eating frequently have some form of oesophageal disease. If on the other hand, vomiting occurs many hours after feeding, but contains undigested food, this suggests gastric retention for whatever cause. In bilious vomiting syndrome dogs always vomit bile in the early morning and will not vomit during the remainder of the day.

The age of the patient is useful in considering the possibility of congenital or acquired disease, while salivation has been observed most frequently in patients with oesophageal or gastric disease. Salivation is also a feature of chronic liver disease in cats. Scavenging, although rarely admitted by the owner, is frequently implicated in dogs and this is caused by irritation and inflammation of the upper digestive tract, and may lead to obstructive changes. Cats on the other hand are fastidious eaters and scavenging is a rare occurrence. It is unusual to observe gastritis alone in either dogs or cats, except in chronic gastric disease; it is much more common for gastritis to be accompanied by enteritis, suggesting a possible infective nature.

Character of the vomitus

This information should not be considered in isolation but related to the other features of dysfunction described above. The materials which may be vomited are few in number, and are of considerable diagnostic value.

'Coffee grounds' appear as brown granules and are produced by the action of gastric acid on fresh blood. In most cases the blood originates from the stomach, and the most likely causes of such bleeding are gastric ulceration, neoplasia or rupture of blood vessels associated with persistent vomiting. If bleeding is severe then black tarry faeces are also likely to be observed. Fresh unchanged blood on the other hand, may occasionally originate from the stomach if it is rapidly vomited. However it is more likely to have originated from the oral cavity, pharynx or oesophagus.

Vomition of undigested food is usually associated with oesophageal disease especially if this occurs a short time after eating, while in gastric disease food may be retained for many hours after eating before vomition occurs. In the latter situation it may appear partially digested. Bile is never observed in vomiting due to oesophageal disease but may be observed in bilious vomiting syndrome where large volumes of bile may be produced. Bile may also be observed wherever persistent vomiting is present. Faecal vomiting is rare and associated with lower intestinal obstruction where the intestinal contents may return to the stomach by reverse peristalsis. Unproductive vomiting may be associated with acute gastritis where vomiting continues even though the stomach is empty. However it may be due to impaction of the stomach with foreign material. The author has seen this situation in dogs which have eaten plastic bags, packaging material and plastic toys which block the pylorus.

Physical examination

This should substantiate the findings of the history and be used to detect any further abnormalities in body systems, or perhaps a lack of any such abnormalities. If the patient is retching then look for signs of foreign bodies or upper respiratory tract infection, such as tonsillitis, enlarged submandibular lymph nodes, pharyngitis or tracheitis. When dysphagia appears to be the problem a thorough check of cranial nerve function should be made to detect where the lesion may be located.

When regurgitation is thought to be present a careful examination of the neck may reveal changes in the cervical oesophagus, while bulging of the oesophagus at the thoracic inlet may occasionally occur in thoracic oesophageal conditions. Examination of the thoracic oesophagus cannot be carried out without radiographic techniques.

Classification

The clinical examination may be summarized in the form of a flow diagram. This shows an approach to investigation which is designed to assist the clinician with any individual case (Fig. 4.2). It is important to emphasize

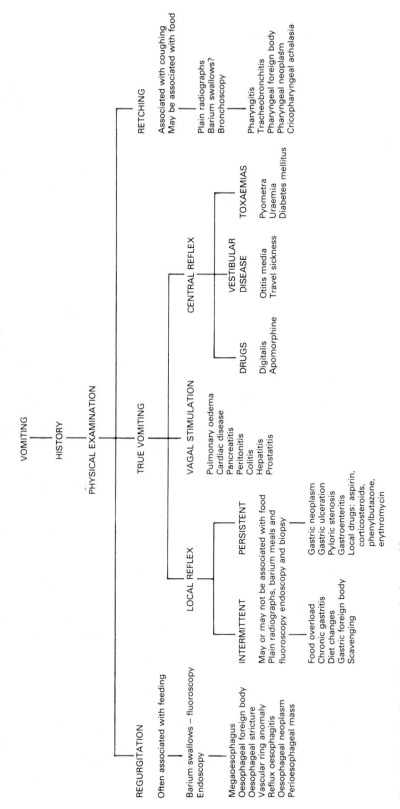

Fig. 4.2 Method of classifying and investigating vomiting.

that there is no ideal system of classifying the cause of vomiting, the flow diagram is only intended as a guide which the authors have found useful in an applied context. Using the classification shown in Fig. 4.2 it can be seen how the clinical examination allows a distinction between retching, regurgitation and vomiting. Once this is made the most effective methods of diagnosis are listed together with the possible diagnosis. When the case falls into the vomiting category, further divisions are made into primary and secondary vomiting based on the clinical findings. Further divisions within these categories can be made using the methods of investigation described. The important point to stress is that one should adopt a line of straightforward elimination of options which can be used in ones own working environment and then apply this to the appropriate cases.

Further investigation

There are several diagnostic procedures which are frequently employed to assist in the investigation of vomiting. Not all the procedures will be required in individual cases, and they should be selected based on the conclusions obtained from the clinical examination. A different approach will be required depending on whether the animal is retching, regurgitating or vomiting. For example, vomiting associated with gastric disease will require the use of radiographs and endoscopy while vomiting due to a toxaemic condition will require biochemical analysis and possibly radiographic studies. In general, the diagnostic procedures most frequently used to assist in the investigation of vomiting include radiology, endoscopy, biochemistry, bacteriology and virology.

1   Biochemistry is important where the clinician feels the problem is not primarily associated with the digestive tract, and may be due to a metabolic disorder.

2   Primary bacterial infections are rare causes of gastritis or gastroenteritis, while viral infections such as parvovirus and distemper, are well-recognized. The identification of viral disease is important, as it helps determine the prognosis and assists the clinician in advising the client regarding vaccination and management of in-contact animals.

3   Radiography is commonly used in the detection of digestive tract disease. In particular the value of barium studies and fluoroscopy cannot be overstated. They may frequently provide a diagnosis and being non-invasive are readily accepted by the client and the patient.

4   The development of endoscopy has also allowed important advances in veterinary gastroenterology. If abnormalities are detected radiographically, endoscopy allows the clinician to examine the oesophagus and stomach in great detail without the need for invasive surgery. In many cases the abnormal tissue can be visualized and biopsy samples collected, allowing a

definitive diagnosis to be made. The main disadvantage of endoscopy is the requirement for general anaesthesia, for patient cooperation and to protect the equipment. In addition it will only detect abnormalities where the mucosa is involved, so lesions of deeper tissues will be less easily identified. In such cases the only procedure available to the clinician is exploratory surgery, but this should only be carried out where there is strong evidence to suggest it will yield diagnostic information, and other less invasive techniques have failed to yield meaningful information or are not available. For many practitioners this may be their only way of following up abnormal radiographs.

Table 4.5 A classification of dysphagias

Oral dysphagia:
    Difficulty in prehension and aboral transfer of food
    Under voluntary control. Cranial nerves, 5, 7 & 12
    Mandibular fracture
    Temperomandibular joint dysfunction
    Craniomandibular osteopathy
    Oral lesions
    Foreign bodies
    Cleft palate
    Eosinophilic myositis/atrophic myositis
    Brain lesion

Pharyngeal dysphagia
    Difficulties in control of food from caudal mouth to oesophagus
    Not under voluntary control. Cranial nerves, 5, 7, 10, 11
    Tonsillar, pharyngeal infections
    Pharyngeal neoplasia
    Foreign bodies
    Soft palate defects
    Polyneuropathy
    Myositis
    Myasthenia gravis
    Brain lesions
    Cricopharyngeal achalasia

Oesophageal dysphagia
    Megaoesophagus
    Vascular ring anomaly
    Oesophageal foreign body
    Oesophageal neoplasia
    Oesophageal stricture
    Perioesophageal mass
    Oesophageal perforation
    Diaphragmatic hernia

Investigation of retching

Where the clinical examination suggests vomiting associated with retching then it is also likely to reveal evidence of submandibular lymph node enlargement, tonsillitis, pharyngitis and tracheitis. There may be additional signs of nasal discharge or coughing. In such cases the retching and subsequent vomiting occur through inflammation of the respiratory tract and the investigation should be directed towards the cause of the infection. This may involve radiological examination of the respiratory tract and culture of bronchial secretions if this is possible.

Occasionally retching may be due to disease of the digestive tract. Dysphagia due to oral or pharyngeal dysfunction or cricopharyngeal achalasia may be present. Neoplasia or foreign body obstruction may lead to mechanical or painful lesions. In all these cases careful observation of eating behaviour will often produce valuable information. An inability to pick up, chew or deliver food to the pharynx, or an inability to synchronize the pharyngeal stages of swallowing may occur. In the case of foreign bodies or neoplasia, food often falls out of the mouth or is retained in the mouth for long periods of time. In the case of nerve damage, the food is moved successfully towards the pharynx but this leads to gagging and retching, resulting in food or fluids being expelled back through the mouth or down the nostrils.

If any of these situations arise then the clinician should examine the cranial nerve function very carefully in order to determine which cranial nerves are damaged (Table 4.5). In addition fluoroscopic examination of the actual swallowing process is very helpful in determining where the failure in the swallowing process originates. Such fluoroscopic examinations are very difficult to carry out and ideally should be recorded on video tape in order to allow careful observation on repeated occasions until the problem can be identified. This is obviously a specialist procedure which requires patient referral to an appropriate centre.

Regurgitation

Regurgitation is commonly associated with disorders of the oesophagus. Plain radiographs of the oesophagus followed by barium swallows are usually the most rewarding methods of diagnosis. Initially plain views should be taken of the cervical and thoracic oesophagus to observe if there are any obvious changes such as radio-opaque foreign bodies, tumour masses or other gross lesions. Plain views of the thorax are also useful in detecting the presence of aspiration pneumonia which is often associated with oesophageal disease.

Assuming this is inadequate for a diagnosis to be made and there is no evidence of oesophageal perforation, the next step is to carry out a barium

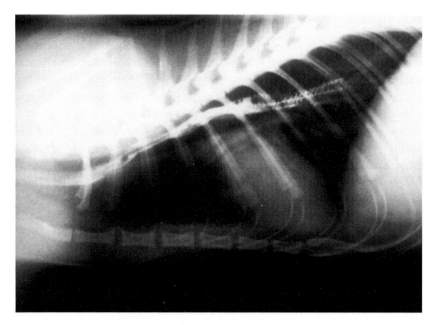

Fig. 4.3 Normal herring bone appearance of the feline oesophagus.

swallow using liquid barium (Micropaque; Nicholas Laboratories) at a dose
rate of 2 ml/kg liveweight. In some cases such as partial obstructions of the
oesophagus, it is quite possible for liquid barium to reach the stomach
without obstruction. It is therefore usual to carry out a further barium
swallow using barium mixed with tinned dog or cat meat. In this case the
amount of barium required is simply that which will give adequate contrast,
but not in excessive amounts making the food unpalatable to the patient.

Barium with food is a very useful way of detecting the presence of
partial obstructions, oesophageal dilation, diverticula and vascular ring
anomaly. If the food and barium reaches the stomach without being retained in
the oesophagus this suggests oesophageal function is intact. It is common to
see small amounts of liquid barium retained in the distal cervical oesophagus
for long periods. Equally the herring bone appearance of the distal thoracic
oesophagus in cats is often highlighted by barium, and is again quite normal
(Fig. 4.3).

If barium reaches the stomach observation by fluoroscopy should be
used to detect possible reflux of gastric contents into the distal oesophagus.
This is the best method of detecting reflux oesophagitis as it is very difficult
to observe on static radiographs. Where fluoroscopy is not available, endoscopy should be employed in order to reach a diagnosis. The distal oesophagus
will be inflamed and often ulcerated while the luminal contents will have a
low pH.

Endoscopy is also useful to observe the tissue damage and assist in the

retrieval of oesophageal foreign bodies, in biopsy collection where oesophageal tumours are suspected, and to detect the presence of stricture and
diverticula.

Investigation of true vomiting

The division of true vomiting into primary conditions of the digestive tract
and those which are secondary should be made at this stage. Of the cases
involving secondary vomiting, the effect of drugs should easily be determined
from the history, and vestibular disease or motion sickness are also easily
recognized. Toxaemic states may be suspected but cannot be diagnosed
from the clinical examination. There may be evidence of polydipsia, polyuria,
pyrexia, halitosis, abnormal behaviour, ketosis, changes in liver and kidney
size and shape or abnormal reproductive function.

Routine haematology, urinalysis and biochemistry should be carried out
in such situations to help reach a diagnosis. Radiographs will be helpful to
confirm changes in the size and shape of the liver or kidneys and to visualize
the uterus.

Where vomiting appears to be primary the investigation will follow a
different course. Radiography and fluoroscopy followed by endoscopy provide
the clinician with powerful diagnostic tools. Exploratory laparotomy is also
indicated where these facilities are not available.

Before an expensive investigation is carried out it should be ensured that
there are no dietary problems such as incorrect or overfeeding especially
in young animals. Although worms are not a common cause of vomiting,
they may be seen in vomitus of young animals. Scavenging dogs are also
more likely to vomit. Locally-acting drugs causing gastritis should also be
ruled out from careful questioning of the owner. Evidence of poor vaccinal
status should be considered together with clinical signs of distemper, hepatitis, leptospirosis and parvovirus infection.

Gastric foreign bodies are difficult to detect on abdominal palpation and
if they are suspected then radiographs with or without barium should be
used to assist the diagnosis. Intestinal foreign bodies and intussusceptions
may be detected on palpation but radiographs are sometimes necessary for
their diagnosis.

Chronic gastritis, gastric neoplasia and ulceration are much more difficult
to diagnose solely on clinical grounds. In these cases radiographs should be
used, followed by a barium meal using barium (Micropaque; Nicholas
Laboratories) at a dose rate of up to 5 ml/kg liveweight. Typical signs are
distortion of the gastric wall, narrowing of the gastric lumen especially in
the antrum or persistent filling defects. In some cases there will be delays in
gastric emptying. Even with fluoroscopy the clinician is often faced with
supporting evidence of primary gastric disease, but no definitive diagnosis.

Further investigation using endoscopy or exploratory laparotomy is required at this stage. There is no doubt that the latter will provide a diagnosis on most occasions while endoscopy may miss lesions not directly associated with the gastric mucosa. However endoscopy is non-invasive and so can be used to eliminate various conditions without subjecting the patient to exploratory surgery. If endoscopy results in a doubtful diagnosis then laparotomy may still be required.

It is important to emphasize that exploratory surgery is not the first diagnostic procedure to employ where gastric disease is suspected. It should be carried out only where there is strong evidence to suggest it will yield a diagnosis. It is also important that the examination is carried out thoroughly as it is very easy to miss lesions or to biopsy an area of normal tissue particularly where a discrete lesion is present.

5/Diseases of the Small Intestine

Macroscopic anatomy

The intestinal tract can be divided into the small intestine and the large intestine. The main function of the small intestine is the digestion and absorption of food, while the large intestine is responsible for the absorption of water, electrolytes and some vitamins. The small intestine commences at the pylorus and terminates at the ileocaecocolic junction. It is divided into three parts; the duodenum, jejunum and ileum (Fig. 5.1).

The pylorus marks the start of the duodenum lying on the right side of the abdomen at the level of the ninth rib. The descending limb moves caudally in contact with the right flank. It terminates just before the pelvic inlet forming a U-bend where the ascending limb moves craniomedially to

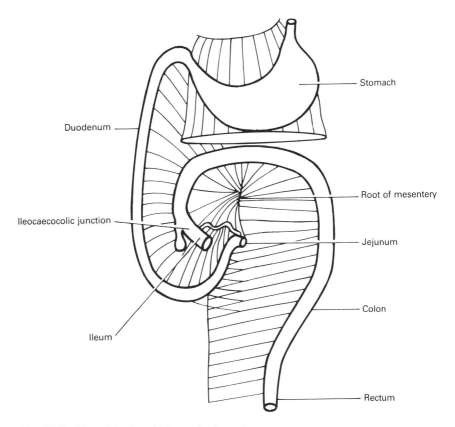

Fig. 5.1 Position of the intestinal tract in the canine.

the level of the sixth lumbar vertebra, close to the root of the mesentery and the left kidney. The duodenum now curves ventromedially forming the start of the jejunum. The two pancreatic ducts and the bile duct open 5 to 8 cm from the pylorus.

The jejunum and ileum form the main part of the small intestine commencing at the ventromedial flexure of the duodenum and terminating at the ileocaecocolic junction. The jejunum and ileum are loosely suspended on a long mesentery which allows the intestine to form loops or coils. There is no clear demarcation between jejunum and ileum.

The small intestine is supplied with blood from branches of the coeliac and cranial mesenteric arteries. Venous drainage is via the gastric and cranial mesenteric veins, into the portal vein and on to the liver. Lymphatic drainage of the duodenum is to the hepatic lymph nodes and from the jejunum and ileum via the mesenteric lymph nodes to the cysterna chyli and the thoracic duct.

Preganglionic parasympathetic and postganglionic sympathetic nerves supply the small intestine. In addition there is an intrinsic autonomic nerve supply between the muscle layers called the myenteric plexus or Auerbach's plexus. Another such intrinsic system lies in the submucosa called Meissner's plexus.

Microscopic anatomy

The wall of the small intestine is similar throughout its length and is composed of outer serosal, muscular, submucosal and mucosal layers.

The serosa is a thin sheet of epithelial cells which is continuous with the parietal peritoneum. The muscular layer is composed of smooth muscle fibres arranged in two distinct layers; an outer longitudinal layer and a thicker inner circular layer. The latter layer forms the ileocaecocolic sphincter. Between the layers lies Auerbach's plexus. The submucosa is mainly composed of elastic fibres and collagen. It is richly supplied with blood vessels, lymphatics and neurones. Large lymphatic nodules called Peyers patches, are found throughout the antimesenteric border of the small intestine; they are most prominent in the distal ileum.

The mucosa is the innermost layer which consists of an epithelial lining, intestinal glands, lamina propria and muscularis mucosae. The epithelial cells are also known as enterocytes. The lining is thrown into large folds called villi which effectively increase the surface area by 10 times. The cells on these villi have small finger-like projections called microvilli which increase the surface area a further 20 times (Fig. 5.2). Between the villi there are large numbers of tubuloalveolar glands secreting into the crypts of Lieberkühn. They produce mucus and protect the duodenal lining from gastric acid.

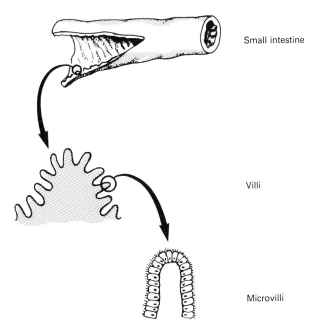

Small intestine

Villi

Microvilli

Fig. 5.2 Method of providing a large surface area for absorption.

The enterocyte layer is only one cell thick and lies on a basement membrane. It is columnar in shape and interspersed with goblet cells and enteroendocrine cells (see below). Cells originate from the crypts of Lieberkühn, which lie at the base of the villi as pore-like openings onto the surface, and slowly migrate up the villi towards the tip, becoming functionally mature on the way. The cells already on the tips slough off and are lost in the faeces (Fig. 5.3). This process is called epithelial renewal and occurs every 4 days (Eastwood 1977). The goblet cells are found in the crypts and on villi and take their name from their shape and the fact that they secrete mucus. Enteroendocrine cells, or argentaffin cells, are wedge-shaped cells lying on the basement membrane between the enterocytes. Many types are now recognized. They are part of a family of cells called the amine precursor uptake and decarboxylation (APUD) cells. They secrete a series of hormones including cholecystokinin, secretin and gastrin (Grube & Forssmann 1979).

The lamina propria forms a layer immediately below the base of each villus and extends into the villus itself. This layer is composed of loose collagen, elastic fibres and reticulin. Blind-ending lacteals or lymphatic ducts lie in the centre of each villus. Submucosal capillaries infiltrate the villus forming a dense network and smooth muscle fibres from the muscularis mucosae enter the villus to assist in contraction of the lymph vessels (Fig. 5.3). Small numbers of mast cells, lymphocytes, fibroblasts and leucocytes, and plasma cells are found in the lamina propria.

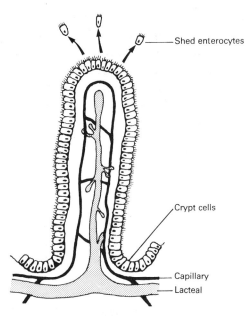

Shed enterocytes

Crypt cells

Capillary

Lacteal

Fig. 5.3 Structure of the small intestinal villus.

Physiology

The function of the small intestine is to complete the digestion of nutrients
and ensure their subsequent absorption into the general circulation. This is
achieved in three phases;
1   Intraluminal digestion involving enzymes produced by the stomach and
exocrine pancreas together with bile.
2   Mucosal digestion involving enzymes associated with the microvilli
which further hydrolyse the products of intraluminal digestion.
3   The absorption of end products into the enterocytes and then into the
capillaries or lacteals.

To aid the digestive process a large volume of water is secreted into the
duodenum which ensures the intestinal contents remain isotonic. This is
only possible because there are pores present between the enterocytes in the
duodenum making it very permeable. The permeability of the small intestine
decreases in the more distal segments and is minimal in the large intestine.

Control of the digestive process is under the influence of neural reflexes
and hormones. The former are mediated from the central nervous system,
through the vagus nerve and are associated with the sight, smell and taste of
food. This stimulates release of gastrin in the stomach with production of
pepsin and acid. The same vagal reflex stimulates release of exocrine pancreatic secretion. Hormonal control of digestion is mediated through
cholecystokinin, secretin and gastrin inhibitory peptide. When acid chyme

reaches the duodenum it stimulates gastrin inhibitory peptide (GIP) which reduces further gastrin secretion. Cholecystokinin is produced by the entero-endocrine cells of the duodenum in response to the presence of fat and amino acids stimulating the release of exocrine pancreatic secretion rich in enzymes. It also inhibits gastrin secretion and contracts the gall bladder which results in bile entering the duodenum. Secretin is also produced from the duodenal enteroendocrine cells in the presence of acid and stimulates the production of exocrine pancreatic secretion low in enzyme and rich in bicarbonate (Argenzio 1980).

Protein digestion

The majority of protein is hydrolysed in the proximal small intestine although the process starts in the stomach (Argenzio 1980). Pepsin in the stomach is a non-specific endopeptidase which splits proteins into smaller peptides. Proenzymes in the pancreatic secretion are activated by duodenal enterokinase when they enter the intestine and trypsin then continues to activate more of itself and other enzymes (Fig. 5.4). Trypsin and chymotrypsin split proteins into smaller peptides while carboxypeptidase A and B cleave terminal amino acids from these peptides. The end result of this intraluminal digestion is some free amino acids but mainly small peptides (Kim & Erickson 1985). Elastase is also present and splits internal bonds of proteins. Nucleic acids are also split by other specific enzymes such as ribonuclease and deoxyribonuclease (Brobst 1980).

Free amino acids can now be absorbed across the small intestine while the larger peptides undergo further digestion by brush border enzymes known as peptidases (Fig. 5.5). While larger peptides are split at the brush border, dipeptides are absorbed into the enterocyte and split by peptidase within the cell. Seven different peptidase enzymes have been recognized to date (Tobey *et al.* 1985). The absorption of amino acids is an energy-dependent active process closely linked to sodium transport, in turn it is

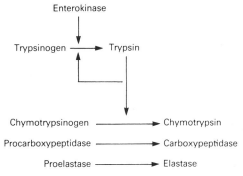

Fig. 5.4 Method of enzyme activation by enterokinase.

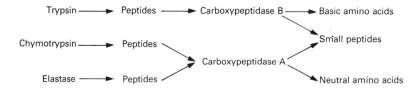

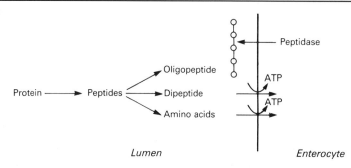

Fig. 5.5 Process of protein digestion and absorption.

thought closely linked to adenosine triphosphatase (ATPase) mechanisms creating a transenterocyte gradient. Different carriers are used for different classes of amino acids. From the enterocyte, amino acids leave the small intestine via the portal circulation. Some may be used by the enterocytes for repair and as an energy source (McDonald *et al.* 1988).

Carbohydrate digestion

Most dietary carbohydrate is composed of starch although smaller amounts of dissacharides such as lactose and sucrose may be present. Other carbohydrate in the diet cannot be digested because the enzymes required are not present in the dog and cat. They include hemicellulose, cellulose and lignin, termed dietary fibre (Argenzio 1980).

Little digestion of carbohydrate occurs until it reaches the small intestine. Starch is composed of amylose linked together by alpha 1−4 bonds and amylopectin linked by alpha 1−6 bonds. Alpha amylase present in pancreatic secretion splits starch into smaller saccharide units by cleaving

Fig. 5.6 Linkage between glucose units in starch.

the alpha 1−4 bonds while being unable to split the alpha 1−6 bonds in starch (Fig. 5.6). The products of this digestion are maltose, maltotriose and limited dextrins with a small amount of free glucose (McDonald *et al.* 1988).

Before absorption can occur the products of alpha-amylase digestion must undergo further digestion by the brush border enzymes, the disaccharidases (Fig. 5.7). These enzymes lie on the microvilli surface together with carrier proteins for absorption of their products. Enzymes include lactase, sucrase, maltase (glucoamylase) and alpha dextrinase (isomaltase). These enzymes are most active in the jejunum and the end products glucose, galactose and fructose, are absorbed into the enterocytes. There are specific carriers present which actively absorb the monosaccharides into the enterocyte. In this way absorption can occur even against a concentration gradient during a large meal (Tennant & Hornbuckle 1980). Sucrose and lactose do not undergo intraluminal digestion but are digested on the brush border by specific disaccharide enzymes and absorbed into the enterocytes.

Fat digestion

Triglyceride forms the bulk of dietary fat which is digested and absorbed with great efficiency. Other ingested fats like cholesterol and phospholipid are less efficiently digested. Triglyceride is classified according to the fatty acid chain length into those with only eight carbon atoms termed short-chain triglycerides (SCT), those with between eight and 12 carbon atoms termed the medium-chain triglycerides (MCT) and those with more than 12 carbon atoms, the long-chain triglycerides (LCT) (Simpson & Doxey

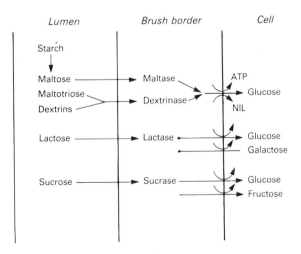

Fig. 5.7 Process of carbohydrate digestion and absorption.

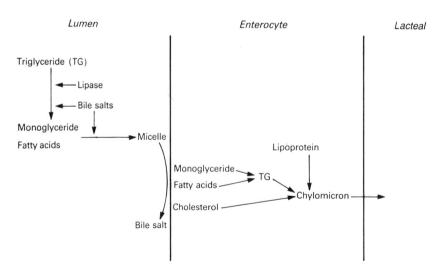

Fig. 5.8 Process of fat digestion and absorption.

1983). The difference in chain length is important when considering the method of digestion and absorption (Simpson 1987).

Intraluminal digestion of LCT requires the presence of lipase and bile salts. The former splits the triglyceride into free fatty acids and monoglyceride while the latter acts as a detergent, providing a water/lipid interface for lipase to digest the fat. An emulsion or micelle is formed by the segmental intestine contractions mixing the fat, lipase and bile salts, forming an emulsion or micelle. The micelle results in the production of very small particles of lipid which create a large surface area for digestion and absorption. Once digestion has occurred the micelle transports the free fatty acids to the brush border for absorption into the enterocyte (Fig. 5.8). Other fat-soluble products such as fat-soluble vitamins are also absorbed in this process. Fatty acids diffuse into the enterocytes passively because of the lipid membrane. To maintain the concentration gradient for this process, fatty acids in the enterocytes are rapidly converted to triglycerides, which are less osmotically active. Triglycerides attach to carrier proteins (lipoproteins), to form chylomicrons, which then leave the enterocytes and enter the lacteals. The formation of chylomicrons improves the solubility of the fat which allows the triglyceride to enter the general circulation, where it is carried to the liver or tissues.

Short- and medium-chain triglyceride are more water soluble than LCT and the process of lipase digestion is thus more efficient. Micelle formation is not essential, and the fatty acids can be absorbed into the enterocyte directly. Once in the cell they reform into triglyceride and are absorbed directly into the portal blood rather than the lacteal. In addition SCT and

MCT can be absorbed intact into enterocytes and then into the portal blood without intraluminal digestion (Simpson & Doxey 1983).

Bile salts are in short supply during a large meal and are therefore conserved by the animal. Once the fat has been absorbed they are re-absorbed into the ileal enterocytes and travel via the portal blood to the liver to be immediately reused. This process is very efficient in the normal dog and is called the enterophepatic circulation of bile salts (Argenzio 1980).

Pathophysiology of diarrhoea

A definition of diarrhoea might be given as faeces which are unformed as a result of increased bulk or fluid content. This may occur as a consequence of several mechanisms:

Osmotic changes

Active secretion

Increased permeability

Altered motility

Most cases of diarrhoea are induced by one of these factors and some cases may involve more than one mechanism at the same time (Moon 1978).

1   Osmotic diarrhoea is most frequently associated with retention of nutrients in the intestinal lumen, e.g. exocrine pancreatic insufficiency, brush border enzyme deficiency or from malabsorption syndromes. In all cases non-absorbed products create an osmotic gradient between the intestine and the plasma, with the movement of fluid from the plasma into the intestine. Carbohydrate exerts the greatest osmotic gradient because bacterial degradation yields organic acids, amines and ammonia which increase the osmotic effect. An important feature of osmotic diarrhoea is that usually it is easily resolved by fasting the animal.

2   In secretory diarrhoea there is active fluid secretion into the lumen of the intestine which is independent of any of the other mechanisms described. Most secretion normally originates from the crypt area while most absorption occurs at the tips of the villi. When secretion becomes greater than absorption, diarrhoea develops. The fluid is normally isotonic and there is a major loss of bicarbonate which causes metabolic acidosis to develop. Active secretion of fluid is mediated through cyclic adenosine monophosphate (cAMP) which is itself driven by hormonal stimulation. Various bacterial toxins will also stimulate this mechanism including those produced by *Escherichia coli*, *Salmonella* spp. and cholera. In addition, bacterial degradation of fat yields hydroxy fatty acids which also stimulate intestinal secretion, as will unabsorbed bile acids, prostaglandins and serotonin. Various intestinal and pancreatic tumours, thyroid carcinoma and conditions causing hypergastrinaemia also induce hypersecretion.

3   Normally there are small pores between the crypt cells which allow fluid

movement into the intestinal lumen. This is a passive process and when it becomes greater than the absorptive capacity of the intestine, diarrhoea develops. Changes in pore size, with a consequent increase in permeability, may occur because: (1) there is increased hydraulic pressure as in cardiac disease or lymphatic obstruction; and (2) inflammation of the intestinal mucosa resulting in physical damage to the mucosa. Most frequently only simple sugars and amino acids are lost but if the damage is severe then large molecular plasma proteins may also be lost giving rise to a protein-losing enteropathy.

4   Many clinicians believe diarrhoea is caused by increased intestinal motility. This is frequently not the case. There are basically two types of intestinal motility: (1) segmentation; and (2) peristalsis. The former is thought to be the primary intestinal motility which mixes chyme and allows efficient absorption of nutrients, whilst peristalsis moves the contents of the intestine towards the rectum. When diarrhoea occurs it is often due to failure of segmentation and thus of mixing and absorption. The peristalsis which occurs is reflexly stimulated by increased volumes of chyme which are moved towards the rectum and voided as diarrhoea.

Introduction to enteritis

Diseases of the small intestine may be conveniently divided into those which are acute and sudden in onset such as canine parvovirus and those which are chronic in nature, such as malabsorption syndromes. As with all classifications there will always be some degree of overlap of conditions. For example, canine parvovirus may start as an acute gastroenteritis but following physical damage to the small intestine chronic enteritis associated with malabsorption may develop.

Acute enteritis may be described as being sudden in onset in a previously healthy animal. It is usually self-limiting with recovery following several days of acute symptoms. Chronic enteritis on the other hand occurs where a dog or cat has persistent or intermittent diarrhoea over a period of weeks or months. The animal is often bright and may lose weight in spite of a good appetite.

In this chapter conditions associated with acute enteritis are discussed (Table 5.1) followed by some of those conditions which are often described as chronic in nature (Table 5.2).

Acute enteritis

Dietary diarrhoea

Dogs in particular will tolerate a wide variety of diets, while cats tend to be

Table 5.1 Differential diagnosis of acute enteritis

Dietary
  Sudden diet changes
  Incorrect diet
  Scavenging
  Overfeeding
  Reduced fibre
  Dietary allergy
  Lactase deficiency

Viral
  Canine parvovirus
  Distemper
  Infectious canine hepatitis
  Feline enteritis
  Rotavirus infection
  Coronavirus infection

Bacterial
  Salmonellosis
  Campylobacteriosis
  Tyzzer's disease
  Miscellaneous bacterial infections

Other
  Haemorrhagic gastroenteritis
  Intestinal obstruction
  Intussusception

fastidious and require a high protein diet. If the diet is changed suddenly, especially from a dried to a tinned food, then diarrhoea often follows for several days which will be self-limiting. Unfortunately most owners on observing the diarrhoea then change the diet, further exacerbating the problem. This leads to episodes of apparent relapsing acute diarrhoea although there is a history of frequent diet changes. Treatment simply involves the selection of a suitable standard diet fed at the correct rates without change or supplementation.

Dogs are frequently fed high carbohydrate diets usually in the form of biscuit, potato or bread. High levels of cereal or potato in the diet, especially if not precooked will often lead to diarrhoea. This is because the carbohydate is not as digestible when uncooked and may reach the distal ileum and colon where bacterial fermentation occurs. The problem should be recognized from a careful history, and is easily corrected by changing the dietary management.

Milk is renowned for causing diarrhoea in adult dogs and occasionally cats, although it is not common in the authors' experience. The problem is often referred to as a 'milk allergy' when in fact it is a 'milk intolerance' and occurs because there is a deficiency of the brush border enzyme lactase. The

Table 5.2 Differential diagnosis of chronic enteritis

Parasitic
    Roundworm infection
    Giardiosis
    Cryptosporidium spp.

Maldigestion
    Exocrine pancreatic insufficiency
    Bile acid deficiency
    Brush border enzyme deficiency

Malabsorption
    Lymphocytic–plasmacytic enteritis
    Gluten sensitivity
    Eosinophilic enteritis
    Lymphangiectasia
    Regional enteritis
    Neoplasia (lymphosarcoma)

Bacterial overgrowth

Endocrine disorders
    Feline hyperthyroidism
    Addison's disease

Toxaemic states
    Renal disease
    Chronic liver disease

Other
    Cardiac disease

---

diarrhoea is sudden and acute but rapidly settles when milk is withdrawn from the diet. The problem is simply treated by removal of milk from the diet. Those adult dogs and cats which tolerate milk in the diet have usually been fed milk since weaning and therefore appear not to develop a lactase deficiency.

Preparation of homemade diets is often associated with enteric problems. Overcooking meat often reduces its digestibility, feeding raw egg introduces trypsin inhibitors and excessive cereals leads to bacterial fermentation in the colon and increased faecal bulk. Feeding fresh meat alone often induces foul-smelling diarrhoea and is also low in calcium. Feeding of tinned meats rich in liver, kidney or heart may also induce diarrhoea in individual cases.

Scavenging can be a major problem and one which is sometimes difficult to detect. It is not uncommon for responsible owners to be totally unaware that their dog is scavenging. In such situations there is recurrent diarrhoea which settles immediately the dog is hospitalized. The problem often recurs as soon as the dog returns to its own environment. Macroscopic examination of the faeces may help to reveal the type of rubbish the dog has eaten.

A further dietary problem may arise from owners simply overfeeding their puppy or kitten with the result that the next meal is ingested before the first meal has undergone complete digestion and absorption. In this situation the previous meal is moved to the colon before complete absorption has occurred, with subsequent bacterial fermentation leading to an osmotic or secretory diarrhoea.

Many diets are low in fibre, leading to low food residues in the distal ileum and colon. This fails to stimulate peristalsis and chyme is retained for long periods in the colon allowing a greater opportunity for bacterial fermentation and subsequent diarrhoea. The inclusion of fibre in the diet will quickly resolve the problem.

True dietary allergies have been described, often manifest by acute relapsing diarrhoea. Other cases present as chronic diarrhoea with other manifestations including dermatitis and chronic otitis. Irish Setters with gluten sensitivity have been described. This may be reversible when a gluten-free diet is fed (Batt *et al.* 1984). Other commercial foods and table scraps have been implicated as possible dietary allergens. Such allergens may cause vomiting and/or diarrhoea and are frustrating to identify, as this can only be achieved by laborious dietary exclusion. Very often the clinician is faced with trying foods which are thought to be rarely implicated in food allergy, in the hope of obtaining a remission of symptoms. Foods such as fresh mutton, rice and chicken are good choices. If the dog responds, then one of the original foods is introduced per week till the offending food is identified. When the offending food is detected it is necessary to determine which component of the food is responsible. It may be protein, carbohydrate, fat or a preservative. Some foods such as soya bean contain trypsin inhibitors which actively prevent the protease enzymes from digesting proteins.

Canine parvovirus

This is a highly contagious epitheliotropic enterovirus with a predilection for rapidly dividing cells. Hence the leucopenia and gastroenteritis seen in adults and myocarditis of puppies (Williams 1988). The first outbreak of acute parvovirus infection occurred in 1978 when dogs were affected in one of two ways: (1) sudden deaths and acute myocarditis in unweaned puppies with a very high mortality rate in affected litters; and (2) weaned puppies and adult dogs showed signs of acute gastroenteritis which was rapidly fatal if left untreated in the early stages. The first syndrome is now rare, and is only seen when totally susceptible unvaccinated dams pick up the infection and pass it to the fetus. After ingestion the virus lodges in the pharyngeal lymphoid tissues and thymus and then establishes itself in the rapidly dividing crypt cells of the intestinal villi. Joint infection with parvovirus has also been documented (Williams 1988).

A very heavy loss of good breeding animals occurred in the early years but the development of acquired immunity followed by vaccination has resulted in a sharp fall in mortality. It is now rare to observe acute myocarditis in puppies but isolated outbreaks and individual cases of gastroenteritis still occur. The problem appears to be worst in stray dogs of poor vaccinal status and in those with low maternal protection or under stress.

Clinical diagnosis

The gastroenteric form usually starts with anorexia and marked depression which is followed by persistent vomiting, initially productive but rapidly yielding only gastric secretion and occasionally blood. Faeces are usually fluid or gelatinous in consistency and red/brown in colour. They have a fetid smell and may contain sloughed mucosal casts. There is frequently tenesmus and severe dehydration rapidly develops. The temperature may be high initially ($103-105°F$) but quickly falls to below normal, so the dog becomes shocked and will die if not treated quickly.

The diagnosis is often suspected on clinical grounds but may be confirmed by haematology, serology and virus isolation. Haematology shows a severe leucopenia and neutropenia with total white cell counts as low as 0.9 $\times$ 109/litre. This level of immunosuppression often results in secondary bacterial infection. Virus may be isolated from the faeces (Else 1980) or faecal haemaglutination may be useful in demonstrating the virus. Fluorescent antibody tests on tissues can also be used to detect the virus. Serology to demonstrate a rising titre is essential. Single estimates of parvovirus titres vary considerably from dog to dog and are not diagnostically reliable. Finally histological examination of small intestinal biopsy samples will reveal villus atrophy and viral involvement of the crypt cells suppressing epithelial renewal. Changes associated with the large intestine are rare.

Treatment

These are real emergencies and require intensive fluid therapy if they are to survive. A compound lactated Ringer solution is required and should be maintained until the dog is observed to be able to retain oral fluids. This may involve intravenous fluids for 4 to 7 days. If fluids are stopped prematurely then the dog will often relapse and die.

All food and oral fluids should be withdrawn. Metaclopramide (Emequell; SmithKline Beecham Pharmaceuticals) should be given intramuscularly at 0.5 mg/kg twice daily and appears to be the only effective method of reducing the vomiting and preventing further exhaustion and electrolyte loss.

Broad spectrum antibiotics in the form of ampicillin (Amfipen; Gist-Brocades Pharmaceuticals) at $5-10$ mg/kg daily by intramuscular injection are required to prevent secondary bacterial infection. Oral fluids and kaolin based preparations should only be started once the dog stops vomiting. Lectade (SmithKline Beecham Pharmaceuticals) should be the oral fluid of choice initially followed by water to maintain fluid balance.

Prevention is much better than cure and this can easily be achieved by adequate vaccination. Where dogs are kept in close confinement, strict hygiene and adequate vaccination are essential. Carrier states do exist which make control more difficult. The virus is very resistant and can last in the environment for up to many months. Sodium hypochlorite or one of the new parvocidal disinfectants should be used to keep environmental contamination low (Williams 1988).

Other canine viral enteritides

Both rotavirus and coronavirus infections have been detected in dogs, but their true role as primary pathogens is still questioned (Murdoch 1986).

Coronavirus is another epitheliotrophic enterovirus which has been implicated in acute enteritis followed by villus atrophy and malabsorption. Enteritis is very similar to that observed with parvovirus so the two conditions can only be differentiated by faecal isolation or serology. Coronavirus may occur simultaneously with parvovirus making it difficult to decide which is the significant pathogen. In coronavirus infection an ocular and nasal discharge may also be present. Treatment is very similar to that for parvovirus infection. Control is more difficult as a vaccine is not available.

Very little is known about rotavirus infection although it has been isolated from dogs with acute enteritis. Unlike parvovirus and coronavirus this virus attacks the cells at the tip of the villi not the crypt cells. The clinical signs are normally less severe than those observed with parvovirus and coronavirus. A watery mucoid diarrhoea lasting some 10 days is observed with little vomiting, anorexia or pyrexia. Treatment is again along the lines used for dogs with parvovirus.

Feline enteritis

Feline enteritis is also known as feline panleucopenia and feline parvovirus infection. In addition to gastroenteritis the virus may cause stillbirths, abortion and fetal resorption in pregnant queens and cerebellar hypoplasia in neonatal kittens. All forms of the condition are seen less frequently because of effective vaccination, but gastroenteritis is still seen in isolated situations. The virus has preference for rapidly dividing cells and following ingestion establishes in the pharyngeal lymphoid tissue prior to dissemination via the circulation to the bone marrow and intestinal crypt cells. The virus can cross the placenta and in early gestation leads to fetal death and resorption. Infection in the second half of gestation may result in cerebellar hypoplasia in neonates.

The virus is very resistant and can survive for up to 1 year in infected premises. Formaldehyde, gluteraldehyde and hypochlorite disinfectants are required to clean infected premises.

Clinical diagnosis

The symptoms may vary from mild enteritis to peracute gastroenteritis and sudden deaths. Following a 2 to 10 day incubation period the first signs observed are lethargy, anorexia and pyrexia. The cat may appear very thirsty, sitting over the water bowl, but often fails to drink. Vomiting starts before diarrhoea and is persistent. Acute abdominal pain is observed and the intestines feel fluid and gas-filled. The temperature often falls if the animal survives more than 3 days and the diarrhoea becomes fluid and contains blood. There is severe dehydration and the mortality rate can reach 75%. Secondary bacterial infection is likely due to the immunosuppression and physical damage to the intestine.

Diagnosis is often based on clinical findings and a history of inadequate vaccination. Examination of oropharyngeal swabs and faeces for virus or serology may be employed to confirm the diagnosis. Histological examination of the intestine reveals dilation of the crypts, destruction of enterocytes and the presence of inclusion bodies in surviving cell nests at the base of the mucosa with epithelial proliferation in surviving areas. Changes are most marked in the ileum.

Treatment

This is very similar to that employed for canine parvovirus infection. Intensive fluid therapy using lactated Ringer's solution followed by dextrose saline should be given intravenously. Oral fluids and food should be withheld until vomiting has stopped. Broad spectrum antibiotics such as ampicillin (Amfipen; Gist-Brocades Pharmaceuticals) are essential as is metaclopramide (Emequell; SmithKline Beecham Pharmaceuticals) as described for canine parvovirus infection. Vaccination of healthy cats using a live vaccine will provide good protection against infection. For pregnant queens and unweaned kittens a dead vaccine is also available.

Other feline viral infections

Feline coronavirus is closely related to feline infectious peritonitis (FIP). It may cause a mild self-limiting diarrhoea in kittens but is not pathogenic to adult cats (Rutgers 1989). A non-fatal acute enteritis may be seen in kittens from weaning to 12 weeks of age. Cross-reaction of serology with FIP is common, making a definitive diagnosis difficult. FIP is thought to be a mutant of enteric coronavirus (Murdoch 1986).

The importance of rotavirus is not entirely clear. The virus has been isolated from cat faeces but it is not necessarily a primary pathogen. It is thought to cause a mild self-limiting enteritis in cats.

Acute bacterial enteritis

Although bacteria are frequently implicated as causing enteritis in dogs and cats, there are very few documented cases. Bacteria such as *E. coli* (toxigenic), *Campylobacter* spp., *Salmonella* spp., *Staphylococcus* spp., *Yersinia* spp. and *Klebsiella* spp., have been documented (Murdoch 1986, Rutgers 1989). The importance of *E. coli* as a cause of acute diarrhoea is still debatable, for even though it may be isolated on faecal culture, it does not confirm the diagnosis. The situation is further complicated by the knowledge that faecal culture does not necessarily reflect the population in the small intestine (Thorne & Gorbach 1978, Zimmer 1983).

Yersinia may give rise to a mild enteritis and lymphadenopathy of the mesenteric lymph nodes together with weight loss. The organism is carried by birds and small mammals and so is more likely to involve cats rather than dogs. Although rare, Tyzzer's disease in kittens due to *Bacillus piliformis* has also been recorded.

Campylobacterosis

Campylobacter jejuni was previously known as *Vibrio* spp. and has only been recognized as a pathogen in man since 1977. It is so common in man that it may overtake Salmonellosis as the commonest cause of food poisoning. The organism is widely distributed throughout the world in animals and birds. No cultural difference has been found between the organism causing human enteritis and that found in pets (Fox *et al.* 1983). Carrier states exist and although dogs and cats may act as a reservoir, it is thought that very few cases of human enteritis originate from household pets (Prescott & Munroe 1983). The main sources of infection include raw milk, undercooked meat, especially poultry, and water (Blaser *et al.* 1979, Williams 1987).

Campylobacter is excreted more frequently from stray dogs than pet-owned dogs and there is a poor correlation between excretion and the presence of diarrhoea (Simpson *et al.* 1988). Excretion is also intermittent and repeated culture may be required for its detection (Burnie *et al.* 1983). The organism is an opportunist and takes advantage of a favourable environment such as those under stress or with concurrent viral infection which allow the organism to establish (Burnie *et al.* 1983). Excretion in cats is variable with surveys revealing from 10.7 to 45% of cats positive on faecal sampling (Blaser *et al.* 1980, Fox *et al.* 1985).

It has been stated that cats rarely have diarrhoea associated with *Campylobacter* (Gruffydd-Jones *et al.* 1980). However we have seen many cases which present with an acute self-limiting infection which lasts some 10 days. Pyrexia, depression, abdominal pain and diarrhoea, occasionally with blood, may be present. Vomiting is not common and mortality rate is low. Flattening of the villi, reduced numbers of goblet cells and infiltration of inflammatory cells are found on histology of the intestine. Relapses appear to be quite common.

When the organism is isolated from faecal samples, treatment with tylosin (Tylan; Elanco Products) at 20 to 40 mg/kg/day orally should be instituted, as it is often successful. Erythromycin at 40 mg/kg for at least 10 days may also be used especially in young animals and is available as a paediatric suspension (Erythroped; Abbott Laboratories).

Salmonellosis

There are over 1800 serotypes of salmonella known to cause food poisoning. Animals and man may carry the organism without showing clinical signs, and excrete it intermittently for months. Salmonella tends to lodge in the mesenteric lymph nodes especially after short-term antibiotics have been given and is then difficult to eliminate (Bell *et al.* 1988). It is an important zoonosis and rivals *Campylobacter jejuni* as the commonest cause of food poisoning, and like Campylobacters the source of outbreaks is often never determined. Many salmonella organisms which cause food poisoning in man may not show signs in dogs or cats, but are simply carried by these species.

The major sources of infection include raw milk, uncooked meat especially poultry, poor slaughterhouse hygiene and use of recycled slaughterhouse waste as animal feed. Human infection attributable to pets is very rare compared with the above sources (Cruikshank 1986).

In one study salmonella was isolated intermittently from the faeces of stray dogs with only 3.8% excreting the organism (Burnie *et al.* 1983). Other surveys however reveal up to 30% excretion in dogs (Boreland 1975). Cats have also been studied and from 159 sampled cats only 2% were positive (Fox *et al.* 1985).

Varying severity of enteric infection has been observed. Subclinical disease is common while clinical disease is more frequent in young, old or debilitated dogs or cats. Cats appear to be more resistant to infection than dogs. Pyrexia, abdominal pain, profuse watery diarrhoea occasionally with blood, together with vomiting may be observed.

Treatment is controversial, as the infection is normally self-limiting, and because of the risk of carrier states and resistance. Unless the dog or cat is severely ill no antibiotics should be used (Hall 1988). Routine screening should be performed until three clear negative faecal samples have been obtained. Non-antibiotic symptomatic treatment may be given as required.

Tyzzer's disease

This is an uncommon disease which has been recorded in mice, rabbits, gerbils, hamsters, dog, foxes, wild cats as well as domestic cats. It is caused by a pleomorphic bacterium, *Bacillus piliformis* which is an obligate intracellular pathogen.

Outbreaks of disease have been recorded in laboratory animals (mice and rabbits especially) where carriers are apparently common. It is not known if the carrier state exists in cats. Morbidity and mortality in cats is greatest in kittens. Stress, immunosuppression, feline leukaemia virus (FeLV), overcrowding and poor hygiene appear to be important in feline outbreaks.

Clinical diagnosis

Clinically in the kitten, Tyzzer's disease may appear like feline panleucopenia. There may be sudden deaths together with kittens which have subnormal temperatures, palor of mucus membranes, tachycardia, dyspnoea, abdominal distention and pain. Vomiting occasionally occurs while profuse diarrhoea is always present and may contain blood. Icterus has been reported in some cases (Jones *et al*. 1985).

Laboratory tests may reveal anaemia, leucopenia, hepatic jaundice and elevated serum alanine aminotransferase levels. Affected cats should be checked for the presence of FeLV and feline immunodeficiency virus (FIV).

Post-mortem examination usually reveals multiple areas of necrosis in the liver, and occasionally periportal fibrosis with proliferation of biliary duct epithelium. The organism is found within hepatocytes. A myocarditis with areas of cardiac muscle necrosis may also be observed with evidence of the organism in the cardiac muscle cells. The intestinal tract may show inflammation and evidence of the organism within the cells.

Treatment

This is very unlikely to be effective so the prognosis must always be extremely guarded. Those that do survive may remain in poor condition and susceptible to infection, ultimately leading to the need for their humane destruction.

Haemorrhagic gastroenteritis (HGE)

This is a condition which is observed in the small and toy breeds of dog, especially the King Charles Spaniel, Sheltie, Pekinese and Poodle. Although dogs of any age may be affected, those between 2 and 4 years of age are most frequently involved. It is not unknown for dogs to have a relapse (15%) at any time in the future. Although the aetiology is not known, there is no evidence of inflammation on histological examination of the intestine. It is generally thought that the cause is an anaphylactic reaction, possibly to bacterial endotoxin. In particular *Clostridium perfringens* has been implicated in some clinical cases.

Clinical diagnosis

There is usually a sudden onset of acute vomiting and diarrhoea which develops to the stage where large amounts of fresh blood are produced. Clients are often very alarmed as they find the dog collapsed and passing quite large amounts of blood. Although mild forms of the condition may occur most are very acute and the dogs rapidly become shocked, dehydrated, collapsed and should be treated as real medical emergencies. Examination will often reveal tachycardia, pallor of mucous membranes, normal to sub-normal temperature, depression and a characteristic fetid smell on the breath.

The condition must be differentiated from parvovirus infection, infectious canine hepatitis, acute pancreatitis and intestinal obstructions which may appear very similar in the early stages. There are no diagnostic tests to confirm the presence of HGE, so differentiation is based on elimination of other conditions. The packed cell volume (PCV) is often greater than 60% with a proportional rise in serum proteins. White cell counts vary considerably and clotting factors may be abnormal.

Treatment

Intravenous fluids, as compound lactated Ringer's solution, should be administered immediately to counter the state of shock and to replace the fluid and electrolyte loss. Broad spectrum antibiotic cover should also be provided, ideally as ampicillin in combination with aminoglycosides, to protect against Gram-positive and -negative bacteria. Corticosteroids may be helpful in those cases which are severely shocked.

The dog should be kept warm, in a quiet and stress-free environment. The response to treatment should be monitored carefully and adjusted as required. Although many cases appear critically ill and the prognosis must always be guarded, it is likely that most cases seen early and given adequate treatment will survive.

Intestinal obstruction

Obstruction is most likely to occur in the small intestine or at the ileocaeco-colic junction and only very rarely in the large intestine. Foreign bodies are most frequently involved but obstruction may be caused by tumours, intus-susceptions, congenital or acquired strictures or paralytic ileus.

Foreign body obstruction is most likely to occur in dogs with a history of eating rubbish or stones. Foreign bodies in cats are rare but when they do occur may involve fish hooks, fish bones or linear foreign bodies such as string. Adenocarcinoma is the most likely tumour to obstruct the intestine as it often grows into the lumen, unlike lymphosarcoma which usually causes annular thickening of the intestinal wall. Intussusceptions most frequently occur at the ileocaecocolic junction with small intestine tele-scoping into the colon.

Clinical diagnosis

Clinical signs depend to some extent on the location of the obstruction. Those which occur in the proximal small intestine are often manifest by acute persistent vomiting with faeces being passed initially often diarrhoeic in nature. Any blood in the faeces is likely to be dark and tarry in con-sistency. Obstructions in the distal small intestine will also cause vomiting, but not so acutely as proximal obstructions. Formed or diarrhoeic faeces will be passed for a short time before ceasing altogether. The authors have observed dogs where partial obstruction has occurred with a history of intermittent vomiting and diarrhoea.

Where an intussusception is present, vomiting may be seen together with the passage of faeces which rapidly become reduced in volume and bloody, resembling redcurrant jelly. Tenesmus is also observed in some cases of intussusception. Adenocarcinomas may partially block the intestine before causing complete obstruction. The clinical signs may therefore vary and may give the impression of a chronic problem rather than a sudden acute obstruction. Ulceration is quite common so that faeces may contain altered or fresh blood.

In all cases the animal will not only exhibit vomiting and diarrhoea but also dehydration, anorexia and depression and may develop abdominal pain. Palpation of foreign bodies can be difficult due to the free movement of intestinal loops in the abdomen. Intussusceptions are often palpable as fairly static hard sausage-shaped structures in a more fixed position. Tumours, if small, may be difficult to palpate in the early stages.

Radiographs will detect radiodense foreign bodies without difficulty, but radiolucent foreign bodies may be missed. However a large gas cap should be visible and possibly evidence of gravel collection within the intestine just proximal to the obstruction (Fig. 5.9). Barium should be used with care

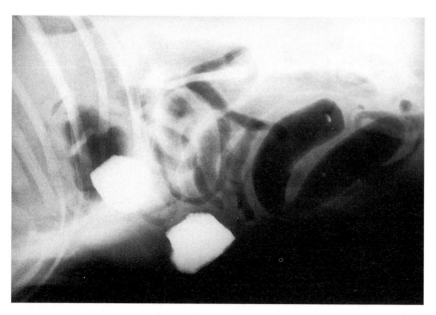

Fig. 5.9 Plain radiograph of small intestinal foreign bodies.

where obstruction is suspected, because if the bowel is perforated, barium
will enter the peritoneum from where it will not be resorbed. In cases where
perforation is suspected Gastrografin (Schering Chemicals) which can be
resorbed should be used; this gives an equally satisfactory contrast.

Treatment

In all the cases described above, surgical intervention is required to correct
the problem. No medical treatment is likely to be successful and the longer
the foreign body lies in the bowel the more likely it is that perforation will
occur with ensuing peritonitis and death. Liquid paraffin should be used
with great care as it may move the foreign body further along the intestine,
only to block at the ileocaecocolic junction.

The removal of adenocarcinomas is quite feasible especially if detected
early before adhesions have formed or metastasis has occurred. Complete
resection of a portion of intestine is feasible in some cases with end-to-end
anastomoses of healthy tissue.

Intussusceptions may be reduced in the early stages before fibrous adhesions have formed. If they are diagnosed late then complete resection of
the ileocaecocolic region with small and large intestine may be required.
End-to-end anastomosis of the small and large bowel is feasible especially if
there is an adequate length of intestine left for normal function.

Chronic small intestinal diseases

Parasitic enteritis

Infestation with roundworms does occur especially in puppies and kittens. Where there is a heavy infestation in a puppy or kitten this may be associated with poor growth, distention of the abdomen and mucoid diarrhoea. They are rarely implicated in causing chronic diarrhoea in adult dogs and cats. The authors have examined faeces from many hundreds of dogs and cats as part of the investigation for chronic diarrhoea but detected roundworms in less than 5% of cases. Migrating larvae may cause damage to the lungs and liver especially if present in large numbers.

Hookworm infestation in the UK usually involves *Uncinaria* spp. which are not blood-sucking like *Ancylostoma* spp. Both may be implicated in causing diarrhoea if present in large numbers, with associated colic and melaena. In addition to these signs if the damage caused to the mucosa is severe, then plasma proteins may be lost into the intestine. Tapeworms even when present in large numbers rarely cause diarrhoea.

Diagnosis of roundworm infestation is made from examination of the faeces for ova. Where evidence of worms is detected, they should be treated and the animal reassessed at a later date, so that parasites can be definitively ruled out of the investigation into chronic diarrhoea.

Treatment

Treatment involves the use of an effective anthelmintic such as fenbendazole (Panacur; Hoechst Animal Health) 20 mg/kg for 5 days or 100 mg as a single dose (Table 5.3). It is more important to ensure the dog and cat population is kept free of worms and this involves regular worming whether evidence of worms is present or not. This is especially true in the case of breeding bitches.

Giardiasis

Giardiasis in dogs and cats is now recognized to be more important than previously considered. Ingested cysts are the main source of infection, following faecal contamination of food. *Giardia* is not host specific so canine and feline infection can affect man (Scarlet-Krunz 1987). In a UK survey *Giardia* cysts were detected in 13.9% of stray dogs' faeces, all of which were carrying the parasite without clinical signs (Simpson *et al.* 1988). The prepatent period following ingestion appears at 4 to 8 days.

The trophozoites attach by means of a sucker to the duodenal mucosa

Table 5.3 Some anthelminthics suitable for the dog and cat

Telmin KH	Mebendazole	Dog/cat	1 × 100 mg bid for 2 days adults
			½ × 100 mg bid for 2 days neonate
Panacur 10%	Fenbendazole	Dog/cat	20 mg/kg for 5 days, or 100 mg as single dose
Piperazine	Piperazine	Dog/cat	500 mg/kg once
Strongid Paste	Pyrantel	Dogs	9 cm paste/4½ kg
Lopatol 100	Nitroscante	Cats	1 × 100 mg/4.4 kg
Lopatol 500	Nitroscante	Dogs	1 × 500 mg/22 lbs

and are therefore rarely observed in the faeces. *Giardia* rarely establishes below the jejunum. Problems occur most frequently in puppies and kittens where large numbers of *Giardia* are present and may alter the gut flora and induce changes to the brush border which lead to chronic diarrhoea and malabsorption.

Clinical diagnosis

Although asymptomatic carriers do exist many dogs and cats will exhibit signs which include the passage of soft, pale and unformed faeces which may appear granular or 'frothy' in appearance. Sometimes faeces are observed to be shiny or greasy due to steatorrhoea. Although individual episodes of diarrhoea may appear acute, there is usually a history of chronic or persistent diarrhoea.

Diagnosis is based on the examination of faeces for the presence of cysts. This must be carried out carefully as many methods are simply unreliable. Direct examination of the faeces may reveal trophozoites but they are often absent. A peroral method of sampling the duodenal juice has been shown to be very reliable (Hall *et al*. 1988). Otherwise an ether extraction method which concentrates the cysts found in faeces should be employed (Ridley & Hawgood 1956).

Treatment

Once a diagnosis has been made, the animal should be treated with metronidazole (Flagyl; RMB Animal Health) at 25 mg/kg bid for 10 days. The faeces should be checked after the course of treatment to ensure that *Giardia* spp. has been eliminated. It is also advisable to inform the owner that *Giardia* is a zoonosis, and that strict hygiene is required during the treatment period.

Cryptosporidia

Cryptosporidia spp. has been associated with enteritis in calves and other farm livestock but is very rare in small animals. A recent survey of stray dogs failed to find any evidence of the organism in faecal samples (Simpson *et al.* 1988). The condition has been reported more in the cat than the dog, especially where the cat is immunosuppressed (Bennett *et al.* 1985).

Clinical signs are those of fluid faeces and dehydration and are especially severe in kittens. Fortunately the condition is usually self-limiting. The organism is most often found in situations of poor hygiene and overstocking. Diagnosis is difficult to obtain and involves the careful examination of faeces for oocysts. Faecal flotation using Sheather's sugar solution or acid fast stains has been employed.

Treatment involves the use of oral sulphonamides at 50 mg/kg/day for at least 10 days.

Bacterial overgrowth

This is a condition seen in man and dogs where bacteria in the small intestine proliferate to abnormally high levels and subsequently interfere with intestinal function. There are few documented cases in dogs, in contrast to the extensive literature written on the subject in man. In the few canine reports *Pseudomonas aeruginosa* (Simpson 1982), *Bacteroides* (Reife *et al.* 1980), *E. coli*, *Enterococcus*, and *Clostridium* spp. (Batt 1983) have been implicated. *Clostridium difficile* has been reported as causing chronic diarrhoea in dogs (Berry & Levett 1986).

The German Shepherd dog appears to be more frequently represented than other breeds, although any breed can be affected. There is no sex predisposition. The aetiology is complex and not fully understood but may involve one of the following: (1) increased gastric pH (above 5) results in ingested bacteria surviving passage through the stomach to the small intestine; (2) extensive use of broad spectrum antibiotics may allow one population of bacteria to survive while others are suppressed; (3) reduced intestinal motility such as in stagnant loop syndrome, paralytic ileus and intestinal obstruction may allow bacteria to proliferate (Pidgeon 1983); and (4) impaired immunity has also been implicated (Whitbread *et al.* 1984). Bacterial overgrowth is often present in dogs with exocrine pancreatic insufficiency, due to the presence of unabsorbed food in the small intestine.

Proliferating bacteria may produce protease enzymes which damage the microvillus structure of the small intestine and destroy the brush border enzymes and carrier proteins (Issacs & Kim 1983). They may also increase lysosomal fragility and lead to loss of mitochondria within enterocytes. Histologically there are rarely any morphological changes present, only biochemical changes. It is also possible that bacteria may deconjugate bile salts leading to steatorrhoea and the presence of bile products in the large intestine. Unabsorbed fats are converted to hydroxy fatty acids which induce large intestinal secretory diarrhoea (Williams 1988). Carbohydrates may be broken down to oligosaccharides which have an osmotic effect in the large intestine (Batt 1987).

Anaerobic bacteria are thought to cause more damage than aerobic bacteria. The former organisms appear to break down the glycocalyx layer which protects the mucosa. This allows luminal contents to damage the brush border proteins and intestinal function (Batt & Hall 1989).

Clinical diagnosis

Clinical signs exhibited by dogs with bacterial overgrowth include chronic intermittent diarrhoea which may or may not be associated with weight-loss and polyphagia. Depressed appetite, coprophagia and flatulance may also be detected. Culture of the faeces is not normally of diagnostic value, and it is often necessary to culture intestinal juice or determine serum folate and vitamin B12 levels. Many bacteria have the ability to synthesize folate and bind B12 in the small intestine. These changes can be measured in the serum to reflect changes in the intestine. Elevated serum folate levels and reduced serum B12 levels are indicative of bacterial overgrowth. Xylose absorption may be abnormal in some cases due to bacterial utilization of the monosaccharide (Simpson 1982), but is equally likely to be in the normal range. Urine nitrosonapthal test may also be positive (Burrows & Jezyk 1983).

Histological examination of intestinal biopsy samples rarely reveals any gross change although some infiltration with lymphocytes and plasma cells may occur. Assay of brush border enzymes will reveal a fall in alkaline phosphatase activity.

Treatment

An attempt should be made to determine the underlying cause, which should be corrected, but in the majority of cases this is never found. Fortunately the changes described above are rarely permanent and following suitable antibiotic treatment normal small intestinal function can be restored. Oxytetracycline 10 mg/kg tid for up to 30 days is required or tylosin 10 mg/kg tid or metronidazole 20 mg/kg/day for the same period may be used (Table 5.4). It is not unusual for relapses to occur, if the underlying cause has not been controlled.

Lymphocytic—plasmacytic enteritis

This is a chronic inflammatory condition of the small intestine characterized by infiltration of the lamina propria by plasma cells and lymphocytes (Tams 1987). Middle-aged dogs of either sex are most susceptible and it

Table 5.4 Drugs employed for the treatment of chronic small intestinal disease

Tylosin (Tylan)	10 mg/kg tid for bacterial overgrowth
	20–40/kg inflammatory bowel disease
Oxytetracycline (Terramycin)	10 mg/kg tid bacterial overgrowth
Metronidazole (Flagyl)	25 mg/kg bid
Prednisolone	1–3 mg/kg/day
Azathioprine (Imuran)	0.3 mg/kg/day for cats
	1–2 mg/kg/day for dogs

appears more common in the German Shepherd dog although any breed can be affected. Similar infiltrations have been observed in other conditions such as bacterial overgrowth and giardiasis.

In the Basenji a complex disease entity exists, characterized by anorexia, occasional vomiting and chronic diarrhoea. Histological changes to the small intestine resemble lymphocytic–plasmacytic enteritis. The condition is thought to have a hereditary basis and may be precipitated by stress. Hypoalbuminaemia and hypergammaglobulinaemia are other hallmarks of the condition (Breitschwerdt *et al.* 1982).

The condition has also been diagnosed in cats which usually only develop a mild form of the condition, and certainly are never as severely affected as the Basenji.

The aetiology of the condition is not understood but may simply reflect a normal intestinal response to antigen such as bacteria, virus or allergen (Williams 1988). This is further substantiated by a resolution of the problem when a hypoallergen diet is fed or where corticosteroids are administered (Tams & Twedt 1981). Antibodies to many antigens have been sought but so far without success (Hayden & Van Kruiningen 1982).

Clinical diagnosis

Three forms of the condition are recognized: (1) dogs presented with chronic vomiting, (2) dogs presented with chronic diarrhoea; and (3) dogs presented with chronic vomiting and diarrhoea.

In addition, evidence of anorexia, halitosis, borborygmi, polydipsia/polyuria and listlessness have been recorded. The signs may be observed to wax and wane and weight-loss occurs especially in advanced cases. Abdominal pain has been observed in some cases manifest as arching of the back or assuming a praying position.

When vomiting occurs it often contains bile, and there is no relationship to feeding, although partially digested food vomited hours after feeding may be observed, indicating disturbed gastric motility. Gastric biopsies are usually normal in such dogs, indicating the need to examine the intestine. It is very important to understand that vomiting may be the *only* sign associated with inflammatory bowel disease, in some cases, and that there may be *no* evidence of diarrhoea.

In the diarrhoeic form faeces are often soft or fluid in nature with increased volume, a foul smell and passed with increased frequency. Although the diarrhoea originates from the small intestine it is important to understand that secondary large intestinal involvement may occur.

In advanced cases depression, weight-loss, dull coat, hepatomegaly, splenomegaly and lymphadenopathy may be detected. Ascites and sub-cutaneous oedema develop when protein-losing enteropathy (PLE) and hypoproteinaemia occur.

In cats the condition has also been recognized, with signs of anorexia, weight-loss and chronic diarrhoea. Vomiting may also be a feature of the condition (Rutgers 1989).

Laboratory investigation reveals a leucocytosis with lymphocytosis and eosinophilia. Hypoproteinaemia with loss of both albumin and globulin occurs and an associated hypocalcaemia. Xylose and fat absorption are often poor and serum folate and B12 may also be depressed. Exocrine pancreatic insufficiency should be considered in the differential diagnosis, but the trypsin-like immunoreactivity value will be normal. Radiographs are singularly unrewarding.

A definitive diagnosis requires a laparotomy and collection of small intestinal biopsy samples. The condition most often affects the duodenum and jejunum, but may involve the ileum, so samples should be collected from all regions. Histological examination will reveal plasma cell and lymphocyte infiltration of the intestinal wall with some degree of villus atrophy in severe cases (Fig. 5.10).

Treatment

As it is considered to be an immune-mediated condition, corticosteroids are frequently used in treatment. Prednisolone is used at 2 to 4 mg/kg/day for 2 weeks followed by 1 to 2 mg/kg/day for a further 2 weeks, reducing to alternate day therapy if symptoms do not recur. Where PLE is present the doses should be higher and for a longer period of time, up to a year in some cases. Where high doses are poorly tolerated, azathioprine (Imuran; Calmic Medicals) can be included, allowing a reduction of 50% in the prednisolone dose. Use azathioprine at 2 mg/kg/day and reduce both drugs as the dog responds to therapy. In cats use 0.3 mg/kg of azathioprine on alternate days. Metronidazole (Flagyl; RMB Animal Health) 10 mg/kg tid can be used to reduce bacterial overgrowth and to reduce any cell-mediated immune response. The dose may be reduced to twice daily and then once daily after 2 weeks. All three drugs may be used in combination in severe cases (Tams

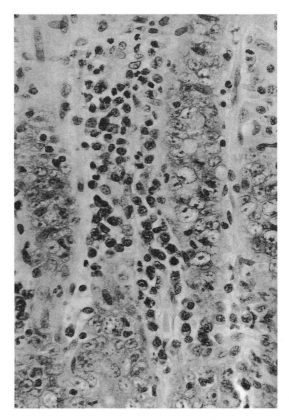

Fig. 5.10 Biopsy of the small intestine showing plasma cell and lymphocyte infiltration of the lamina propria.

1987). tylosin (Tylan; Elanco Products) has also been shown to be an effective antibiotic in this condition (Van Kruiningen 1976).

Where vomiting is present, metaclopramide (Emequell; SmithKline Beecham Pharmaceuticals) at 0.5 mg/kg, 30 min before food is often helpful. Where colitis is present then prednisolone may have to be supplemented by Salazopyrin (Pharmacia) 20 mg/kg, twice daily with or without azathioprine.

The most important features of the diet are that it should be low in fat and non-allergenic. Such diets include Hills d/d or Waltham selected protein diet. A good vitamin mineral supplement is essential and if additional energy is required medium chain triglyceride (MCT) such as coconut oil should be used at 1 to 2 ml/kg liveweight (Williams 1988).

Eosinophilic enteritis

This is a chronic inflammatory condition of the digestive tract which may involve only the small intestine or may also involve the stomach or large intestine (Williams 1988). There appear to be more cases reported in German Shepherd dogs although other breeds may also be affected. The aetiology is thought to be an allergic reaction to food components (Quigley & Henry 1981) or internal parasites such as *Toxocara canis* (Hayden & Van Kruiningen 1973). It has been reported in both dogs and cats although it is not as common as lymphocytic−plasmacytic enteritis. In cats the eosinophil infiltration may be more extensive and involve tissues outwith the digestive tract.

It is thought the eosinophils are attracted to the intestine by a chemotactic factor produced from intestinal mast cells which suggest a type 1 hypersensitivity reaction has occurred. However chemotactic factor is also released by T lymphocytes and complement so there may be an Arthus reaction or delayed cell-mediated hypersensitivity involved (Franklin *et al.* 1986)

Clinical diagnosis

The clinical signs depend on the severity of the condition in the individual dog or cat. In dogs many cases are mild leading to chronic diarrhoea and variable weight loss. In severe cases hypoproteinaemia develops due to the loss of plasma proteins into the intestine, resulting in subcutaneous oedema, ascites and hydrothorax. In these cases weight-loss and diarrhoea are severe. If the large intestine is involved, fresh blood and tenesmus are often observed. Where the stomach is involved vomiting will also be a feature and may occasionally contain blood. Although the appetite is initially normal this will change and anorexia will develop. Cats are most frequently involved in middle age and exhibit vomiting and diarrhoea often with blood present and are almost always anorexic. Hepatomegaly, splenomegaly and lymphadenopathy may also be seen in cats (Rutgers 1989).

Diagnosis may be confirmed by examination of whole blood for a persistent eosinophilia together with examination for evidence of hypoproteinaemia. A definitive diagnosis requires a laparotomy to collect small intestinal biopsy samples. Histological examination will reveal heavy infiltration of eosinophils throughout the wall of the intestine and involve the mesenteric lymph nodes (Quigley & Henry 1981). Careful examination for evidence of parasitic involvement should also be carried out, particularly for signs of *Toxocara canis* larva.

Treatment

As with lymphocytic−plasmacytic enteritis, there appears to be an immune basis to the problem. Therefore treatment usually involves the use of prednisolone at 2 to 4 mg/kg/day for at least 4 weeks, followed by a period of reduced dosage. The addition of azathioprine (Imuran; Calmic Medical Division) may be required in severe cases. Tylosin has been shown to be effective in treating the condition (Van Kruiningen 1976). If evidence of parasitic involvement is present then an anthelmintic which is effective against adults and larvae should be included. It is advisable to consider changing the diet to a hypoallergenic diet such as Waltham selected protein diet or Hills d/d diet. Where the severe form of the condition is present, the prognosis must be guarded, but in mild forms the prognosis is reasonable, especially if the dietary change is maintained after the initial treatment has been completed. Treatment of cats is similar but likely to be less successful.

Gluten sensitive enteropathy

The terms 'sprue' and 'coeliac disease' have been used to describe a similar condition seen in man. The condition recognized in the dog is due to a product of gluten digestion which is toxic to mucosal cells and elicits an immune response. Crypt mitosis is depressed and so epithelial renewal is reduced resulting in villus atrophy (Lorenz 1980). Familial sensitivity to gluten has been detected in the Irish Setter and appears to have a hereditary basis. It involves young dogs up to 1 year-old, where partial villus atrophy and malabsorption have been detected. The condition appears to be corrected when the dogs are placed on a gluten-free diet but relapses when a gluten diet is reintroduced. Biochemical studies of the brush border have shown a deficiency in aminopeptidase N which will result in a reduced degradation of gluten, leading to hypersensitivity. Increased intestinal permeability has also been detected (Batt & Hall 1989). Only puppies fed cereal-based diets were observed to have histological and biochemical changes to the small intestine. These included partial villus atrophy, lymphocyte infiltration, reduced levels of alkaline phosphatase and aminopeptidase N, and finally increased permeability (Hall & Batt 1988).

Clinical diagnosis

The condition should be suspected in young Irish Setters which exhibit signs of weight-loss or failure to thrive in association with chronic intermittent diarrhoea. They are often between 4 and 7 months of age. Diagnosis is further confirmed by low serum folate levels but normal B12 levels suggesting a proximal small intestinal malabsorption. There is often reduced xylose absorption. A definitive diagnosis is made from biopsy of the duodenum and jejunum where partial villus atrophy, lymphocyte infiltration and loss of brush border enzymes are detected.

Treatment

Affected dogs should be placed on a gluten-free diet and maintained on this once symptoms have disappeared. This means the diet must be free of cereal products and when such a diet is instigated the histological changes in the small intestine slowly reverse and clinical signs disappear. Rice-based foods and tinned meat should be used rather than cereals such as wheat and maize. A low fat diet is also helpful and a good vitamin mineral supplement should also be provided. In severe cases prednisolone and tylosin should be given in a similar manner to that used in lymphocytic–plasmacytic enteritis.

Regional enteritis

Regional enteritis is also known as granulomatous enteritis and Crohns disease in man. Although recorded in the dog (DiBartola *et al*. 1982) and the cat (Van Kruiningen *et al*. 1983) it is rare compared with the number of cases seen in man. The aetiology for this inflammatory condition of the intestine is not known although it has been associated with *Trichuris* larvae (DiBartola *et al*. 1982). Male dogs appear most frequently involved especially those under 4 years of age. The condition is progressive and involves the ileum and possibly the caecum and colon. Segments of affected intestine lie next to segments of normal intestine. There appears to be some association between regional enteritis and perianal fistulas in some dogs.

Clinical diagnosis

Both dogs and cats present with diarrhoea often containing fresh blood and mucus. Faeces are small in volume and tenesmus is often present, especially where the terminal colon is involved. Occasionally patients will vomit and exhibit abdominal pain. Weight-loss is a feature especially in advanced cases and in all cases the signs may wax and wane.

Laboratory investigation may reveal an eosinophilia, and hypoprotein-aemia in advanced cases. The only method of obtaining a definitive diagnosis is the biopsy of affected sections of intestine and lymphoid tissue at laparotomy. Histologically there is involvement of all layers which are thickened and contain cellular infiltrates. Large numbers of eosinophils, plasma cells, lymphocytes, multinucleate giant cells and macrophages are seen. The regional lymph nodes are similarly affected.

Treatment

The use of corticosteroids, azathioprine and tylosin have all been advocated at doses similar to those for lymphocytic–plasmacytic enteritis. Surgical resection of affected intestine has also been carried out in cases where the changes are not extensive. In all reported cases the outcome has been death or euthanasia, therefore the prognosis must be considered very guarded indeed.

Lymphangiectasia

This is a serious condition of the small intestine which results in a protein-losing enteropathy. Although rare in the dog it is said to be seen more commonly in Yorkshire Terriers (Williams 1988) and as a hereditary disease in the Norwegian Lundehunds (Flesja & Yri 1977). The aetiology is not known although a congenital (primary) or acquired (secondary) obstruction to the intestinal lymphatic drainage is implicated. Secondary cases may include right-sided heart failure, constrictive pericarditis, neoplastic or inflammatory obstructions to the lymphatics or granuloma formation of mesentric lymph nodes (Burns 1982). Most cases are frequently found to be secondary to chronic inflammatory bowel disease (Williams 1988). Gross dilation of the lacteals and deeper lymph vessels occurs and there is said to be reduced immunoglobulin A (IgA) levels and consequently more chance of secondary infection occurring (Suter *et al.* 1985). Chyle leaks out of the dilated lacteals leading to a serious loss of plasma protein and thus hypoproteinaemia (Burns 1982).

Clinical diagnosis

The main symptoms observed are chronic diarrhoea associated with weight-loss and frequently subcutaneous oedema, ascites and hydrothorax due to hypoproteinaemia. The appetite may initially be intact but as the condition advances anorexia develops.

Diagnosis is based on the observation of hypoproteinaemia (both albumin and globulin fall), lymphopenia, poor fat and xylose absorption tests, and reduced serum folate and B12 levels. A microcytic anaemia may occasionally occur. Confirmation of protein loss into the intestine can be made using radiolabelled albumin given intravenously, and the faeces monitored for 3 days for radioactivity (Barton *et al.* 1978).

In the Norwegian Lundehund there is inflammation associated with lymphangiectasia but there is no leucopenia nor obvious site of lymphatic obstruction. Lymph nodes are usually small and unreactive. No dietary basis has been found for the condition and there is thought to be an immunodeficiency or hypoplasia of the lymphatic system.

Laparotomy and biopsy of the small intestine is required to obtain a definitive diagnosis. Gross examination of the mesentery will reveal dilated lymphatic vessels and lymphadenopathy. Histologically there are dilated lacteals and other lymphatic vessels and some evidence of inflammation

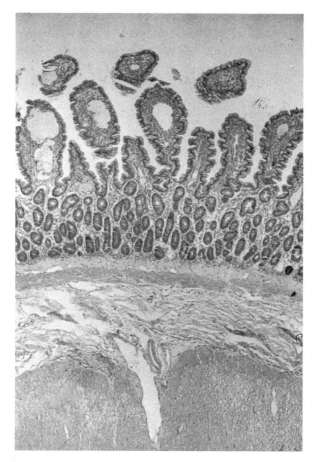

Fig. 5.11 Histological section of small intestine showing dilated lacteals from a dog with lymphangiectasia.

(Fig. 5.11). Partial villus atrophy and crypt hyperplasia may also be seen (Batt & Hall 1989).

Treatment

The prognosis is very difficult to predict as some dogs respond very well to treatment while others totally fail to respond. The cases which are diagnosed early appear to have a greater chance of being successfully treated than advanced cases. There is no way of determining which outcome will occur before treatment is initiated. Where there is evidence of heart disease or obstruction, this should be treated. In idiopathic forms prednisolone at 2 mg/kg/day together with tylosin 10 mg/kg bid should be given. Long-chain triglyceride (LCT) is formed into chylomicrons and released into the lacteals. In lymphangiectasia this results in lymphatic hypertension and so further protein loss. So in addition a low fat diet such as Hills i/d or Waltham low fat diet should be fed. If additional fat is required for energy this can be given as medium-chain triglyceride (MCT) which is absorbed into the portal blood and not the lymphatic system. An adequate vitamin/mineral supplement should be added because fat absorption is impaired.

Intestinal neoplasia

Around 60% of intestinal tumours occur in the small intestine (Tomlinson *et al.* 1982). They include lymphosarcoma, adenocarcinoma, adenoma, leiomyosarcomas. Lymphosarcoma is the commonest tumour observed in dogs and cats followed by adenocarcinoma (Head & Else 1981). Tumours may result in malabsorption, obstruction, bacterial overgrowth or protein-losing enteropathy. Lymphosarcoma is seen mainly in young animals while adenocarcinomas is seen in the middle to old-age group.

Lymphosarcomas may cause malabsorption and protein-losing enteropathy, but rarely cause intestinal obstruction because of the intraluminal nature of their growth. Clinically the dog or cat exhibits chronic intermittent diarrhoea with a slow onset of weight-loss and variable appetite. Cats suspected of this condition should be examined for FeLV, as up to 30% may be positive. Diagnosis is based on signs of hypoproteinaemia including subcutaneous oedema, ascites and hydrothorax, and detecting malabsorption

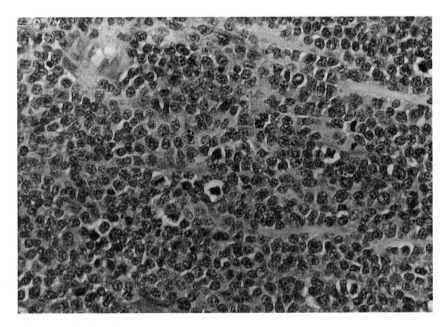

Fig. 5.12 Histological section from the small intestine of a dog with lymphosarcoma.

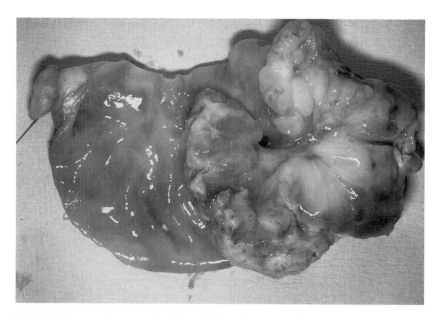

Fig. 5.13 Macroscopic appearance of a small intestinal adenocarcinoma.

from reduced xylose and fat absorption. Biopsy of the small intestine especially the ileum will reveal grossly thickened intestinal walls and generalized lymphocyte infiltration which includes the mesenteric lymph nodes (Fig. 5.12). The prognosis is poor in all cases, but chemotherapy can be attempted using vincristine (Oncovin; Eli Lilly & Co.), cytosine arabinoside (Cytosar; Upjohn), cyclophosphamide (Endoxana; Boehringer Ingelheim) and prednisolone in combination. This regime has been adopted for treatment of multicentric lymphosarcoma and leukaemias but there are no reports of successful use of this treatment in intestinal lymphosarcoma.

Adenocarcinoma is seen most frequently in the duodenum and large intestine. Siamese cats and generally those over 11 years appear to be most frequently affected (Rutgers 1989). There is proliferation of a segment of the intestine which grows into the lumen causing signs of obstruction (Fig. 5.13). Mucosal ulceration develops leading to the presence of observable amounts of blood in the faeces. Other clinical signs may include vomiting and anorexia. The condition is one of slow insidious onset with an acute terminal phase. Often the tumour is well-advanced at the time of diagnosis and may involve other loops of intestine, adhesions or metastasis to other tissues. Radiographs are often helpful in making a diagnosis. The prognosis must be very guarded, but if there are no signs of spread then surgical excision can be successfully carried out.

References

Argenzio R.A. (1980) Comparative physiology of the gastrointestinal system. In: *Veterinary Gastroenterology*. N.V. Anderson (ed.), Lea & Febiger, Philadelphia, 172–198.

Barton C.C., Smith C., Troy G., Hightower D. & Hood D. (1978) The diagnosis and clinicopathological features of canine protein-losing enteropathy. *Journal of American Animal Hospital Association*, **14**; 85–91.

Batt R.M. (1983) Bacterial overgrowth associated with a naturally occurring enteropathy in the German shepherd dog. *Research in Veterinary Science*, **35**; 42–46.

Batt R.M. (1987) The effects of intestinal bacterial overgrowth on mucosal enzymes and absorption in the dog. In: *The Veterinary Annual*. C.S.G. Grunsell, F.W.G. Hill and M.E. Raw (eds), Scientechnica, Bristol, 188–195.

Batt R.M., Carter M.W. & McLean L. (1984) Morphological and biochemical studies of a naturally occurring enteropathy in the Irish setter: A comparison with coeliac disease in man. *Research in Veterinary Science*, **37**; 339–346.

Batt R.M. & Hall E.J. (1989) Chronic enteropathies in the dog. *Journal of Small Animal Practice*, **30**; 3–12.

Bell J.L., Palmer S.R. & Payne J.M. (1988) *The Zoonoses*. Edward Arnold, London.

Bennett M., Baxley D., Blundell N., Gaskell D.J., Hart C.A. & Kelly D.E. (1985) Cryptosporidiosis in the domestic cat. *Veterinary Record*, **116**; 73–74.

Berry A.P. & Levett P.N. (1986) Chronic diarrhoea in dogs associated with Clostridium difficile infection. *Veterinary Record*, **118**; 102–103.

Blaser M.J., Craven J., Powers B.W., LaForce F.M. & Wang W.L. (1979) Campylobacter enteritis associated with unpasteurised milk. *American Journal of Medicine*, **67**; 715–718.

Blaser M.J., LaForce F.M., Wilson N.A. & Wang W.L. (1980) Reservoirs for human Campylobacterosis. *Journal of Infectious Diseases*, **141**; 665–669.

Boreland E.D. (1975) Salmonella infection in dogs and cats, tortoises and terrapins. *Veterinary Record*, **96**; 401–402.

Breitschwerdt E.B., Waltman C., Hagsted H.V., Ochoa R., McClure J. & Barta O. (1982) Clinical and epidemiological characterisation of a diarrhoeal syndrome in Basenji's. *Journal of American Veterinary Medical Association*, **180**; 914–920.

Brobst D.F. (1980) Pancreatic function. In: *Clinical Biochemistry of Domestic Animals*. J.J. Kaneko (ed.), Academic Press, New York, 259–282.

Burnie A.G., Simpson J.W., Lindsay B. & Miles R.S. (1983) The excretion of Campylobacters, Salmonellae and *Giardia lamblia* in the faeces of stray dogs. *Veterinary Research Communications*, **6**; 133–138.

Burns M.G. (1982) Intestinal lymphangiectasia in the dog: A case report and review. *Journal of American Animal Hospital Association*, **18**; 97–105.

Burrows C.F. & Jezyk P.F. (1983) Nitrosonapthal test for screening of small intestinal diarrhoeal disease in the dog. *Journal of American Veterinary Medical Association*, **183**; 318–322.

Cruikshank J.G. (1986) Salmonella and Campylobacter infections — An update. *Journal of Small Animal Practice*, **27**; 673–681.

DiBartola S.P., Rogers W.A., Boyce J.T. & Grimm J.P. (1982) Regional enteritis in two dogs. *Journal of American Veterinary Medical Association*, **181**; 904–908.

Eastwood G.L. (1977) Gastrointestinal epithelial renewal. *Gastroenterology*, **72**; 962–975.

Else R.W. (1980) Fatal haemorrhagic enteritis in a puppy associated with a parvovirus infection. *Veterinary Record*, **106**; 14–17.

Flesja K. & Yri T. (1977) Protein-losing enteropathy in the Lundehund. *Journal of Small Animal Practice*, **18**; 11–23.

Fox J.G., Moore R. & Ackerman J.I. (1983) Canine and feline Campylobacterosis, Epidemiology and clinical and public health features. *Journal of American Veterinary Medical Association*, **183**; 1420–1425.

Fox J.G., Ackerman J.A. & Newcomer C.R. (1985) The prevalence of Campylobacter jejuni in random source cats used in biomedical research. *Journal of Infectious Diseases*, **151**; 743–744.

Franklin R.T., Jones B.D. & Feldman B.F. (1986) Medical conditions of the small intestine. In: *Canine and Feline Gastroenterology*. B.D. Jones (ed.), W.B. Saunders, Philadelphia, 161–202.

Grube D. & Forssmann W.G. (1979) Morphology and function of the enteroendocrine cells. *Hormone and Metabolism Research*, **11**; 589–606.

Gruffydd-Jones T., Marston M. & White E. (1980) Campylobacter jejuni enteritis from cats. *Lancet* ii; 366.

Hall E.J. (1988) Primary treatment of small intestinal disease. In: *The Veterinary Annual*. C.S.G. Grunsell, F.W.G. Hill & M.E. Raw (ed.), Scientechnica, Bristol, 226–231.

Hall E.J. & Batt R.M. (1988) Challenge studies demonstrate gluten sensitivity of a naturally occurring enteropathy in Irish Setter dogs. *Gastroenterology*, **94**; A167.

Hall E.J., Rutgers H.C. & Batt R.M. (1988) Evaluation of the peroral string test in the diagnosis of canine giardiosis. *Journal of Small Animal Practice*, **29**; 177–183.

Hayden D.W. & Van Kruiningen H.J. (1973) Eosinophilic gastroenteritis in German Shepherd dogs and its relationship to VLM's. *Journal of American Veterinary Medical Association*, **162**; 379–384.

Hayden D.W. & Van Kruiningen H.J. (1982) Lymphocytic-plasmacytic enteritis in German shepherd dogs. *Journal of American Animal Hospital Association*, **18**; 88–96.

Head K.W. & Else R.W. (1981) Neoplasia and other allied conditions of the canine stomach and feline intestine. In: *The Veterinary Annual*. C.S.G. Grunsell, F.W.G. Hill & M.E. Raw (eds), Scientechnica, Bristol, 190–208.

Issacs P.E. & Kim Y.S. (1983) Blind loop syndrome and small bowel bacterial contamination. *Clinical Gastroenterology*, **12**; 395–414.

Jones B.R., Johnstone A.C. & Hancock W.S. (1985) Tyzzers disease in kittens with familial primary hyperlipoproteinaemia. *Journal of Small Animal Practice*, **26**; 411–419.

Kim Y.S. & Erikson R.I.T. (1985) Role of peptidases of the human small intestine in protein digestion. *Gastroenterology*, **88**; 1071–1073.

Lorenz M.D. (1980) Canine malabsorption syndrome. *Compendium of Continuing Education for Practising Veterinarian*, **2**; 885–892.

McDonald P., Edwards R.A. & Greenhalgh J.F.D. (1988) Digestion. In: *Animal Nutrition*, 4th edition. Longman Scientific & Technical, Essex, 130–157.

Moon H.W. (1978) Mechanisms in the pathogenesis of diarrhoea: A review. *Journal of American Veterinary Medical Association*, **172**; 443–448.

Murdoch D.B. (1986) Diarrhoea in the dog and cat. I Acute diarrhoea. *British Veterinary Journal*, **142**; 307–316.

Pidgeon G.L. (1983) Chronic disorders of the exocrine pancreas, small bowel and large bowel. *Veterinary Clinics of North America*, **13**; 541–550.

Prescott J.F. & Monroe D.L. (1983) Campylobacter jejuni enteritis in man and domestic animals. *Journal of American Veterinary Medical Association*, **181**; 1524–1530.

Quigley P.J. & Henry K. (1981) Eosinophilic enteritis in the dog: A case report with a brief review of the literature. *Journal of Comparative Pathology*, **91**; 387–392.

Reife S.P., Goldstein J. & Alpo D.H. (1980) Effects of secreted *Bacteriode* proteases on human intestinal brush border hydrolysis. *Journal of Clinical Investigation*, **66**; 314–322.

Ridley D.G. & Hawgood B.C. (1956) The value of formol-ether concentration of faecal cysts and ova. *Journal of Clinical Pathology*, **9**; 74–76.

Rutgers H.C. (1989) Diarrhoea in the cat. *In Practice*, **11**; 139–148.

Scarlet-Krunz J.M. (1987) Potential and newly recognised pet associated zoonoses. In: *Current Veterinary Therapy IX*. R.W. Kirk (ed.), W.B. Saunders, Philadelphia, 1087–1091.

Simpson J.W. (1982) Bacterial overgrowth causing intestinal malabsorption in a dog. *Veterinary Record*, **110**; 335–336.

Simpson J.W. (1987) Fat absorption in dogs and its diagnostic value in exocrine pancreatic insufficiency and malabsorption. In: *The Veterinary Annual*. C.S.G. Grunsell F.W.G. Hill & M.E. Raw (eds), Scientechnica, Bristol, 319–323.

Simpson J.W. & Burnie A.G. (1988) Campylobacter excretion in canine faeces. *Veterinary Record*, **112**; 46.

Simpson J.W., Burnie A.G., Miles R.S., Scott J.L. & Lindsay D.I. (1988) Prevalence of Giardia and Cryptosporidium infection in dogs in Edinburgh. *Veterinary Record*, **123**; 445–447.

Simpson J.W. & Doxey D.L. (1983) Quantitative assessment of fat absorption and its diagnostic value in exocrine pancreatic insufficiency. *Research in Veterinary Science*, **35**; 249–251.

Suter M.M., Palmer D.G. & Schen K.H. (1985) Primary intestinal lymphangiectasia in three dogs. A morphological and immunological investigation. *Veterinary Pathology*, **22**; 123–130.

Tams T.R. (1987) Chronic canine lymphocytic-plasmacytic enteritis. *Compendium on Continuing Education for the Practicing Veterinarian*, **9**; 1184–1194.

Tams T.R. & Twedt D.L. (1981) Canine protein losing enteropathy syndrome. *Compendium on Continuing Education for the Practicing Veterinarian*, **3**; 105–114.

Tennant B.C. & Hornbuckle W.E. (1980) Gastrointestinal function. In: *Clinical Biochemistry of Domestic Animals*. J.J. Kaneko (ed.), Academic Press, New York, 283–337.

Thorne G.M. & Gorbach S.C. (1978) Enteroxogenic *Escherichia coli*: Detection and importance in diarrhoeal disease of children. *Journal of American Veterinary Medical Association*, **173**; 592–595.

Tobey M., Heizer W., Yek R., Haang T. & Hefner C. (1985) Human intestinal brush border peptidases. *Gastroenterology*, **88**; 913–926.

Tomlinson M.J., McKenzie P.J. & Nordine R.A. (1982) Colonic adenocarcinoma with cutaneous metastasis in a dog. *Journal of American Veterinary Medical Association*, **180**; 1344–1345.

Van Kruiningen H.J. (1976) Clinical efficacy of tylosin in canine inflammatory bowel disease. *Journal of American Animal Hospital Association*, **12**; 498–501.

Van Kruiningen H.J., Ryan M.J. & Shindel N.M. (1983) Classification of feline colitis. *Journal of Comparative Pathology*, **93**; 275–295.

Whitbread T.J., Batt R.M. & Gaithwaite G. (1984) Relative deficiency of IgA in the German Shepherd dog: A breed abnormality. *Research in Veterinary Science*, **37**; 350–352.

Williams D.A. (1987) Campylobacterosis. *Journal of American Veterinary Medical Association*, **193**; 52–53.

Williams D.A. (1988) Chronic small intestinal disease of the dog and cat. In: *Proceedings of a Course in Small Animal Gastroenterology and Nutrition*. New Zealand Veterinary Association, 133–150.

Zimmer J.F. (1983) Clinical management of acute gastroenteritis including virus induced enteritis. In: *Current Veterinary Therapy VIII*. R.W. Kirk (ed.), W.B. Saunders, Philadelphia, 1171–1176.

6/Diseases of the Large Intestine

Anatomy of the large intestine

Macroscopic anatomy

The large intestine consists of the caecum, ascending colon, transverse colon, descending colon, rectum and anus (Fig. 6.1). Such an anatomical division is useful when viewing radiographs or carrying out an endoscopic examination.

The caecum is vestigial and has no recognized function in the dog and cat. The colon of the dog and cat is relatively short (0.2 to 0.6 m) compared

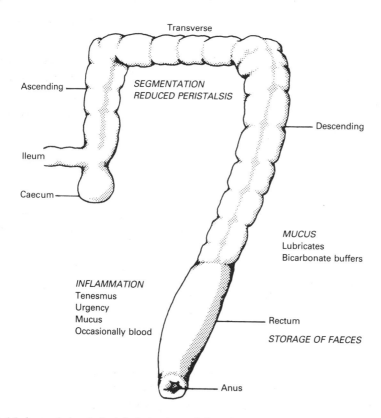

Fig. 6.1 Anatomical and physiological aspects of the colon.

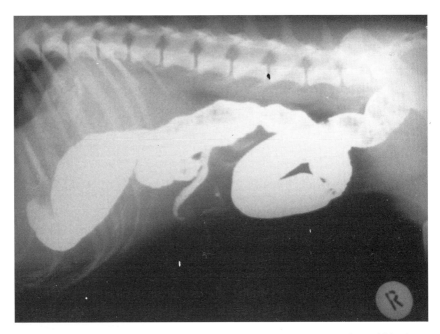

Fig. 6.2 Sigmoid flexure of the descending colon highlighted by liquid barium within the colon.

with herbivores, which reflects a difference in function between the species. The ascending colon is only 2 to 8 cm long and follows a cranial direction from the ileocaecocolic junction on the right side of the abdomen, to the right colonic flexure, just caudal to the stomach. The colon then traverses to the left side of the abdomen, as the transverse colon, as far as the left colonic flexure. The colon is then directed caudally towards the pelvic inlet as the descending colon. This is the longest section of the colon and is continuous with the rectum at the pelvic inlet.

The colon normally assumes the shape of a large question mark although its position can vary considerably in individual cases. It is not uncommon for the normal descending colon to have a 'sigmoid flexure' just cranial to the pelvic inlet, similar to that found in the human colon (Fig. 6.2).

The rectum starts at the level of the pelvic inlet and runs through the pelvic canal to the anus. The anus merges with the perineal skin marking the end of the digestive tract.

Microscopic anatomy

The microscopic structure of the colon is similar throughout its length. Within the outer serosal layer lies a muscular layer, submucosa and inner mucosa. The serosa is a thin sheet of transparent connective tissue which is continuous with the parietal peritoneum. Within the serosa the muscle layer is composed of the outer longitudinal fibres and inner circular muscle fibres. The submucosa comprises connective tissue, blood vessels, lymphoid tissue and nerves. The submucosal blood vessels are normally visible through the thin mucosa on endoscopic examination. The mucosa is lined by a single layer of columnar epithelial cells, which also line the deep invaginations known as the mucosal crypts. Interspersed between the columnar cells are large numbers of goblet cells. The surface of the mucosa is smooth without villi.

Physiology of the large intestine

The colon has three main functions: the absorption of water, absorption of electrolytes and the storage of faeces. Most of the water and electrolytes are absorbed in the ascending and transverse colon, while the storage of faeces occurs in the descending colon and rectum.

Colonic motility is a complex but highly organized process which is essential for the normal functions described above. The remnants of a meal normally reach the colon within 5 h and the transit time in the colon may vary from 1 to 3 days.

There are two types of colonic motility: segmented contractions and peristaltic contractions. Segmented contractions are the result of contraction of the circular muscle fibres and are designed to ensure adequate mixing of the luminal contents with very little propulsion along the colon. This is the primary contraction of the colon and assists in the absorption of water and electrolyte.

Peristalsis moves the luminal contents along the colon towards the rectum. In the dog and cat, retrograde peristalsis also occurs and is used to ensure the contents are not moved too quickly towards the rectum. Retroperistalsis occurs most frequently in the ascending colon where most of the water and electrolyte is absorbed (Burrows & Merritt 1983). Powerful peristaltic waves also occur and move the faecal material from the transverse colon towards the rectum where it is stored. The main stimuli for colonic motor activity are an increase in intraluminal pressure or distension of the colon. Distension stimulates both segmented and peristaltic contractions. This explains why bulking agents in the diet such as fibre assist in treating both diarrhoea and constipation. In diarrhoea they encourage segmented contractions thus improving absorption, and in constipation they promote peristalsis, ensuring the colon is evacuated regularly.

The colon has a resting electrical rhythm called the 'slow wave' activity originating from a pacemaker in the mid-colonic region. When this is stimulated either by hormones such as cholecystokinin or by autonomic neurological stimulation, the slow-wave activity increases resulting in a 'spike potential' and this is associated with muscle contraction.

Coordination of muscle contraction occurs because of the organized slow-wave activity. There are two types of spike potential. The first occurs at the same speed as the slow-wave activity, around 5 cycles/min. The muscle contractions associated with this spike potential are segmented contractions and retroperistalsis. The second type is associated with bursts of spike potentials which last up to 20 min and are associated with mass peristalsis moving faecal material towards the rectum. These latter spike potentials are often called 'migrating' spike potentials and are blocked by the action of atropine and lost in inflammatory disease. Thus in colitis there is usually a decrease in motility, and not hypermotility as is frequently suggested.

There is powerful neurological control of colonic motility via the parasympathetic and sympathetic nervous systems. These systems appear to regulate the myenteric plexus of the colon. The parasympathetic fibres stimulate colonic motility while the sympathetic (adrenergic) fibres inhibit colonic activity. Gastrointestinal hormones also play a part in the control of colonic function. Cholecystokinin and gastrin are thought to act on the colon following ingestion of a meal to stimulate colonic motor activity in addition to their other functions (Snape *et al.* 1978).

Absorption of water by the large intestine is important in maintaining homoeostasis. This is especially true if there is small intestinal diarrhoea, when the colon compensates for absorptive failure in the small intestine. This 'reserve capacity' is important in helping the dog and cat to control water loss from the gastrointestinal tract. Water absorption occurs passively following active salt reabsorption, which is an energy-dependent process requiring glucose. This process creates very large concentration gradients between the lumen and the mucosal cells. The absorption of volatile fatty acids and ammonia contributes further to the concentration gradient.

The tight junctions between the columnar cells are very effective at preventing 'leakage' of salt and water back into the colon. If this barrier is damaged by inflammatory disease or toxic agents then the bowel becomes permeable and watery diarrhoea develops (Rask-Madsen & Jenson 1973). Potassium absorption and secretion is regulated by the colon through carrier-mediated receptors on the mucosal cells. Chloride is also actively absorbed from the colon although there may be some exchange of chloride and bicarbonate. This may be important in maintaining a pH of 6.5 in the colon.

No digestion or absorption of ingested nutrients occurs in the colon. Volatile fatty acids (VFAs) are produced in large amounts in the colon from bacterial fermentation. These VFAs are actively absorbed together with salt. If this process is interrupted VFAs stay in the colonic lumen and create a powerful osmotic force, drawing water into the lumen and thus creating diarrhoea.

The colon contains large numbers of bacteria, the majority of which are anaerobic organisms such as *Bacteroides*, *Lactobacillus*, *Clostridia* and *Streptococcus* spp. These bacteria carry out many actions including conversion of long-chain triglycerides (LCT) to hydroxy fatty acids which are a potent cause of secretory diarrhoea. Castor oil contains the hydroxy fatty acid, ricinoleic acid which also creates a secretory diarrhoea (Binder 1973). Cholic acid is converted to deoxycholic acid and may act to cause a secretory diarrhoea if it reaches the colon.

There is considerable ammonia production by bacteria in the large intestine. This is of little importance in the normal animal as the ammonia is converted to urea in the liver and excreted via the kidney. If there is severe liver disease or portosystemic shunting of blood, the ammonia exerts a powerful effect on the central nervous system known as hepato-encephalopathy.

Bacteria in the colon are also responsible for the conversion of sulpha-salazine to sulphapyridine and 5-aminosalicylate; the latter is a powerful anti-inflammatory agent used in the treatment of colitis. The colonic goblet cells also produce large amounts of mucus which is an important lubricant for easier passage of faeces. It is produced by stimulation of the mucosa by the presence of faeces and by nervous stimulation.

Concepts of colonic disease

Failure to absorb water, electrolytes or store faeces occurs in colonic disease and is usually manifest as diarrhoea or constipation. Up to 50% of chronic diarrhoea cases may be attributed to colitis (Burrows 1980). In the authors' experience colitis is common in dogs but not in cats. There are several symptoms which are particularly associated with disease of the colon namely; diarrhoea, tenesmus, dyschezia, haematochezia, vomiting and constipation.

Diarrhoea occurs in colonic disease following a failure to absorb water and electrolytes. It may also occur where there is a failure in colonic motility particularly segmented contractions. Although the character of the diarrhoea will vary depending on the type and severity of colonic disease, there is usually increased frequency, tenesmus and reduced volume of faeces, which are often soft-to-liquid in nature. Mucus is often present and occasionally fresh blood will be detected if there is ulceration of the colon.

Tenesmus or straining to pass faeces often occurs in colitis especially where the caudal part of the colon or rectum is involved. In severe diarrhoea, residual tenesmus without passage of faecal material is common. Tenesmus is often a feature of constipation where an impaction of the colon occurs with very hard faeces.

Dyschezia or pain on defaecation must be differentiated from tenesmus. Pain on defaecation is most often associated with lesions in the rectum and anus. Conditions such as constipation, anal stricture, neoplasia and inflammatory conditions of the rectum, anal sacs and anus may give rise to pain.

Haematochezia or blood in the faeces is quite common in colonic disease. Blood is usually fresh, lying on the surface of the faecal bolus when the anus or rectum is involved. When the ascending colon is involved the blood may be changed to a dark colour or mixed with the faeces, rendering them almost black depending on the amount of haemosiderin present. The fresher the appearance of the blood the more likely it is to have originated from the caudal part of the large intestine.

Vomiting occurs in approximately 30% of dogs with colonic disease. This is not usually associated with feeding, but may suggest to the clinician that gastroenteritis is present. However gastritis is *not* present in such cases and vomiting occurs for one of two reasons: either because of absorbed toxins affecting the chemoreceptor trigger zone in the medulla or because of stimulation of colonic receptors following inflammation or distention leading to stimulation of the vomiting centre through the vagus nerve (Bush 1985).

Constipation occurs where there is reduced frequency of defaecation or impaction of the colon with hard faeces and failure to pass faeces. Patients often exhibit tenesmus and dyschezia when constipated. There is a direct correlation between the duration of faecal retention in the colon and the development of constipation. Retention of faeces promotes increased resorption of water which in turn leads to drier and harder faeces which are more difficult to pass. Mechanical obstruction from material such as bone fragments may also occur in dogs.

Acute colitis

Introduction

In a clinical context the difference between acute colitis and chronic colitis is, in many respects, only a difference in the duration of time the condition has been present. As with all forms of colitis, the inflammation leads to disruption of colonic function; namely disruption in the absorption of water and electrolytes. In addition there may be reduced colonic segmented contractions.

Acute colitis is relatively common in dogs but is much more unusual in cats. The aetiology is rarely detected although dietary influences may be important. In particular the effects of scavenging and ingestion of abrasive foods such as bone may be important causes. Bacterial infection especially involving *Salmonella* and *Campylobacter* spp. should be considered together with heavy infestations of *Trichuris vulpis*.

Clinical diagnosis

The onset of clinical signs is usually sudden with profuse watery diarrhoea often containing mucus and occasionally blood. Vomiting may be present as may pyrexia and abdominal pain. Dehydration occurs most frequently when vomiting and diarrhoea are both present, and is unusual with diarrhoea alone. Tenesmus and urgency are often reported by the owner as is nocturnal defaecation.

It is important to examine the faeces for evidence of bacterial infection and for parasites. Occasionally and especially when there is pyrexia, a neutrophilia will be observed. Assuming there is no evidence of infection or parasitism, endoscopy usually reveals the mucosa to be inflamed, with a 'granular' appearance and loss of visualization of submucosal blood vessels. Ulceration may be observed.

Histopathological examination of affected gut reveals varying levels of acute mucosal and submucosal inflammation characterized in the early stages by oedema and polymorphonucleocyte infiltration. Increasing numbers of plasma cells and lymphocytes occur in more advanced or longer standing cases. Goblet cell hyperplasia may also occur (Fig. 6.3).

Treatment

Treatment should be based on eliminating the underlying cause if this can be found. Where evidence of endoparasites such as *Trichuris* spp. is detected the patient should receive 5 days' treatment with fenbendazole (Panacur; Hoechst Animal Health) at a dose rate of 20 mg/kg/day. Where *Salmonella* spp. are detected and the patient is pyrexic, then antibiotic sensitivity should be obtained and a suitable antibiotic administered systemically. *Campylobacter* spp. may often be isolated from cases of acute colitis but this is usually an opportunist organism, which should still be eliminated using either erythromycin at 40 mg/kg/day or tylosin 40 mg/kg/day for 5 days (Murdoch 1986).

Correction of fluid balance must be considered in the initial stages of treatment if there is any evidence of dehydration. Otherwise with the idiopathic form, treatment should involve the use of sulphasalazine (Salazopyrin; Pharmacia) at 20 to 40 mg/kg/day in divided doses (Bush 1985). This drug is only activated in the colon by action of bacteria pro-

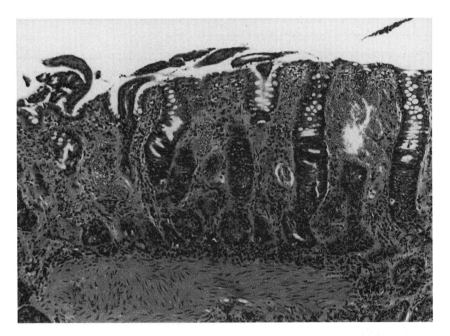

Fig. 6.3 Inflammatory changes observed on histological examination of a dog with acute colitis.

ducing sulphapyridine and 5-aminosalicylic acid. The latter component is considered to be responsible for the improvement in colitis.

Idiopathic colitis

Introduction

This form of colitis is now considered to be one of the commonest causes of chronic diarrhoea in the dog (Bush 1985) and appears to be much less common in the cat (Rutgers 1989). However, there is a report of six cases of lymphocytic–plasmacytic colitis in cats (Nelson *et al.* 1984). It may be better described as a syndrome rather than a specific condition as there are many possible aetiological agents which may be responsible for the changes in the colon. Idiopathic colitis appears to affect any breed of dog and cat with no age or sex predisposition. However, cases appear to be more common in German Shepherd dogs, Rough Collies and Labradors.

Unfortunately it is still unusual to determine the cause in the majority of cases of idiopathic colitis, hence the term, but occasionally a specific diagnosis is obtained. In this respect mycotic colitis has been recorded in cats due to *Aspergillus* spp. (Bolton & Brown 1972).

The authors consider that dietary factors may be very important in the aetiology of colitis, because of the response noted to dietary management without drug therapy. Other aetiological agents include *Trichuris vulpis* infection, *Salmonella* spp. and *Campylobacter* spp. Idiopathic colitis may also develop as a sequel to gastroenteritis, secondary to small intestinal disease (especially where bile or fat enters the colon), secondary to systemic toxaemia (e.g. uraemia) or as a component of an immune-mediated disease. Parasitic colitis, histiocytic colitis and granulomatous colitis (which are discussed later in this chapter) may in fact be more specific manifestations or more advanced forms of idiopathic colitis. Further study is required in this area to determine the true aetiology of the majority of idiopathic colitis cases.

Clinical diagnosis

Usually patients with idiopathic colitis are bright and show few signs of ill health. Appetite is often good, and there is little evidence of weight-loss in the early stages. Vomiting is observed in 30% of cases; as explained earlier, there is no primary gastric involvement causing the vomiting.

The owner will often report a profuse watery diarrhoea which contains mucus. Blood is seen in less than 20% of cases, as ulceration is not a feature of this condition (Nelson *et al.* 1984). Tenesmus and urgency are variable and dependent on inflammation involving the distal colon and rectum. Usually the faeces are passed in small but frequent amounts. Patients often posture on several occasions but pass only small amounts of faeces. There is rarely evidence of abdominal pain, dyschezia, or dehydration.

Investigation should start by examination of a faecal sample for evidence of infection or endoparasites. Radiographs including barium studies are often unrewarding unless there are gross changes affecting the mucosa. A definitive diagnosis requires endoscopy and biopsy of the colon.

Endoscopy of the colon requires careful preparation or the technique will be unrewarding (Table 6.1). The patient should be starved overnight and receive a warm water enema first thing in the morning. Following successful evacuation of faeces this should be repeated within an hour. The clinician should be aware of the fact that enemas may induce hyperaemia of the colonic mucosa. General anaesthesia is not required for this procedure, and a combination of acepromazine (ACP; C-Vet) at 0.05 mg/kg and buprenorphine (Temgesic; Reckitt & Colman) at 0.01 mg/kg, both given intramuscularly, provides adequate sedation and analgesia. The patient should be laid in left lateral recumbency, and the tip of the endoscope lubricated prior to insertion through the anus. Little resentment occurs once this has been achieved and careful examination of the colon can normally proceed without difficulty.

In idiopathic colitis, macroscopic findings on endoscopy may include

Table 6.1 Preparation of the patient for colonoscopy

1 Fast the patient for 12 h
2 Administer a warm water enema
3 Repeat enema after initial evacuation of bowel
4 Administer a suitable sedative
5 Place patient in left lateral recumbency
6 Carry out endoscopic examination

loss of visualization of submucosal blood vessels and thickening of the mucosa which may assume a granular appearance. It is only rarely that signs of ulceration are observed but it is much more common for the mucosa to be friable and bleed easily on passage of the endoscope. The colon may be difficult to dilate and persistent muscle contraction may be observed as the endoscope is passed up the colon.

Multiple biopsy samples should ideally be collected from the rectum, descending, transverse and ascending colon both from apparently normal and obviously diseased sites. Although it is very likely that change in the colon will be diffuse in the majority of cases, focal lesions do occur and would be missed without thorough visual examination and multiple biopsy collection. It is important to emphasize that biopsy samples should be collected even if the mucosa appears normal.

Histopathology will reveal numerous goblet cells, with infiltration of the

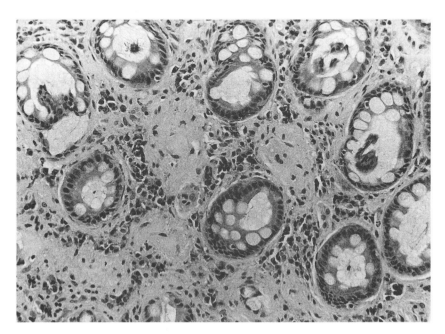

Fig. 6.4 Histological changes in idiopathic colitis.

lamina propria with inflammatory cells such as polymorphonucleocytes, lymphocytes and plasma cells (Fig. 6.4). Fibrosis will be observed to a variable degree especially where the condition is advanced or has been present for some weeks.

Treatment

The drug of choice in the treatment of idiopathic colitis is sulphasalazine (Salazopyrin; Pharmacia) at 20 to 40 mg/kg in divided doses. Treatment is often required for at least one month and relapse is relatively common unless the underlying cause is found and removed. The main side effect in dogs is keratoconjunctivitis sicca or dry eye, but this is not common. This condition appears to be due to the sulphapyridine component of sulphasalazine although there is reference to 5-aminosalicylic acid causing dry eye (Barnett & Joseph 1987). A new drug has become available which contains no sulphapyridine, so reducing the risk of side effects. The drug called mesalazine (Asacol; Pharmacia) may be given at 10 to 20 mg/kg. In cats side effects include anorexia and anaemia, and they must be observed for signs of salicylate toxicity. The oral dose of sulphasalazine used in cats should be 25 mg/kg/day (Rutgers 1989).

In a few cases withdrawal of the drug immediately results in relapse, and in such cases the patient may need to be maintained on a low maintenance dose.

Occasionally dogs will not respond to sulphasalazine alone and prednisolone should therefore be included at 1 mg/kg/day. The authors have observed cases which have not responded to either of these regimes, but have responded to metronidazole (Flagyl; RMB Animal Health) given orally at 30 mg/kg/day for dogs and 15 mg/kg/day for cats (Chiapella 1986). In addition to being an antibacterial drug, it also suppresses cell-mediated immunity. It is the latter function which appears to be beneficial in idiopathic colitis.

Dietary management in idiopathic colitis may be of great importance, with various reports suggesting success in treatment of the condition using diet alone. Some 30% of cases appear to respond well to restricted protein diets such as Hills d/d or Waltham selected protein diet. Cats appear to have responded well to lamb, horsemeat and boiled rice or Hills c/d diet (Nelson *et al.* 1984). Dry cereal-based diets should be avoided as they exacerbate the signs of colitis (Burrows 1988). However the inclusion of bran to selected protein diets may help to restore normal colonic motility. Until more is known about the importance of diet in idiopathic colitis it is advisable to use one of the above regimes as it may significantly reduce the risk of relapse. In all cases the diet should be fed in at least two meals per day.

Prognosis for this condition should always be guarded as the risk of relapse is quite high, about 30% of cases requiring further treatment. This requirement basically reflects our poor knowledge of the true aetiology in many cases. If dietary factors prove to be important in the aetiology of idiopathic colitis, then the prognosis may be greatly improved in the future, by formulation of exclusion diets.

Parasitic colitis

Introduction

Both hookworms and whipworms may cause colitis, but they are much less common in the UK than they are in the USA (Bush 1985). The clinical picture is similar to that presented in idiopathic colitis with the following exceptions.

Where whipworms (*Trichuris vulpis*) are involved there is usually increased mucus production as a result of marked goblet cell hyperplasia with blood rarely present in the watery diarrhoea. Where hookworms are involved, the diarrhoea is usually mucoid and contains blood and there is marked weight-loss.

In both cases faecal worm egg counts should be carried out, but eggs are not always detected as adults release eggs intermittently. A high circulating eosinophil count may be present in some cases. Endoscopy and biopsy of the colon will assist in making a diagnosis.

Treatment

For both whipworms and hookworms a broad spectrum anthelmintic such as fenbendazole (Panacur; Hoechst Animal Health) should be given orally for 5 days using 20 mg/kg/day. Where there is marked inflammatory reaction, this should be supplemented by a course of sulphasalazine tablets at the dose rate already described.

Histiocytic colitis

Introduction

This is a rare condition which has only been recorded in Boxers (Kennedy & Cello 1966) and French Bulldogs (Van der Gaag *et al.* 1978), and is particularly common in young female dogs. It has also been reported in cats (Van Kruiningen & Dobbin 1979). The aetiology is not known but appears to be familial and differs from idiopathic colitis by the presence of histiocytes and mucosal ulceration. Various other aetiologies have been suggested including deficiency of lysosomal enzymes, failure of macrophages to degrade ingested foreign material, and the presence of chlamydial organisms within macrophages (Van Kruiningen 1975).

Clinical diagnosis

The history and clinical signs are similar to those described for idiopathic colitis, except that the diarrhoea often contains fresh blood as well as mucus. The dogs may have a variable appetite and some evidence of weight-loss (Ewing & Gomez 1973). There is rarely evidence of dehydration, pyrexia or abdominal pain (Kennedy & Cello 1966).

Diagnosis is based on the typical history and clinical picture together with clinical chemistry and endoscopy. A leucocytosis and hypoalbumin-aemia and hypergammaglobulinaemia may be detected. Endoscopy of the colon will reveal thickening of the mucosa, loss of visualization of submucosal blood vessels, ulceration and excess mucus production (Ewing & Gomez 1973). Confirmation of the diagnosis is obtained from histological examination of biopsy samples which reveal heavy mucosal infiltrations of PAS-positive histiocytes in addition to other inflammatory cells such as plasma cells and lymphocytes (Fig. 6.5).

Treatment

Most cases respond to treatment using sulphasalazine (Salazopyrin; Pharmacia) at 20 to 40 mg/kg/day in divided doses and tylosin (Tylan; Elanco Products) 20 mg/kg bid orally for 3 to 4 weeks. The successful treatment of a feline case of histiocytic colitis has been reported (Van Kruiningen & Dobbin 1979). In this case tylosin followed by tetracycline and chloramphenicol was used orally for 7 months, after which intestinal function returned to normal. Unfortunately relapses are common once treatment has stopped. In these cases treatment may be required for life, either as low doses of the above drugs or therapy which is used intermittently when relapse is observed.

Granulomatous colitis

Introduction

Granulomatous colitis is also known as regional enteritis or Crohns' disease; it affects both the ileum and large intestine (Ewing & Gomez 1973). The aetiology is unknown and may present as either a focal or diffuse lesion. It may simply reflect an advanced form of idiopathic colitis and has some of the features seen in histiocytic colitis of Boxers.

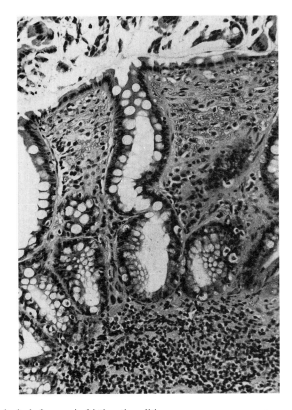

Fig. 6.5 Histological changes in histiocytic colitis.

Clinical diagnosis

Where the colon is involved the patient is usually presented with a history of fluid faeces, often containing fresh blood and occasionally mucus. Pyrexia and partial anorexia are observed, although dehydration is rare. Bloody diarrhoea, vomiting and weight-loss were reported in one feline case (Van Kruiningen *et al.* 1983).

In severe cases especially those involving the distal colon and rectum, inflammatory changes lead to healing by fibrosis which in turn leads to fibrous tissue scarring and stricture formation. In these cases constipation, tenesmus, dyschezia and haematochezia may be observed.

Where the diffuse form of the condition is present, then the amount of blood present in the colon may be extensive, and the dog may lose weight and become hypoproteinaemic due to a true protein-losing enteropathy (Bush 1985). Leucocytosis and mild anaemia may be detected. Endoscopy is the most effective method of obtaining a diagnosis. The mucosa is thickened and ulcerated with fissures which bleed readily. These lesions may be diffuse throughout the colon or isolated to one small focal region. Thus the entire colon must be examined before this condition can be excluded.

Biopsy of affected gut will reveal surface ulceration with large numbers of lymphocytes and plasma cells, macrophages or giant cells, involving all the layers of the colon. The submucosa may be thickened by early granulation tissue with large numbers of macrophages and granulomas. Lymphoid hyperplasia and thickening of the muscle layer has also been described (Van Kruiningen *et al.* 1983).

Treatment

If the lesion is focal and accessible then surgical resection of the affected bowel is the most effective method of treatment. When the lesion is diffuse, the treatment usually involves the use of sulphasalazine and prednisolone together with tylosin at the dosages already described.

The prognosis in all cases is poor as relapses are common even in those cases where surgical resection has been carried out. Until the underlying cause can be determined it is unlikely that the prognosis will improve.

Eosinophilic colitis

Introduction

Eosinophilic colitis is part of a complex which may affect the stomach, small intestine or large intestine of both dogs and cats (Theran 1968, Moore 1983). The condition may present as an acute or chronic form and may involve all or part of the gastrointestinal tract. The cause is not known but parasitic or allergic reactions are considered likely (Rutgers 1989). Unfortunately this must be considered as an oversimplification as many cases do not respond to hypoallergen diets or anthelminthics. Until more precise information is obtained, it would be better to consider this to be an immune-mediated colitis. In cats a more severe form may occur in which there is eosinophilic infiltration involving the spleen, liver, kidneys and heart, as well as the gastrointestinal tract (Moore 1983).

Clinical diagnosis

Dogs or cats will present in a similar manner to those with idiopathic colitis, except that haematochezia is often present together with a high circulating eosinophil count (eosinophilia: more than $1500/mm^3$). Dyschezia, tenesmus and urgency have also been reported, especially where the distal colon is involved.

Diagnosis is based on the clinical picture dominated by persistently high circulating eosinophil count, and confirmed following endoscopy of the colon and collection of biopsy samples.

Macroscopically the colon will have slightly thickened mucosa with evidence of ulceration or will bleed easily when touched with the endoscope. Biopsy samples will reveal very large numbers of eosinophils within the mucosa and underlying tissues.

Treatment

Eosinophilic colitis should initially be treated by worming the dog or cat with fenbendazole (Panacur; Hoechst Animal Health) at 20 mg/kg orally for 5 days. In addition the patient should be placed on a selected protein diet such as Hills d/d diet or Waltham selected protein diet. These two procedures will occasionally eliminate the possible aetiological agent.

It is usual to supplement the above treatment with a course of oral prednisolone at 1 to 2 mg/kg/day (Sherding 1980, Moore 1983) together with tylosin (Tylan; Elanco Products) at 20 mg/kg bid (Rutgers 1989). This therapy should be maintained for 1 month, at which time the prednisolone should be withdrawn slowly and the tylosin stopped. The prognosis is generally good and relapses are less likely than with other cases of chronic colitis. In cats the situation is somewhat different, as both forms carry a much more guarded prognosis (Moore 1983, Rutgers 1989).

Irritable bowel syndrome

Introduction

There appear to be a significant number of dogs, but not cats, which exhibit signs similar to idiopathic colitis, but following investigation show no evidence of inflammation (Bush 1985). There are no inflammatory changes detected on biopsy nor any abnormality on blood chemistry or faecal analysis. These dogs have non-inflammatory intestinal disease which is thought to be physiological rather than pathological in origin, and involves altered motility of the intestinal tract. Stress appears to be an important factor in the manifestation of clinical signs.

In the authors' experience this condition is primarily seen in the larger breeds of dogs; it is associated with working dogs under training and dogs which are excitable or nervous. It appears to be associated with the individual's relationship to its environment rather than the situation being particularly stressful. The problem does occur in the non-working dog where there is some other form of environmental stress. Examples of these stress factors include death of the owner, changes of environment, a new baby or a new dog in the household. The diagnosis of irritable bowel syndrome (IBS) must be used with caution, as there is no definitive diagnostic test to confirm its presence and there is a real danger of overdiagnosis based on clinical features alone because these clinical signs are similar to other forms of colitis. It is therefore very important to diagnose this condition through a process of exclusion.

Clinical diagnosis

Dogs are presented with intermittent but acute episodes of diarrhoea which is usually watery and mucoid in nature. The history will reveal poor response to treatment using drugs for colitis. Borborygmi, flatus, abdominal pain and tenesmus may be observed. Haematochezia and weight-loss are not features of the condition and if present should suggest an alternative diagnosis.

Diagnosis can only be made by ruling out all other pathological causes of colonic disease. It is therefore essential to carry out the usual tests to rule out other causes of colonic disease, including faecal analysis, blood chemistry, endoscopy and biopsy of the colon.

On endoscopy it may be difficult to dilate the colon which is often coated with thick tenacious mucus but otherwise shows no signs of abnormality. Multiple biopsy collection and examination must be carried out to confirm the absence of pathological changes.

Treatment

There are several drugs which may be of value in this condition. The choice of drug depends on the individual case, giving consideration to the following: (1) the dog's character, (2) the ability to remove the stress factor; and (3) the degree to which clinical signs such as diarrhoea are present.

Where the dog's temperament is very excitable or nervous the use of acetylpromazine (ACP; C-Vet) at 0.05 mg/kg orally will provide some control of the behaviour, without inducing sedation. This has proved of great value in these selected cases and does not have to be given for a protracted period of time, as young excitable dogs often grow out of the condition.

Where the stress factor can be removed this should be the method of choice in all cases. Training is one such situation which has been identified where diarrhoea can be stopped or induced based on the amount of training being carried out. Household stress factors are often difficult to identify and harder to remove. In such cases, diphenoxylate (Lomotil; Gold Cross Pharmaceuticals) at 0.05 to 0.1 mg/kg bid or loperamide (Imodium; Janssen Pharmaceutical) at 0.05 to 0.1 mg/kg, as motility modifiers have proved very useful (Chiapella 1986). These drugs are thought to restore normal segmented contractions and so improve colonic function.

Dietary fibre has also been valuable in the treatment of this condition. By increasing the dietary fibre the faecal bulk is increased and the dogs colonic motility patterns are improved. Fibre (Nutrifyba; Sanofi Pharma) is given at ½ to 2 teaspoonfuls/day in food depending on body size.

The prognosis must be guarded in all cases as they are susceptible to relapses throughout their lives. Even if one stress factor is removed another may take its place. Thus it is usual for a dog to require treatment intermittently throughout its life.

Constipation

Introduction

Constipation may be defined as infrequent, or the absence of, defaecation, with passage of very hard faeces, tenesmus and reduced faecal volume (Burrows 1986). It is quite common in dogs and cats and must be differentiated from a state of megacolon for which it may be mistaken. Animals with megacolon are constipated but animals with constipation may not have megacolon.

Constipation will occur in any condition which prevents the passage of faeces through the rectum and anus. The list of possible aetiologies is very large and includes diseases of the colon, rectum and anus together with secondary causes such as orthopaedic or prostatic disease (Table 6.2). In all cases the main feature is retention of faeces which leads to further water absorption, making the faeces drier and harder, and so more difficult to pass. In constipation, peristalsis is initially increased, but rapidly becomes reduced as the colon becomes hypomotile. Degeneration of nerves may occur and megacolon may develop (Burrows 1986).

Clinical diagnosis

Animals are usually presented with a history of failing to pass faeces for several days with associated tenesmus, anorexia and even intermittent vomiting. Vomiting occurs due to vagal stimulation of the vomiting centre through colonic distention. Dehydration may occur in advanced cases and this is associated with depression and lethargy. Palpation of the abdomen will reveal a large descending colon full of faeces. More detailed physical examination should be carried out in order to determine the underlying cause. In particular signs of excessive coat casting, ectoparasites, prostatic disease and orthopaedic problems should be considered. Rectal examination is an extremely important part of the physical examination. It helps in establishing the presence of faeces in the rectum, stricture formation, perineal hernia, anal gland disease or pelvic narrowing. The anal tissues may be swollen and oedematous and partial rectal prolapse may be seen in advanced cases where tenesmus has been a feature.

Diagnosis is based on the above examination and from radiographs of the abdomen which will reveal the presence of a large faecal mass in the colon.

Treatment

It is essential that the underlying cause is corrected if the animal is to respond to treatment and not suffer frequent relapses. The immediate constipation should be treated using enemas. Enemas may be proprietary or warm water, soapy, saline or liquid paraffin and should be given at body temperature to prevent shock. The aim should be to soften the faecal mass and promote colonic motility, but in many cases the faecal mass may be so hard that manual break down and removal is required. This is painful and should be carried out under general anaesthesia (Burrows 1986). If dehydration is present this should be corrected using intravenous fluid therapy prior to administration of the anaesthetic.

Once the underlying cause has been corrected and the constipation cleared it is important to initiate preventive measures. Dogs should not receive any bones in the future. Cats should be restricted from hunting or treated regularly with liquid paraffin at 5 to 25 ml bid orally to stop fur and hair accumulation. Ectoparasitism should be kept under control and regular grooming carried out. Bulk-forming agents (e.g. Peridale granules and capsules; Arnolds Veterinary Products) may be used to assist the formation of soft, easily-passed faeces and to promote peristalsis. Fibre (Nutrifyba, Sanofi Pharma) may be added to the diet at ½ to 2 teaspoonfuls/day in food, especially where the food is of low residue.

Table 6.2 Aetiological agents of constipation

Impaction of colon with bone, hair or fur
Low residue diets
Pseudocoprostasis
Pelvic injury and narrowing
Perineal hernia
Anal or rectal tumours
Prostatic disease
Orthopaedic conditions — failure to posture
Rectal stricture
Anal gland disease
Rectal foreign body
Megacolon
Feline dysautonomia

Pseudocoprostasis

Introduction

Pseudocoprostasis occurs in both dogs and cats particularly those which have long hair around the perineal region. If the dog or cat has diarrhoea or is infrequently groomed, faecal soiling builds up eventually creating a faecal mass so great that it interferes with defaecation and physically blocks the anal opening. Once the anus is blocked defaecation becomes impossible and constipation develops.

Clinical diagnosis

The patient may be presented with a history of diarrhoea followed by difficulty or inability to pass faeces. Tenesmus and frequent attention to the perineal region may also be reported. Examination of the perineal region will reveal a large faecal mass over the anus. In the summer months it is not uncommon for such animals to be affected by 'strike' with large numbers of maggots in the skin around and under the faecal mass.

Treatment

Treatment involves the removal of the faecal mass which is often painful and may have to be carried out under sedation or general anaesthesia. Careful removal of the faecal mass is achieved by clipping away the hair between the skin and the faecal mass, which is slowly folded back to reveal the perineal tissue. The skin under the mass is often very inflamed and secondarily infected. In addition maggots lying next to the skin and burrowing into the skin may be found and these should be carefully removed. As the anus is uncovered it is not unusual for the faeces retained in the rectum to be forcibly expelled due to colonic contraction thus relieving the constipation.

Once the mass has been removed all the hair in the perineal region should be clipped back. The animal should be given an Elizabethan collar to prevent self-damage, and antibiotics given parenterally.

Table 6.3 Aetiology of megacolon

Congenital	Degeneration of myenteric plexus
Acquired	Retention of faeces leading to colonic atony
	Neoplasia of rectum or anus
	Pseudocoprostasis
	Perineal hernia
	Feline dysautonomia

It is not uncommon for the condition to recur if steps are not taken to advise the owner how to prevent similar problems. The hair around the perineum must be kept short and the dog regularly groomed. Treatment for diarrhoea must be carried out. Owners should routinely examine the perineum to observe early stages of faecal build-up and remove any accumulated faeces to prevent pseudocoprostasis.

Megacolon

Introduction

Although the aetiology of megacolon is not known, the condition may be divided into congenital cases where there is aplasia of the ganglia in the myenteric plexus of the colon, and acquired cases where the condition is secondary to an underlying cause or is truely idiopathic (Webb 1985, Bright *et al.* 1986) (Table 6.3). Megacolon is not the same as constipation, the former condition occurring because of loss of motor function and resultant inability to expel faeces. No evidence has been found to suggest that failure of relaxation of the anal sphincter is the primary problem in megacolon. It appears that prolonged retention of faeces which occurs in constipation may lead to degeneration of colonic nerves in acquired megacolon (Burrows 1986). In cats, megacolon may be associated with the Key–Gaskell syndrome which is now rare in the UK. In this condition there is urinary retention, megaoesophagus, dry mucous membranes and dilatation of the pupils in addition to megacolon (Sharp *et al.* 1984).

Clinical diagnosis

The history and physical examination of animals with megacolon are similar to those of animals with constipation. Anorexia, depression, intermittent vomiting, failure to pass faeces and sometimes tenesmus are observed. In some cases the animal may be presented because of faecal incontinence which appears to be an 'overflow' problem. A history of recurrent episodes of so-called constipation may be reported with failure to respond to treatment. Abdominal palpation often reveals a large firm mass which may be recognized as the colon. The rectum is often found to be empty on examination (cf. constipation).

Diagnosis is based on the clinical examination and the radiographic features revealing a grossly enlarged colon. The colon may be so grossly distended with faeces, that it appears to take up most of the abdomen (Fig. 6.6). Urinary retention and megaoesophagus should be eliminated in affected cats.

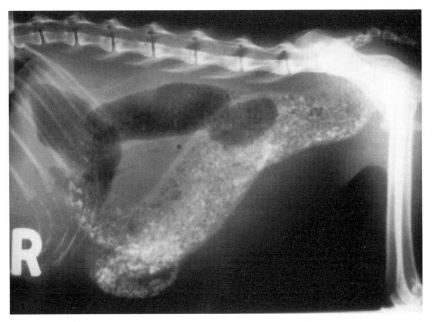

Fig. 6.6 Plain lateral radiograph of a megacolon.

Treatment

The prognosis in megacolon must be very guarded as it is rarely possible to restore colonic motor function in congenital or long-standing acquired cases. The colon may be emptied in a similar manner to that described for constipation. Thereafter steps should be taken to prevent the colon retaining faeces. Peridale granules (Arnolds Veterinary Products) may assist, as may prophylactic use of high fibre diets or liquid paraffin. However, in most cases medical treatment fails and surgical removal of the colon should be considered (Webb 1985). Normally this procedure involves removal of the bowel segment from the proximal ascending colon to the pelvic inlet. The remaining portion of ascending colon is anastomosed to the rectum (Bright *et al.* 1986). If the rectum is left intact then the animal may retain continence and be able to live a reasonably normal life, although diarrhoea may persist in some cases (Burrows 1988).

Colonic tumours

Introduction

The most common tumours of the colon in the dog and cat are polyps, adenocarcinomas and lymphosarcomas, although other types do occur (Head & Else 1981, Crow 1985). Factors which are thought to predispose to colonic and rectal neoplasia include low fibre diets, slow colonic transit times, high levels of bile and fat in the colon, and the presence of long-standing severe colitis (Crow 1985).

Polyps are usually benign and occur most frequently in the distal colon or rectum. They tend to be space-occupying causing local obstruction to the passage of faeces. Occasionally they are associated with subsequent development of adenocarcinomas.

Lymphosarcoma usually occurs as a diffuse tumour of the colon although focal lesions do occur. They rarely cause obstruction, but thickening of the colonic wall results in interference with motility and absorption.

Adenocarcinomas often appear as focal lesions which tend to be proliferative and lead to obstruction of the colon. Ulceration is common as is secondary infection. The consequence of infection and inflammation is fibrous tissue formation and ultimately stricture formation. The commonest site for adenocarcinoma is said to be the distal colon and rectum, with metastasis to the sublumbar lymph nodes (Crow 1985).

Clinical diagnosis

Clinical signs accompanying development of intestinal tumours are often vague, insidious and slowly progressing, although in a few cases sudden clinical onset is described (Head & Else 1981). Patients may have a history of diarrhoea or constipation depending on the type of tumour present, the stage of development, and location — whether diffuse, focal or obstructive. Adenocarcinomas are usually space-occupying so present with tenesmus, dyschezia, haematochezia and possibly diarrhoea. Lymphosarcomas are generally diffuse and involve the majority of the colon and cause chronic diarrhoea which rarely contains blood. Polyps are generally space-occupying, obstructive and result in tenesmus, passage of ribbon-like faeces, occasionally with haematochezia, especially when they ulcerate. Occasionally they cause apparent constipation and dyschezia.

With advanced colonic neoplasia, weight-loss and vomiting may occur together with the symptoms indicated above. Such changes may be due to' the advanced colonic disease or to metastasis affecting the function of other tissues. Stricture formation may also occur where inflammation is severe and attempts at healing induce fibrosis.

Diagnosis is achieved by radiographic examination of the colon using barium or double contrast studies which may reveal the classic 'apple core' filling defect seen with adenocarcinomas (Fig. 6.7), or a diffuse abnormality of the colonic mucosa as seen with lymphosarcoma (Fig. 6.8). Where tumours have metastasized the sublumbar lymph nodes may be enlarged (Crow 1985). Unfortunately radiographs will not detect all colonic neoplasms and even when they do detect abnormalities, endoscopic examination with biopsy sampling is essential to confirm the diagnosis and offer a prognosis.

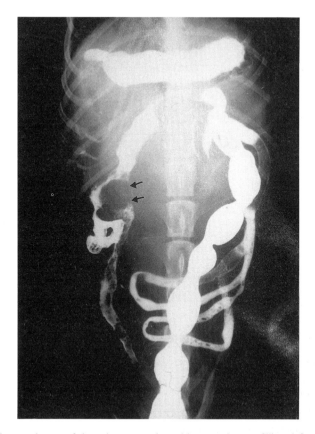

Fig. 6.7 Adenocarcinoma of the colon presenting with an apple core filling defect (arrowed).

Endoscopy reveals ulceration, general thickening of the mucosa, or space-occupying lesions. Multiple biopsy samples including apparently normal and abnormal tissues should be taken. This ensures a representative assessment of the colon and any tumour present and allows a decision to be made regarding the most effective method of treatment.

Treatment

Where adenocarcinoma is diagnosed in the early stages it may be successfully removed by resection of the affected part of the colon. However, if the rectal tissues are involved, this becomes a difficult proposition and attempts at resection may lead to faecal incontinence. Where the adenocarcinoma is well-established and metastasis has occurred to the sublumbar lymph nodes and other tissues, the prognosis is very guarded and chemotherapy in addition to surgery should be instituted.

Polyps are usually operable and even when they occur in the rectum

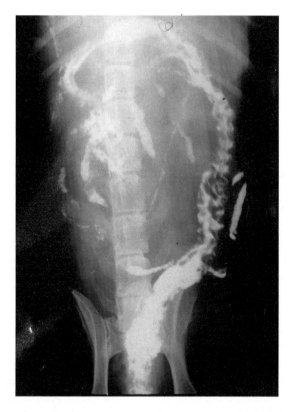

Fig. 6.8 Barium column showing gross mucosal changes in a case of colonic lymphosarcoma.

they may be removed using proctoscopy and diathermy. It is important to submit the polyp for histopathological analysis as some may prove to be early carcinomas.

Lymphosarcoma is rarely responsive to therapy especially as it tends to be diffuse and involve the majority of the colon. Cats with lymphosarcoma should be checked for evidence of feline leukaemia virus (FeLV) a positive result indicates a very grave prognosis.

Rectal stricture

Introduction

Stricture formation is most often detected in the rectum or anus of the dog but is uncommon in cats in our experience. The aetiology is rarely determined although trauma, previous surgery and neoplasia may be possible factors involved in their development (Seim 1986). Some may be truly idiopathic or congenital aplasias. In any event there is physical damage to the colon resulting in healing by fibrosis which causes difficulty in the passage of faeces. Further tenesmus and passage of faeces breaks down the fibrous tissue leading to exacerbated inflammatory reaction and further fibrous tissue production. This vicious cycle continues until the dog has marked scarring and stricture resulting in dyschezia.

Clinical diagnosis

Dogs are usually presented with a history of dyschezia and tenesmus and the faeces passed are often small in diameter or ribbon-like in character. Fresh blood is often observed on the surface of the faeces. Rectal examination is a very important part of the physical examination and may be resented but confirms a severe restriction to the diameter of the rectum or anus by a narrow band of fibrous tissue. Once the presence of a stricture has been confirmed an attempt should be made to determine the cause of the problem. This is particularly important if a tumour is present.

Treatment

Correction of the underlying cause should be attempted wherever possible. In most cases this is not found and manual dilation of the stricture is carried out under general anaesthesia. Postoperatively, bulking agents such as Peridale granules (Arnolds Veterinary Products) are used to assist in the passage of soft faeces. Anti-inflammatory drugs such as prednisolone at 1 mg/kg/day may be used to assist in reducing the inflammation and the development of fibrosis. The prognosis must be very guarded as stricture formation recurs in 1 to 2 months in most cases. Surgical resection of the stricture can be attempted but is difficult to carry out and often results in faecal incontinence which is rarely acceptable to the client (Seim 1986).

Rectal prolapse

This is a very rare condition in the dog and cat which is usually associated with persistent tenesmus due to some other cause, so it is not a definitive diagnosis (Seim 1986). It may occur in kittens with diarrhoea, but usually resolves once the diarrhoea is brought under control. Tumours, colitis, parasitism, prostatic disease, perineal herniation and constipation may all be implicated in the generation of rectal prolapse.

Clinical diagnosis

Diagnosis is not difficult to establish but care is needed to differentiate the prolapse from an intussusception (Seim 1986). This can be determined by gentle digital examination of the tissues. A gloved finger inserted between the anal wall and the prolapse will fail to pass any distance into the rectum where a prolapse is present but will pass a long distance into the rectum if an intussusception is present.

Treatment

Treatment really depends on the underlying cause of the problem. This must be corrected if the rectal prolapse is not to recur. Reduction of the prolapse and application of a purse string suture may be used to prevent immediate recurrence while the underlying cause is corrected. Such a suture should be removed after 3 days (Seim 1986). Where the tissues are badly traumatized or where reduction has failed to resolve the problem, resection may be required. The prognosis in general with this condition is poor as prolapse often recurs or because there is a more serious underlying cause, such as adenocarcinoma of the rectum.

Anal sac disease

Introduction

Disease of the anal sacs is very common in dogs and appears to have no age predisposition. The condition may be more common in the small breeds such as Poodles, West Highland White Terriers and Pekinese, rather than the larger breeds of dog. The incidence of anal sac disease is lower in cats and is usually due to impaction although secondary infection and abscessation may also occur. The aetiology is unknown in the majority of cases, although there are several predisposing factors such as low residue diets, changes in viscosity of anal sac secretion and diarrhoea.

Clinical diagnosis

The symptoms vary from dog to dog and with the severity of the problem. There is usually a history of licking and biting at the tail, rubbing the bottom along the ground, tail chasing and even behavioural changes such as suddenly jumping and biting at the hind quarters or flanks. In severe cases pyrexia, anorexia and depression may be observed. Occasionally the dogs lick excessively at the hind quarters producing an acute moist dermatitis.

Physical examination will reveal swollen sacs and rectal examination and attempted expression of the sacs will cause some degree of discomfort. The discharge is usually thick dark brown and foul smelling in impacted sacs and bloody, purulent material where abscessation is present. In the latter case the abscesses are particularly painful and often point to the perineal skin.

Treatment

With impacted anal sacs, expression is usually adequate for relieving the symptoms. The diet should be checked and corrected where necessary, perhaps by the inclusion of bulking agents such as Peridale granules (Arnolds Veterinary Products) or dietary fibre (Nutrifyba; Sanofi Pharma).

Where the sacs are infected, expression under sedation or general anaesthesia may be required. Once the sacs have been thoroughly emptied they should be flushed out with dilute antiseptic solution and finally filled with an antibiotic preparation. The authors prefer to use quick release intramammary preparations for this purpose, infused along the anal sac duct. Where the sacs have pointed to the exterior and discharged, the sites should be thoroughly cleaned and sacs flushed out with antiseptic solution. Antibiotic should again be infused into the sacs. The openings should be kept patent to allow them to discharge for several days. Systemic antibiotics may be justified in these cases and, because Gram-negative organisms are often involved, culture and sensitivity should be carried out in order to determine the most appropriate antibiotic.

Where the problem of anal sac disease is recurrent, surgical removal should be performed.

Anal tumours

Introduction

Tumours of the anal tissue are most frequently benign adenomas but occasionally lipomas, melanomas and leiomyomas occur. Very occasionally malignant tumours such as squamous cell carcinomas, malignant melanoma and adenocarcinomas occur. Anal tumours are most common in old dogs and rare in cats. They may all ulcerate and become secondarily infected. They rarely cause difficulty in defaecation or pain on defaecation unless advanced. Adenomas are hormone-induced, hence their appearance most frequently in old male dogs. They can grow slowly and insidiously to large sizes in some dogs although when multiple they do induce mechanical difficulties in defaecation and are frequently traumatized. Oestrogens suppress the adenomas, while testosterone stimulates their growth. Adenocarcinomas of the glands in the anal sacs are aggressive malignant tumours predominantly in the bitch.

Clinical diagnosis

Owners usually report the dog is paying a lot of attention to the perineal region together with evidence of swelling and bleeding around the anus.

Diagnosis is made on the location, typical character of the lesions and biopsy of the tumours.

Malignant tumours, although rare, present with varying degrees of swelling. They often ulcerate and are invasive with poor circumscription and involvement of deeper structures. Biopsy is the most effective method of confirming the diagnosis. Adenocarcinomas of the anal sac glands are often associated with pseudohyperparathyroidism (Burrows 1988), and a paraneoplastic syndrome with abnormal calcium metabolism may ensue.

Treatment

Although adenomas do respond to oestrogen therapy, its long-term oral use may lead to bone marrow suppression. Injections of oestrogens directly into the tumour bring about a rapid reduction in the size of the tumour at lower doses. This should be followed by castration and surgical excision of the tumours.

Treatment of malignant tumours really depends on very early detection prior to metastasis to other tissues. If surgical removal is carried out early, the prognosis may be quite good. However in advanced cases or inaccessible tumours the surgical excision required is so extensive that faecal incontinence often occurs. In either case if any tumour cells are left following surgery they tend to grow more aggressively and so the prognosis in malignant disease must be very guarded.

References

Barnett, K.C. & Joseph, E.C. (1987) Keratoconjunctivitis sicca in the dog following 5-aminosalicylic acid administration. *Human Toxicology*, **6**; 377–383.

Binder H.J. (1973) Faecal fatty acids — mediators of diarrhoea. *Gastroenterology*, **65**; 847–850.

Bolton G.R. & Brown T.T. (1972) Mycotic colitis in a cat. *Veterinary Medicine and Small Animal Clinics*, **63**; 978–981.

Bright R.M. Burrows C.F. Goring R. Fox S. & Tilmont L. (1986) Subtotal colectomy for treatment of acquired megacolon in the dog and cat. *Journal of American Veterinary Medical Association*, **188**; 1412–1416.

Burrows C.F. (1980) Diseases of the colon, rectum and anus. In: *Veterinary Gastroenterology*, N.V. Anderson (ed.), Lea & Febiger, Philadelphia, 553–592

Burrows C.F. (1986) Constipation. In: *Current Veterinary Therapy IX*. R.W. Kirk (ed.), W.B. Saunders, Philadelphia, 904–908.

Burrows C.F. (1988) Diseases of the canine and feline colon and anorectum. In: *Proceedings of a Course in Small Animal Gastroenterology and Nutrition*. New Zealand Veterinary Association, 225–258.

Burrows C.F. & Merritt A.M. (1983) The influence of alpha cellulose on the myoelectrical activity of the proximal canine colon. *American Journal of Physiology*, **245**; G301–G306.

Bush B.M. (1985) Colitis in the dog. In: *The Veterinary Annual*. C.S.G. Grunsell, F.W.G. Hill & M.E. Raw (eds), Scientechnica, Bristol, 337–347.

Chiapella A. (1986) Diagnosis and management of chronic colitis in the dog and cat. In: *Current Veterinary Therapy IX*. R.W. Kirk (ed.), W.B. Saunders, Philadelphia, 896–903.

Crow S.E. (1985) Tumours of the alimentary tract. *Veterinary Clinics of North America*, **15**; 577–596.

Ewing G.O. & Gomez J.A. (1973) Canine ulcerative colitis. *Journal of American Animal Hospital Association*, **9**; 395–406.

Head K.W. & Else R.W. (1981) Neoplasia and allied conditions of the canine and feline intestine. In: *The Veterinary Annual*. C.S.G. Grunsell, F.W.G. Hill & M.E. Raw (eds), Scientechnica, Bristol, 190–207.

Kennedy P.C. & Cello R.M. (1966) Colitis of Boxer dogs, *Gastroenterology*, **51**; 926–929.

Moore R.P. (1983) Feline eosinophilic enteritis. In: *Current Veterinary Therapy VIII*. R.W. Kirk (ed.), W.B. Saunders, Philadelphia, 791–793.

Murdoch D.B. (1986) Diarrhoea in the dog and cat. I Acute diarrhoea, *British Veterinary Journal*, **142**; 307–316.

Nelson R.W., Dimperio M.E. & Long G.G. (1984) Lymphocytic–plasmacytic colitis in the cat. *Journal of American Veterinary Medical Association*, **184**; 1133–1135.

Rask-Madson J. & Jenson B. (1973) Electrolyte transport capacity and electrical potentials of the normal and the inflamed human rectum *in vivo*. *Scandinavian Journal of Gastroenterology*, **8**; 169–173.

Rutgers H.C. (1989) Diarrhoea in the cat. *In Practice*, **11**; 139–148.

Seim H.B. (1986) Disease of the anus and rectum. In: *Current Veterinary Therapy IX*. R.W. Kirk (ed.), W.B. Saunders, Philadelphia, 916–921.

Sharp N.J.H., Nash A.S. & Griffiths I.R. (1984) Feline dysautonomia (The Key–Gaskell Syndrome) a clinical and pathological study of forty cases. *Journal of Small Animal Practice*, **25**; 599–615.

Sherding R.G. (1980) Canine large bowel diarrhoea. *Compendium on Continuing Education for the Practicing Veterinarian*, **2**; 279–290.

Snape W.J., Matanazzo S.A. & Cohen S. (1978) Abnormal colonic myoelectrical and motor responses to eating in ulcerative colitis. *Gastroenterology*, **74**; abstract.

Theran P. (1968) Eosinophilic gastroenteritis. In: *Current Veterinary Therapy III*. R.W. Kirk (ed.), W.B. Saunders, Philadelphia, 514–515.

Van der Gaag I., Van Toorenburg J., Voorhoot G., Happe R.P. & Aalps. R.H.G. (1978) Histiocytic ulcerative colitis in a French Bulldog. *Journal of Small Animal Practice*, **19**; 283–290.

Van Kruiningen H.J. (1975) The ultrastructure of macrophages in granulomatous colitis in Boxer dogs. *Journal of Veterinary Pathology*, **12**; 446–459.

Van Kruiningen H.J. & Dobbin W.O. (1979) Feline histiocytic colitis *Veterinary Pathology*, **16**; 215–222.

Van Kruiningen H.J., Ryan M.J. & Shindell N.M. (1983) The classification of feline colitis. *Journal of Comparative Pathology*, **93**; 275–294.

Webb S.M. (1985) Surgical management of acquired megacolon in the cat. *Journal of Small Animal Practice*, **26**; 399–405.

7/Investigation of Chronic Enteritis

Introduction

Disease of the gastrointestinal tract is one of the commonest reasons for consulting a veterinary surgeon, only equalled by dermatological conditions. Many acute diarrhoeas are self-limiting, requiring symptomatic treatment for a successful outcome. Only when this fails and subsequent changes of treatment fail, should the problem be defined as chronic diarrhoea. Any diarrhoea which persists longer than 3 to 4 weeks may be classed as chronic. These cases rarely self-cure but require investigation in order to obtain a definitive diagnosis and allow a specific treatment to be instigated. Obtaining a definitive diagnosis is also important because it allows a more accurate prognosis to be given.

Continual symptomatic treatment of chronic diarrhoea is rarely successful, and leads to a disappointed owner and considerable cost, for no observed improvement. It is therefore important to recognize a chronic problem and discuss it with the owner, indicating the need for a proper investigative approach. Although an investigation may be expensive, it is cheaper in the long term compared with weeks or months of repeat consultations and different courses of treatment which fail to solve the problem.

Any investigation must be soundly based, using previous experience and current knowledge of conditions which commonly affect the intestine. Such an investigation must be based on a detailed history and thorough physical examination, to ensure nothing obvious is missed and all relevant data collected.

The clinical examination should allow a decision to be made as to whether the problem is systemic (metabolic) or primarily digestive in origin. If the latter is suspected, the history will often allow a further division to be made, as to whether the diarrhoea is of small or large intestine origin. It is very unusual for both small and large intestinal disease to be present at the same time. Possible exceptions might include regional enteritis, eosinophilic enteritis and lymphosarcoma. Such a division will reduce the differential diagnosis by at least 50%. Having made these divisions, a more detailed investigation will be required to determine the exact cause of the diarrhoea which usually falls into one of the following categories; functional, malabsorptive, inflammatory, or neoplastic problems.

History

It is essential that this part of the clinical examination is carried out in detail, not only with regard to the digestive tract but also with regard to the other body systems. In this way the veterinarian will be able to make the distinction between the presence of systemic disease or digestive disorder. Even though a history may have been taken originally it is important to conduct a new detailed history if possible using a standard proforma, especially if this is a second opinion case (Table 7.1). In addition to assessing the patient for systemic disease the history should be designed to determine if a primary digestive problem originates from the small or large intestine. This can be done by questioning the owner on the subjects shown in Table 7.2.

Many cases of chronic diarrhoea are due to dietary problems, for example owners may change the diet suddenly resulting in an episode of diarrhoea. This makes the owner change the diet back to that originally fed, only to find the symptoms persist, and this often leads owners to try feeding a light diet in order to assist in the control of diarrhoea. If the diet had not been changed suddenly or the change had been maintained, instead of 'chasing' the problem, the diarrhoea would probably have resolved. Changes of diet from dry to tinned foods, overfeeding puppies and kittens, and scavenging are common causes of chronic diarrhoea. So the history should determine the type, amount and any change in diet which may have occurred. Diarrhoeas which persist after 24 h starvations are often secretory or inflammatory in origin while starvation usually leads to cessation of an osmotic diarrhoea.

It is important to check that the problem is genuinely chronic in nature by ensuring there has been adequate time given for the initial treatment to work. Chronic diarrhoea with an associated weight-loss is usually suggestive of a serious progressive problem. Intermittent diarrhoea indicates the patient has the ability to produce formed faeces and may therefore have a functional disorder compared with the patient with persistent diarrhoea resulting from a pathological lesion in the gut or associated organs.

Ravenous appetite, especially if there is associated pica, suggests an exocrine pancreatic insufficiency (EPI) or malabsorption syndrome. Where the appetite is very good but the animal loses weight, this again suggests a maldigestion/malabsorption problem. In advanced malabsorption, anorexia may be observed and weight-loss increases. A normal appetite with no associated weight-loss points to a functional diarrhoea or large intestinal problem.

Faecal character is very valuable to the clinician. Faeces of increased bulk, pale in colour, watery or soft, foul smelling with no fresh blood suggest a small intestinal problem. Faeces which are small in volume,

Table 7.1 Method of recording the history and physical exmination

---

Gastrointestinal Investigation

Name: .... Case No:...... Breed:............ Age:...... Sex:......

Vaccinal Status:............................... Worming Status: ....

Previous History:...

Present History: Duration: .... Symptoms:....................................

Diet 1. Type: ....   Amount: ....   Time: ....

Diet 2. Type: ....   Amount: ....   Time: ....

Appetite: ....   Dysphagia: ....   Scavenging: ....   Coprophagia:...........

Vomiting

Retching: ....   Regurgitation: ....   True Vomiting:.........   Salivation: ....

Intermittent: ....Persitent: ....

Bile: ....   Food: ....·...   Blood: ....   Other: ....

Association with food:..

Time of Vomiting: ....

Faeces

Formed:.............   Soft: ....   Cow pat: ....   Liquid:...............

Intermittent: ....   Persistent: ....   Borborygmi: ....   Flatus: ....

Volume:..............   Frequency: ....   Tenesmus:............   Blood/Mucus: ....

Behaviour: ....   Fitting: ....   Collapsing: ....

Weight Changes: ....

PDPU: ....

Respiratory. Cough:.....   Dyspnoea: ....   Discharges: ....   Exercise tol: ....

Bright: ....   Depressed: ....   Lethargic:.....................

Skin Changes. Pruritis: .....   Scurfy: ....   Dull: ....   Alopecia:.......   Inflamed: ......

Locomotor. Ataxia: ....   Lameness: ....   Paraphlegia: ....   Muscle Wasting: ....

Oestrus: ....   Other pets: ....   Owner: ....

Physical examination: ....

---

passed very frequently and contain fresh blood or mucus indicate a large intestinal condition (Table 7.2). Flatus indicates bacterial fermentation of intestinal contents and usually is suggestive of small intestinal disease, particulary EPI or malabsorption. Where there is blood in the faeces this suggests that an inflammatory, ulcerative or neoplastic lesion is present. Mucus alone supports a functional diarrhoea or non-inflammatory problem.

Table 7.2 Differentiation between small and large intestinal diarrhoea

Symptom	Small intestine	Large intestine
Faecal volume	Increased	Normal or reduced
Faecal frequency	Increased	Markedly increased
Faecal urgency	Rare	May be present
Faecal tenesmus	Rare	Often present
Faecal blood	Rare	May be present
Faecal mucus	Rare	Often present
Steatorrhoea	Common	Rare
Dyschezia	Rare	May be present
Flatus/borborygmi	Common	Rare
Vomiting	May be present	May be present
Weight-loss	Common	Rare
Halitosis	May be present	Rare

Urgency and tenesmus, frequent squatting and moving while posturing are features of large intestinal disease.

Vomiting in association with diarrhoea does not always indicate gastroenteritis is present, as 30% of dogs or cats with colonic disease may vomit. Where there is no primary oesophageal or gastric disease, vomiting associated with intestinal disease usually suggests an inflammatory process involving the small or large intestine.

Working dogs and those under training may exhibit diarrhoea which will often resolve when such work or training is stopped. This is a typical form of functional or stress-related diarrhoea seen in dogs. It can also occur in pet dogs where there is a change in the household such as a new child, change of home, kennelling or other stress factor. The diarrhoea is often intermittent, mucoid and accompanied by little weight-loss and may be associated with work. This is similar to irritable bowel syndrome (IBS) seen in man.

Although infectious agents and internal parasites are not common causes of chronic diarrhoea, they should be considered at this stage especially if the patient originates from a farm or boarding establishment and has not been vaccinated or treated for worms.

Physical examination

It is very important to follow up the collection of a history with a thorough physical examination. This will help to determine if a systemic problem exists and provide positive information regarding the patient's bodily condition, state of hydration and general demeanour. The animal should be examined for evidence of thickened intestinal loops, abdominal pain or fluid/gas-filled intestine. Dogs with EPI or malabsorption often have dry scurfy coats, and may have a characteristic smell similar to dogs with seborrhoea.

Where there is a primary digestive problem it is very unusual to be able to make a diagnosis from the clinical examination alone. Even where the clinical examination strongly supports a possible diagnosis, some additional tests will be required before a diagnosis can be reached. The clinical examination does offer the clinician an inexpensive way of determining in which direction the problem should be investigated and so reduces the differential diagnosis and cost of subsequent investigation (Fig. 7.1).

Systemic disease

Where the history and physical examination reveal additional symptoms to those of chronic diarrhoea, then systemic disease should be considered. This possibility should be investigated prior to assessing digestive function. The most likely systemic diseases which may give chronic diarrhoea as a major sign include; hypoadrenocorticalism, hyperthyroidism, liver disease, renal disease and cardiac failure.

Hypoadrenocorticalism or Addison's disease may present with vomiting, diarrhoea, abdominal pain, polydipsia/polyuria and lethargy, all of which may wax and wane. The diarrhoea is often intermittent and may or may not contain blood. The cause of diarrhoea is not known but is reversed by administration of glucocorticoids. Vomiting may be truly gastric in origin or may be due to oesophageal regurgitation, as dogs with Addison's disease may have oesophageal dilation. Microcardia, bradycardia and reduced size of pulmonary vasculature may be detected. Laboratory tests should include measurement of sodium and potassium, adrenocorticotrophic hormone (ACTH) response test and investigation for neutropenia, lymphocytosis and relative eosinophilia. The ECG will usually reveal peaked T waves, reduced P waves, increased PR interval, prolonged QT, decreased R wave, increased QRS duration and occasional extra systoles.

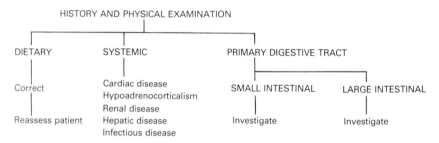

Fig. 7.1 Conclusions which may be drawn from the clinical examination.

Hyperthyroidism is very rare in the dog but is a common problem in elderly cats. Generally there is an increased metabolic rate and catecholamine level. The clinical signs include; polyphagia, weight-loss, hyperactivity, polydipsia/polyuria, vomiting, diarrhoea and tachycardia. Vomiting occurs and is thought to be as a result of direct stimulation of the chemoreceptor trigger zone (CTZ) by thyroid hormone. Diarrhoea is common and is thought to be due to increased food intake (polyphagia), reduced exocrine pancreatic secretion, intestinal hypermotility and malabsorption. Steatorrhoea is a common finding on faecal examination. Laboratory findings include erythrocytosis, macrocytosis and increased inorganic phosphorus, bilirubin and liver enzymes. Serum T3 and T4 levels are often elevated although T3 is sometimes normal. If in doubt a thyroid-stimulating hormone (TSH) response test can be carried out.

Chronic liver disease may present with chronic diarrhoea together with signs of polydipsia, polyuria, vomiting, weight-loss, ascites, hydrothorax and subcutaneous oedema. Diarrhoea may be due to deficiency in bile acids leading to steatorrhoea. Hypoproteinaemia is often present in advanced disease and must be differentiated from renal and gastrointestinal causes. Assessment of liver enzymes and function tests will confirm the presence of liver disease (see Chapter 9).

Chronic renal disease may lead to chronic vomiting and diarrhoea together with other signs such as polydipsia/polyuria, weight-loss, anorexia and halitosis. In renal disease it is thought that gastrin may be retained leading to increased levels of gastric acid which in turn may cause gastric and duodenal ulceration. In addition azotaemia acts directly on the chemoreceptor trigger zone to cause vomiting and interferes with epithelial renewal in the digestive tract, resulting in interference with gastrointestinal function. Laboratory assessment of blood urea, creatinine, calcium and phosphorus, together with a detailed urine analysis will confirm the diagnosis.

Congestive heart failure can cause chronic diarrhoea, which is due to poor venous return to the heart. In addition it is known that secondary lymphangiectasia can be caused by right-sided cardiac failure. In both these cases a variable degree of protein-losing enteropathy (PLE) may be present. Clinical signs should again point to the heart, rather than a primary intestinal disorder. Signs of coughing, exercise intolerance, tachycardia, cardiac murmur or arrythmias, ascites and hydrothorax may be present.

Investigation of chronic intestinal disease

If the clinical examination suggests there is a primary problem associated with the intestinal tract, the next stage is to ensure there is no underlying dietary problem that can be corrected. It is important to establish which part of the intestine is involved as the approach to investigating small intestinal diarrhoea is completely different from that for large intestinal diarrhoea, due to their differing functions (Fig. 7.2). For this reason they will be discussed separately.

Whether the patient is hospitalized to carry out the investigation or not is dependent on facilities available in the practice. Ideally the patient should be hospitalized, as sometimes the diarrhoea may resolve on admission where a strict dietary and exercise control has been established. If the patient can eat normally and pass normal faeces this indicates either the presence of a functional/stress-related diarrhoea or a dietary/scavenging cause, which has gone unnoticed by the client. The dog or cat should be discharged to the owner on the same strict hospital routine, in order to determine if the problem recurs when only the environment has been changed. This approach ensures an expensive and time consuming investigation is not carried out unless essential.

Small intestinal investigation

If the patient continues to have diarrhoea once hospitalized an investigation should be instigated. This should start with a blood profile followed by detailed faecal analysis (Fig. 7.3).

Blood parameters

To assist in ruling out systemic disease as described above, a blood profile should be collected. Routine haematology, serum alanine aminotransfer-

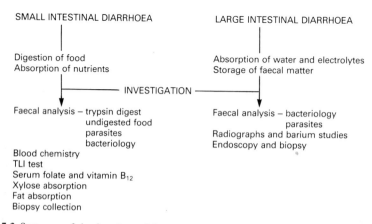

Fig. 7.2 Summary of the functions of the small and large intestine, together with the investigative procedures available.

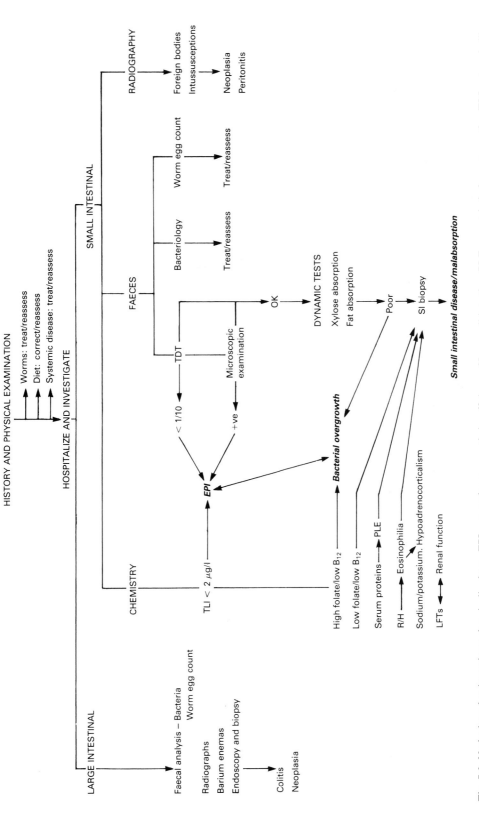

Fig. 7.3 Method used to investigate chronic diarrhoea. EPI = exocrine pancreatic insufficiency, SI = small intestine, PLE = protein-losing enteropathy, TLI = trypsin-like immunoreactivity test, LFTS = liver function tests, R/H = routine haematology.

ase (SALT), serum alkaline phosphatase (SAP), bile acids, blood urea, cholesterol, serum proteins, sodium and potassium should be measured. Lymphopenia may be associated with lymphangiectasia, neutrophilia with inflammatory bowel disease and eosinophilia with parasitic, allergic or eosinophilic enteritis. Raised cholesterol levels are seen in liver disease while lowered cholesterol occurs in EPI or malabsorption. Hypercalcaemia may occur in lymphosarcoma while hypocalcaemia occurs in hypoalbuminaemia.

Where hypoproteinaemia is detected by the presence of ascites, hydrothorax and subcutaneous oedema the cause must be determined. There are really only three possible causes which include advanced liver disease, renal disease or protein-losing enteropathy. At present the usual method of confirming PLE is by ruling out the other two causes. If liver and kidney function are normal then it is highly likely that hypoproteinaemia is due to protein loss through the intestine. As a general guide, there is loss of albumin and globulin in PLE, while only albumin is lost in liver and kidney disease. The definitive test for PLE is the intravenous injection of Cr-labelled albumin with daily measurement of faeces for radioactivity (Barton et al. 1978).

Radiography

Radiographs are basically of little diagnostic value in the investigation of small intestinal conditions. Even barium studies rarely point out any obvious abnormality. They are very rarely included in the standard work up unless there is a suspicion of obstruction due to foreign body or neoplasia.

Feline variations

The physiology of and the conditions affecting the feline digestive tract differ from the canine. Small intestinal problems are more common than large intestinal problems in cats compared with dogs and EPI is very rare in cats compared with dogs. The investigation of chronic diarrhoea in cats should follow that used for dogs with the inclusion of feline leukaemia virus/feline immunodeficiency virus (FeLV/FIV) in the routine blood profile and more careful examination for Giardia in faecal samples.

Faecal analysis

If the faecal examination is to be of value it is essential that the dog is placed on a meat and biscuit diet and that at least two faecal samples are analysed. Faecal samples and not swabs should be collected for bacteriological examination for the presence of Salmonella and Campylobacter which are both intermittently excreted. Where they are detected the patient should be treated and reassessed, in order to determine if the infection was the cause of the diarrhoea or whether there is some other underlying problem present. Similarly a worm egg count should be carried out and if positive, the patient should be reassessed once a course of anthelminthics has been given. This 'rule out' policy will ensure no confusion occurs as the investigation precedes through a logical sequence of tests. Trypsin digest tests should be carried out in *conjunction* with a microscopic examination of the faeces. Only if there is low or nil trypsin titres *and* the presence of undigested food (starch, fat and muscle fibres), should a tentative diagnosis of EPI be made. Using either test individually will always lead to false positive and negative results, but when combined as described above, false results should not occur (Simpson & Doxey 1988).

TLI test

If EPI is suspected following faecal analysis it will be necessary to carry out a trypsin-like immunoreactivity test (TLI) before a definitive diagnosis can be made (Williams & Batt 1983). This test requires a single fasted serum sample for TLI measurement using radioimmuno assay. In the past the *N*-benzoyl-L-tyrosyl-*p*-amino benzoic acid (BT−PABA) test was used for this purpose, but has yielded false positive results and has been superseded by the TLI test. The basis of the test relies on the fact that normally the exocrine pancreas in man and dogs liberates a trypsin-like substance into the blood which can be measured. When there is a deficiency of exocrine tissue the level of this trypsin-like substance falls and the level of the fall can act as a measure of exocrine pancreatic function. Normal values for the dog are greater than 5 µg/l and values less than 2.5 µg/l indicate EPI. Values between 2.5 and 5 µg/l are inconclusive and the dog should be retested one month later. The test has not yet been evaluated for the cat.

Intestinal function tests

Where faecal screening and TLI has yielded no diagnostic information, exocrine pancreatic disease can be ruled out and intestinal function tests should be carried out. These tests include serum folate and B12 estimations, together with xylose and fat absorption tests. It is necessary to carry out all these tests, as in individual cases it is possible to have abnormal folate and B12 results but normal xylose absorption or fat absorption and vice versa. Therefore if one test is used alone the result may be normal when in fact other tests performed at the same time may have yielded evidence of abnormality.

Serum vitamin tests

Serum folate and B12 are water-soluble vitamins which are plentiful in the diet and deficiencies are rare. Any fall in serum levels is almost entirely due to abnormal small intestinal function (Table 7.3). Folate occurs in the diet as a conjugate, namely folate polyglutamate, and is deconjugated at the jejunum brush border, where folate monoglutamate is absorbed on specific receptor sites. The vitamin cannot be absorbed in the ileum, so low levels suggest malabsorption involving the proximal small intestine. On the other hand, some bacteria can synthesize folate, so that high levels are indicative of bacterial overgrowth. Acid and pepsin in the stomach release cobalamin from the dietary protein and link it to R protein at low pH. Once in the duodenum, pancreatic secretion releases the R protein and secretes intrinsic factor which attaches to cobalamin and carries the vitamin to specific receptors in the ileum where absorption of B12 occurs. Vitamin B12 cannot be absorbed in the proximal small bowel. Low levels indicate either malabsorption in the ileum or bacterial overgrowth, as some bacteria utilize B12 (Williams 1987).

Not all cases of bacterial overgrowth lead to changes in serum folate and B12 levels and faecal culture is of little value as the population changes are only present in the small intestine. In an attempt to get round this, another indirect method has been developed, called the nitrosonapthal test (Burrows 1983). The excretion of 4-hydroxyphenylacetic acid and derivatives is measured in urine; they are the product of bacterial degradation of tyrosine in the small intestine. Unfortunately this test may also yield false results although it still acts as a useful screening test.

Xylose absorption test

Xylose is a pentose sugar which if given orally is absorbed without prior digestion in the jejunum. Xylose is absorbed by passive diffusion in the jejunum by a non-energy-requiring process, and so is slower than absorption of glucose. It must be absorbed in the jejunum because it requires a pore size

Table 7.3 (a) Values for serum and vitamin B12 in normal dogs, and (b) association between abnormal serum folate and vitamin B12 levels and small intestinal diseases

(a) Normal values:	
Serum folate	3.5 to 8.5 μg/l
Serum vitamin B12	215 to 500 μg/l
(b) Abnormal levels	
Low folate and low vitamin B12	Proximal and distal small intestinal disease
Low folate and normal vitamin B12	Proximal small intestinal disease
High folate and low vitamin B12	Bacterial overgrowth

of 8×10^{-4} µm, while the pores in the ileum are only 4×10^{-4} µm. Where there is small intestinal disease present the pore size is often reduced so xylose cannot be absorbed. Therefore xylose measures the functional state of the jejunum; it does not detect specific malabsorptive states but a reduced absorptive surface area. In bacterial overgrowth xylose may be rapidly degraded leading to poor xylose absorption curves (Goldstein *et al.* 1970). Normally there is very little xylose in the blood and following oral dosage of 0.5 g/kg liveweight the blood levels should increase to a peak at around 120 min, of greater than 3 mmol/l, in dogs (Hill *et al.* 1970) and between 1.5 and 2.3 mmol/l in cats (Sherding *et al.* 1982) (Fig. 7.4).

Fat absorption test

Fat absorption has been measured for many years using a method which relied on visual assessment of plasma turbidity following oral dosing with vegetable oil (Anderson & Low 1965). This was very subjective and allowed no comparison between patients. For this reason a quantitative method, measuring serum triglyceride post feeding of vegetable oil, has been developed (Simpson & Doxey 1983). A resting triglyceride value is obtained and the patient fed 3 ml/kg liveweight of vegetable oil. Normally the serum triglyceride value will increase to three times the resting value by 3 h post feeding (Fig. 7.5). Dogs with EPI have significantly lower resting triglyceride values and show no increase in value following oral vegetable oil. Repeating the test with added lipase will confirm if this flat response is due to deficiency of lipase or malabsorption. Rarely the poor fat absorption curve will be due to bile acid deficiency and this can be determined by repeating the test with added bile acids, when fat absorption immediately improves (Simpson & Van den Broek 1989).

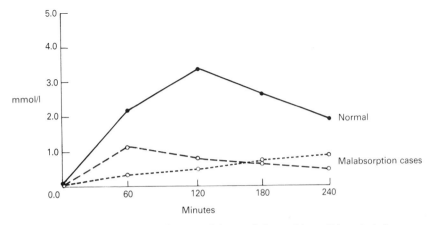

Fig. 7.4 Xylose absorption curves for normal dogs and those with small intestinal disease.

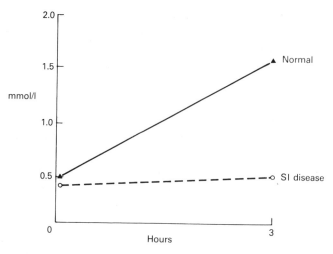

Fig. 7.5 Fat absorption curves for normal dogs and those with small intestinal disease.

Biopsy

These intestinal function tests only indicate there is some degree of mal-absorption present. The only way a definitive diagnosis can be made is following invasive surgery and collection of intestinal biopsy samples. Intes-tinal function tests should be used to provide strong evidence to support the need for a laparotomy, which ensures the surgery is *only* carried out when actually required. In all cases where a laparotomy is carried out, the intestine should be biopsied even if it appears normal, as many of the changes are microscopic and cannot be seen with the naked eye. Full thickness biopsy samples of the duodenum, jejunum and ileum together with a mesenteric lymph node should be collected. The author finds the 4 mm skin biopsy punch (Stiefel Laboratories) very suitable for this purpose. Great care is required where the patient is hypoproteinaemic as these patients are poor anaesthetic risks, immunodeficient and have reduced powers of healing. Although the biopsy procedure may be necessary to offer a definitive diagnosis, it is important to advise the client of the risks involved. In all cases the collection of biopsy samples not only provides a definitive diagnosis but also provides an accurate prognosis.

Large intestinal investigation

The large intestine is not involved in digestion and absorption of food but in the secretion and absorption of water and electrolytes. Diarrhoea develops when there is: (1) an overall secretion of fluid and electrolytes into the colon rather than a net absorption, (2) reduced segmented contractions, with retained peristalsis moving contents more rapidly to the rectum leading to increased desire to defaecate; and (3) abnormally high bacterial populations causing breakdown of food residues and interference with colonic function. Many individual cases are multifactorial and the pathogenesis is generally poorly understood.

The clinician will have decided that a large intestinal problem is present from the character of the faeces and the presence of tenesmus and urgency. The first step in the investigation should be detailed faecal analysis which includes examination for parasites, bacteria and protozoa but not undigested food or trypsin which are not indicated in large intestinal diarrhoea. The presence of *Campylobacter*, *Salmonella*, *Giardia* or *Trichuris* spp. should be considered significant. Such cases should be treated and reassessed following treatment. Where inflammatory bowel disease is suspected, staining faecal mucus with methylene blue may identify leucocytes (Harris *et al.* 1972). Tests for occult blood are rarely employed because there is a high incidence of false positive results.

Where no diagnostic information is forthcoming from faecal analysis the clinician can carry out radiographic examination of the colon. Plain radiographs will only indicate gross changes while barium studies may indicate obstructions, stricture, intussusceptions or filling defects. The authors have found barium enemas of little value as evacuation of the colon is time consuming and difficult to carry out and effective filling of the colon with barium is also difficult. For this reason we advocate use of oral barium which is followed down through the small intestine to the colon, confirms normal ileocaecocolic emptying and then highlights the colon satisfactorily in most cases. It is less stressful on the patient and provides as much information as barium enemas.

With increasing frequency the use of endoscopic examination of the colon is being carried out. It allows visualization of the colon and the collection of biopsy samples from obviously abnormal tissue or multiple biopsies from random sites, without recourse to invasive surgery. Histological examination of biopsy samples allows the clinician to detect microscopic changes which are not visualized. In addition to being non-invasive, this procedure is simple to carry out and saves a considerable amount of time and money in conducting radiographic examinations which may subsequently require endoscopy anyway. This procedure is now used routinely. Preparation using warm water enemas to empty the large intestine is essential.

Most colonic diseases are diffuse and biopsy of the descending colon is usually adequate for the purpose of making a diagnosis in 80% of cases in our experience. However focal lesions do occur and endoscopy of the entire colon should be carried out whenever possible. Normally three to five biopsy samples are adequate for this examination, and should be quickly mounted on cardboard prior to fixing in 10% formal saline.

Biopsy samples which reveal only hyperplasia of the colon, with no cellular infiltration usually indicate the problem is more proximal, and checks should then be made on the caecum and small intestine. Dogs with clinical signs of colitis but normal biopsy results, usually have stress or IBS-type functional diarrhoea. Such dogs are often excitable, nervous or hyper-active in addition to having chronic diarrhoea. In idiopathic colitis there is rarely evidence of ulceration on endoscopy, although the mucosa may bleed easily on being touched by the endoscope. Biopsy samples reveal varying levels of infiltration by plasma cells, lymphocytes and mild fibrosis. With histiocytic colitis in addition to the findings for idiopathic colitis, there are ulcers and histiocytes present. Eosinophilic colitis is recognized by the high proportion of eosinophils in the biopsy samples. Tumours such as adeno-carcinomas are discrete and macroscopic, while lymphosarcoma is more diffuse. In each case biopsy samples will reveal the presence of neoplastic cells.

Summary

There are very few cases of chronic diarrhoea which cannot be diagnosed if a careful systematic investigation is carried out. However in a small proportion of cases, having carried out such an investigation no obvious abnormality will be found. This simply reflects our inability to detect the underlying cause of some forms of intestinal disease. Some of these cases may have functional/stress-related diarrhoea which is similar to the irritable bowel syndrome recognized in man. At present the only method of diagnosing this condition is by ruling out everything else. On endoscopy dogs with IBS show marked contraction of the colon which contains large amounts of tenacious mucus.

The importance of dietary allergens has been established in causing some skin conditions but not as a cause of diarrhoea. It is highly likely some chronic diarrhoea cases will be due to dietary allergies but more research is required before their identity is known. At present hypoallergen diets rely on chicken, mutton and rice as being allergen free. This may be the case but some dogs may have allergies to these as well as preservatives, and even these diets fail to work.

Other undiagnosed cases may be due to failure in detecting parasites which are often difficult to find in faecal samples. In these cases instigation of a low fat diet and course of broad spectrum anthelminthics is necessary.

It is important to emphasize that the aim of the gastroenterologist is to make a specific diagnosis whenever possible, so an accurate prognosis and treatment may be given. Symptomatic treatment is no substitute for a definitive diagnosis, following careful investigation, as such therapy often fails and leads to disappointment and a disillusioned client.

References

Anderson N.V. & Low D.G. (1965) Juvenile atrophy of the canine pancreas. *Animal Hospital*, **1**; 101–109.

Barton C.L., Smith C., Troy G., Hightower D. & Hood D. (1978) The diagnosis and clinicopathological features of canine protein-losing enteropathy. *Journal of American Animal Hospital Association*, **14**; 85–91.

Burrows C.F. (1983) Nitrosonapthal test for screening of small intestinal diarrhoeal disease in the dog. *Journal of American Veterinary Medical Association*, **183**; 318–322.

Goldstein K., Karacadag S. & Wirts C.W. (1970) Intraluminal small intestinal ultilisation of d-xylose by bacteria. A limitation of the d-xylose absorption test. *Gastroenterology*, **59**; 380–386.

Harris J.C., Dupont H.L. & Harnick R.B. (1972) Faecal leucocytes in diarrhoeal illness. *Annals of Internal Medicine*, **76**; 697–703.

Hill F.W.G., Kidder D.E. & Frew C. (1970) A xylose absorption test for the dog. *Veterinary Record*, **87**; 250–255.

Sherding R.G., Stradley R.P., Rogers W.A. & Johnson S.E. (1982) Bentriomide-xylose test in healthy cats. *American Journal of Veterinary Research*, **43**; 2272–2273.

Simpson J.W. & Doxey D.L. (1983) Quantitative assessment of fat absorption and its diagnostic value in exocrine pancreatic insufficiency. *Research in Veterinary Science*, **35**; 249–251.

Simpson J.W. & Doxey D.L. (1988) Evaluation of faecal analysis as an aid to the detection of exocrine pancreatic insufficiency. *British Veterinary Journal*, **144**; 174–178.

Simpson J.W. & Van den Broek A.H.M. (1989) Deficiency of bile salts causing steatorrhoea and weight-loss in two dogs. *Journal of Small Animal Practice*, **30**; 567–569.

Williams D.A. (1987) New tests of pancreatic and small intestinal function. *Compendium on Continuing Education for the Practicing Veterinarian*, **9**; 1167–1174.

Williams D.A. & Batt R.M. (1983) Diagnosis of canine exocrine pancreatic insufficiency by the assay of serum trypsin-like immunoreactivity. *Journal of Small Animal Practice*, **24**; 583–588.

8/Diseases of the Exocrine Pancreas

Anatomy

The pancreas is a pink lobulated gland comprising left and right lobes merging with the body. It lies deep to the pylorus and the duodenum, giving the gland a V-shape. This makes physical and radiological examination of the pancreas very difficult.

The left lobe of the pancreas lies in the greater omentum and crosses the abdominal cavity from the body to the left kidney. It is shorter and thicker than the right lobe. The right lobe of the pancreas lies in the mesoduodenum and on the medioventral surface of the descending duodenum. The lobe is longer and thinner than the left lobe (Fig. 8.1). There are considerable variations in the duct system but normally there is one duct from each lobe of the pancreas which fuse to form a Y-shape within the pancreas. The single duct then leaves the pancreas to enter the duodenum at the minor duodenal papilla. There is often a second duct draining the left lobe of the pancreas and entering the duodenum close to the bile duct at the major duodenal papilla.

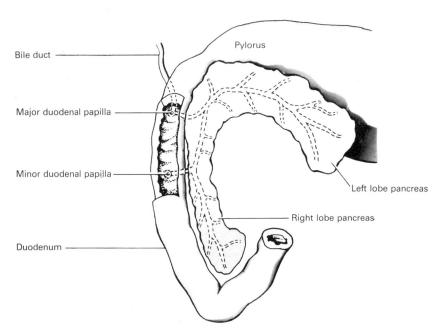

Fig. 8.1 Topographical anatomy of the pancreas.

The pancreas receives blood via the coeliac and cranial mesenteric arteries. Venous drainage is via the pancreaticoduodenal vein and the portal vein. The gland is supplied with both sympathetic and parasympathetic nerves. Pain is a feature of acute pancreatitis and this is mediated through the autonomic nerves and is often referred to the thoracolumbar region.

Over 90% of the pancreas is composed of exocrine tissue which is a compound tubuloacinar gland similar to the salivary glands. A thin connective tissue capsule surrounds the gland with trabeculae which infiltrate the gland, forming lobules. This framework carries the blood vessels and nerves to the glandular tissue. Lobules are composed of acinar secretory units which mark the end of the duct system, giving the appearance of a bunch of grapes. The secretory units are composed of a single line of acinar cells on a reticular basal membrane. Vagal fibres are found at the base of the acinar cells, and within the acinar cells lie large numbers of zymogen granules and they contain the enzyme secretions which bud off at the apical surface to enter the duct system. Leading from these secretory units lie the centroacinar cells which continue as the intercalated ducts carrying secretion away from the secretory units towards the duodenum via the interlobular ducts and collecting ducts.

Randomly distributed throughout the exocrine tissue are islands of cells called the islets of Langerhans. These islets contain specialized cells surrounded by a reticular framework and have a rich vascular supply. There are several cell types present, the alpha cells which produce glucagon, beta cells which produce insulin and delta cells producing somatostatin.

Physiology

Regulation of exocrine pancreatic secretion is mediated through three stimuli; the cephalic, gastric or intestinal phases. The cephalic phase involves the sight, smell and taste of food which stimulates pancreatic secretion via the vagus nerve. Acetylcholine is released at the basal membrane of the acinar cells directly stimulating secretion. The vagus also stimulates release of gastrin from the gastric mucosa which in turn stimulates the production of gastric acid and pancreatic secretion. The pancreatic secretion is rich in enzyme and low in water and bicarbonate.

The gastric phase stimulates pancreatic secretion through two processes: (1) distention of the stomach with food releases gastrin which stimulates gastric acid and pancreatic secretion; and (2) the vagus nerve is also stimulated by gastric distention with food and this directly stimulates pancreatic secretion.

The intestinal phase involves only hormonal stimulation. The presence of acid chyme in the intestine stimulates secretin release from the duodenal mucosa, resulting in the production of pancreatic secretion rich in bicarbonate, to neutralize the acid. On the other hand, the presence of protein or fat stimulates release of cholecystokinin which stimulates the pancreas to produce an enzyme-rich secretion.

There are other gastrointestinal hormones which interact in these mechanisms, but their true function is not clear at this time. Calcium is important as a cofactor in pancreatic secretion. It is important in the activation of proteases and lipase and is involved in the activity of acetylcholine, gastrin and cholecystokinin.

Pancreatic secretion is very similar to plasma with the exception of large amounts of bicarbonate. The specific gravity ranges from 1.010 to 1.030 and has a pH of 8. The volume produced is 70 ml/kg/day in the dog. Most enzymes are produced and stored in the inactive form, with the exception of amylase and lipase (Anderson 1973).

The exocrine pancreas produces several important enzymes necessary for the digestion of chyme. Trypsinogen is activated by enterokinase secreted by the duodenal mucosa. Once activated it will activate more of itself and the other proenzymes found in the exocrine secretion (see Fig. 5.4). All the enzymes produced by the exocrine pancreas require an alkaline medium to function. If acid chyme is not neutralized then lipase is irreversibly inactivated while the other enzymes are reversibly inactivated (Williams 1988).

Trypsin, chymotrypsin, elastase and carboxypeptidase are all involved in the digestion of proteins creating smaller peptides. Final digestion of peptides occurs on the brush border of the small intestine by peptidases and the resultant amino acids are then absorbed (see Chapter 5).

Alpha amylase is not produced in the zymogen granules and is inactive until calcium and chloride ions are present. It is important in the digestion of starch. It produces maltose, maltotriose, limited dextrins and some glucose. Final digestion of saccharides occurs at the brush border by action of the disaccharidase enzymes. Glucose, fructose and galactose are then absorbed across the mucosa.

Although lipase is not secreted in the zymogen granules it remains inactive until co-lipase is released from the zymogen granules to activate the enzyme. Once activated, lipase is responsible for the digestion of dietary fat. Colipase is a low molecular weight protein which is not a true enzyme, but is required to facilitate the surface interaction of lipase, bile salts and lipid, so that fat digestion can take place. The result of lipase action is the production of free fatty acids and monoglyceride. No further digestion occurs at the brush border and these components are absorbed across the mucosa with the aid of bile salts.

The pancreas must protect itself from autodigestion and this is achieved by the presence of various mechanisms. Firstly enzymes are stored in zymogen granules which protect the acinar cells, and they remain inactive until they reach the duodenum. Secondly there are trypsin inhibitors in the acinar cells themselves, such as pancreatic secretory trypsin inhibitor (PSTI). Thirdly there are protease inhibitors present in the extracellular fluid as alpha-1-antitrypsin and alpha-2-macroglobulin to protect the tissues and plasma in the event of enzyme leakage out of the cell. They bind with the leaked protease, irreversibly inhibiting enzyme activity (Hall *et al*. 1988).

Acute pancreatitis

Acute pancreatitis is thought to account for some 66% of pancreatic disease while diabetes mellitus, neoplasia and exocrine pancreatic insufficiency account for only 33% (Anderson 1973). In our opinion the incidence of acute pancreatitis in the UK is much less than that observed in North America. Factors which cause confusion regarding the incidence include: (1) the difference between the clinical picture and that observed in experimental models, (2) the variation in views expressed in the extensive literature; and (3) the difficulty in making a definitive diagnosis. Oedematous pancreatitis occurs initially, which may spontaneously resolve. However if sudden vascular or anoxic events occur together with enzyme activation then acute necrotizing pancreatitis develops (Williams 1988).

There appears to be no breed or sex predisposition although more cases are said to occur in the Dachshund, Yorkshire Terrier and Miniature Schnauzer than in other breeds (Drazner 1986). Cats are very rarely affected, although low grade chronic pancreatitis is sometimes detected as an incidental finding at post mortem (Owens *et al*. 1975) and there may be a link between cholangiohepatitis and chronic pancreatitis (Williams 1988). The aetiology of acute pancreatitis is still poorly understood even though there are various agents recognized as being implicated in some cases (Strombeck & Feldman 1983). Basically there is activation of digestive enzymes within the pancreas, the aetiological agents responsible for this activation of trypsin are not known. Recently it has been suggested that lyososomal enzymes and zymogens become mixed in the acinar cell allowing activation of trypsin, but it is still not clear why this occurs (Williams 1988).

There is little doubt that high fat diets (greater than 60%) are associated with acute, pancreatitis (Strombeck & Feldman 1983). Dogs maintained on high calory diets especially if also overweight and receiving little exercise, are much more commonly affected. Such high fat diets result in increased enzyme production by the pancreas and also make acinar cell membranes unstable (Creutzfeldt & Schmidt 1970).

Any traumatic situation such as road traffic accidents, kicks or surgical manipulation of the pancreas, can cause acute pancreatitis.

Hypercalcaemia created by intravenous calcium salts has been recorded as inducing acute pancreatitis in a dog (Neuman 1975). Such levels: (1) cause vasculitis in the microcirculation of the pancreas, (2) cause protein precipitation within the pancreatic ducts; and (3) assist in the activation of enzymes. Hypercalcaemia may occur because of hyperparathyroidism, lymphosarcoma, vitamin D toxicosis or bone tumours.

Drugs have also been implicated in the aetiology of acute pancreatitis. Sulphamethazole, azathioprine, chlorthiazide diuretics, chlorpromazine and corticosteroids have all been implicated (Creutzfeldt & Schmidt 1970). Cushing's syndrome results in high circulating cortisol levels, and acute pancreatitis has been associated with this condition (Drazner 1986). Corticosteroids cause proliferation of ductal epithelium and increase enzyme production and the viscosity of pancreatic secretion. Tetracyclines have been observed to initiate pancreatitis in cats (Williams 1988).

Hyperlipaemia may predispose to acute pancreatitis or indeed acute pancreatitis may create hyperlipaemia. The circulating lipid levels may cause fat embolism which in turn causes ischaemia of the pancreatic tissues, and in addition lipid may cause physical damage to the capillaries where lipoprotein lipase in endothelial cells digests lipid, producing free fatty acids which cause the capillary damage (Hall et al. 1988).

Infectious agents such as viruses have also been implicated in acute pancreatitis. Parvovirus has a direct action on the pancreatic tissues and in addition may cause intestinal stasis and so allow reflux of duodenal contents into the pancreatic duct. Reflux may contain enterokinase and bacteria both of which may play important roles in inducing pancreatitis. Reflux into the pancreatic duct is common in man but is now thought to be rare in dogs except in the case of parvovirus infection (Hall et al. 1988).

Any situation which causes hypovolaemia or redistribution of blood from the splanchnic tissues such as occurs when catacholamines are released, will lead to pancreatic ischaemia. Stimulation of the spinal nerves following thoracolumbar surgery, may cause hypotension. Equally in those cases of disc lesions where surgery is not employed, corticosteroids are often used with effect described above.

It is now thought that immune-mediated disease may be important in acute pancreatitis. Following an initial episode of acute pancreatitis there may be exposure of cytoplasmic contents to the immune system leading to the production of autoantibodies against pancreatic tissue. The low grade continual destruction of exocrine tissue may ultimately lead to exocrine pancreatic insufficiency. This is thought to involve a type III Arthus reaction and type IV cell-mediated immune response (Hall et al. 1988).

For acute pancreatitis to occur it is necessary for one of several situations to be present: (1) an actively secreting gland, (2) development of duct obstruction; and (3) degeneration of cell membranes with enzyme activation. Most cases of acute pancreatitis are interstitial (oedematous) while the most fatal form is acute necrotizing pancreatitis. The former is also more common in cats, while the latter occurs more often in dogs.

Fixation of complement may cause degeneration of the cell membranes so allowing extracellular fluid to enter the cells. Trypsinogen stored in the cells is activated by either calcium, bile salts or enterokinase. Once trypsin is activated it is able to activate more of itself and two other important enzymes, namely elastase and phospholipase A. Elastase digests the elastic fibres of blood vessels leading to haemorrhage, thrombosis and ischaemia, and in addition it also digests interstitial connective tissue. Phospholipase A on the other hand digests acinar cell membranes thus allowing further enzyme release. It is common for this process to cause acute inflammation and pain which in turn causes hypovolaemia and shock to develop.

Trypsin also activates kallikreinogen and this activates bradykininogen which causes marked vasodilation, a fall in blood pressure and poor venous return to the heart. Add to these changes the fluid lost by vomition and diarrhoea, and it is not surprising that dehydration and hypovolaemia rapidly develop, followed by shock (Fig. 8.2). Bradykinin also causes pain and increases the migration of white blood cells to the pancreas. The vasodilation causes exudation in the pancreas which in turn releases more enzyme and bradykinin, so a self-perpetuating cycle develops. This process is further compounded by the presence of myocardial depressent factor (MDF) produced by the pancreas, which acts on the heart to cause reduced

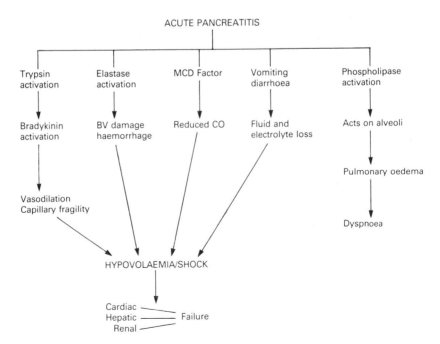

Fig. 8.2 Some aspects of the pathogenesis of acute pancreatitis. MCD = myocardial depressant factor, CO = cardiac output, BV = blood vessel.

cardiac output (Fig. 8.2). The result is major circulatory collapse and a rapidly-developing irreversible shock.

Amylase and carboxypeptidase, are also released but play a very small role in the development of acute pancreatitis. Lipase does cause fat necrosis. There are protease inhibitors present in the extracellular fluid and pancreatic tissue which prevent trypsin activation. They are attached to alpha globulins and include alpha-2-macroglobulin and alpha-1-antitrypsin which transfers trypsin to alpha-2-macroglobulin and PSTI (Hall *et al.* 1988). Where there is large scale release of enzyme the inhibitors are rapidly overwhelmed and remaining active enzyme is free to carry out extensive tissue destruction.

Pancreatic hypoxia which develops due to the ischaemia and hypo-volaemia, makes a favourable environment for Clostridial organisms which are frequently found in the pancreatic duct. Secondary bacterial infection rapidly develops and leakage of this infection into the peritoneum leads to septic peritonitis.

Hypocalcaemia has been observed in acute pancreatitis, and this may result in the development of hypocalcaemic tetany, so compounding the clinical signs already observed. Low serum calcium is thought to occur because of sudden high glucagon release which stimulates the thyroid to produce calcitonin.

The final process in this cascade of events which is called acute pancreatitis is the development of disseminated intravascular coagulation (DIC) (Hardy & Johnson 1980). Activation of the intrinsic clotting mechanism occurs, together with release of a large amount of tissue thromboplastin (of which the pancreas is a rich source), and trypsin activation of prothrombin and the fibrinolytic system. So there is promotion of the clotting process and fibrinolysis at the same time. Complement activation already described activates the intrinsic pathway, and to all this is added the effects of bradykinin which causes capillary fragility and permeability (Drazner 1982).

The end result is a complex chain of events which leads to irreversible shock and DIC and this is why there is such a high mortality. If the dog survives, then subclinical 'smouldering' pancreatitis may continue, with a progressive loss of exocrine function and occasionally endocrine function. The subclinical condition may be punctuated by acute flareups which are often thought to be isolated events, rather than clinical manifestations of a subclinical state.

Clinical diagnosis

Acute pancreatitis may manifest itself in varying levels of severity. The acute form of the condition is more common and will often be fatal if not rapidly recognized. The mean duration of illness is 4 days, although cases have continued for 10 days. Commonly there is a recent history of a large or fatty meal, together with an overweight dog. Anorexia, depression, dehydration, abdominal pain, and vomiting and diarrhoea occur in 90% of cases. Vomiting occurs through stimulation of the vomiting centre via the vagus nerve (Strombeck & Feldman 1983). Pain is frequently manifest as arching of the back, boarding of the abdomen and grunting on expiration. The abdomen often enlarges with gas and ascitic fluid. Diarrhoea is observed in 54% of cases and may become haemorrhagic. Dehydration is often marked and the animal becomes rapidly weak and may collapse in shock. There is a poor capillary refill time and pallor of the mucous membranes. Jaundice is more common in cats due to the common pathway taken by bile and pancreatic secretion, while it is rare in the dog. If it does occur in the dog this is often due to cholangiohepatitis.

In 46% of cases pyrexia is present due to the pain, pyrogen release and secondary bacterial infection, but once hypovolaemia and shock develop the temperature often falls below normal.

Less frequently other signs may complicate the situation. Hypocalcaemic tetany may develop. Dyspnoea, cyanosis and pulmonary oedema may occur as a result of phospholipase A digesting the alveolar membranes and surfactant. Bradykinin adds to this effect by increasing capillary fragility and permeability. Hyperglycaemia may occur either due to diabetes mellitus or surges in glucagon release from the islet cells. Terminally there may be signs of haemorrhage seen on mucous membranes and blood in the faeces and vomitus, due to the development of DIC.

The main differential diagnosis includes haemorrhagic gastroenteritis (HGE), gastrointestinal foreign bodies, intussusception, hepatitis and rupture of the intestine, bladder or gall bladder.

Pancreatic biopsy is rarely carried out because of the patient's critical state of health. If ascites is present then paracentesis will reveal an exudate which is often rich in amylase and lipase. There is often a poor correlation between laboratory findings and the degree of pancreatic tissue damage. There is no single diagnostic test which will yield a definitive diagnosis (Strombeck & Feldman 1983). It depends on the clinical findings, radiographic evidence and laboratory results.

Routine haematology often reveals a high packed cell volume (PCV), indicating dehydration, while the white cell count is elevated with a neutrophilia and a shift to the left. A degenerative shift to the left indicates an overwhelming infection (Cornelius 1976). Check the blood urea and creatinine levels and relate to the urine specific gravity. Where there is azotaemia and a specific gravity above 1.025 this suggests the problem is prerenal due to hypovolaemia but if the specific gravity is less than 1.020 then the azotaemia may be renal in origin. Prerenal uraemia is common due to hypovolaemia and shock, but enzyme activity may damage the renal tubules and result in renal uraemia. It is therefore important to check the urine in each individual case.

A high serum alkaline phosphatase value may indicate bile duct obstruction, or the presence of Cushing's syndrome which has induced acute pancreatitis in the first place. High total bilirubin with a majority being conjugated would also support obstruction to the bile duct.

Ultimately it is necessary to examine the serum amylase and lipase levels. There is considerable debate as to the value of these parameters. However if both the levels excede three times the resting values, they may be considered significant. Serum amylase is not pancreas-specific but lipase is much more specific. The latter correlates well with post-mortem diagnosis of acute pancreatitis (Strombeck *et al.* 1981). Unfortunately elevations in both amylase and lipase may occur in hepatic or renal disease. Elevations in serum trypsin-like immunoreactivity (TLI) which is more frequently associated with detection of exocrine pancreatic insufficiency may be of diagnostic value (Williams 1987).

If there is evidence of petecheal haemorrhages then check the prothrombin time, platelet count, fibrin degradation products (FDP) level and fibrinogen level. This will confirm if DIC is present.

Radiographic examination of the abdomen may be diagnostically useful. In the majority of cases there is a ground glass appearance in the cranial abdomen, especially in the right epigastric region. The stomach will appear empty and gas-filled. Retention of barium in the stomach is common and laparotomy is often carried out because of suspect gastric outlet obstruction. The duodenum is often filled with gas and may have thickened walls, show irregular motility and be displaced to the right or dorsally on repeated exposure. Occasionally the colon will be displaced caudally.

Prognosis

With oedematous pancreatitis, clinical signs may not be observed because it may be subclinical. Such cases carry a reasonable prognosis, especially if the process of the pancreatic damage can be halted. With acute necrotizing pancreatitis as described above the prognosis is very guarded. Patients die from complications such as renal failure but alpha-2-macroglobulin deficiency is a major cause of death and is related to the amount of free trypsin in the circulation. If the patient survives the first 48 h, then recovery is likely. However in this initial period complications such as DIC, bacterial peritonitis, hypocalcaemia and irreversible shock may cause death.

After the initial period, recovery is likely but the prognosis is still guarded as subclinical pancreatitis may continue and ultimately result in exocrine pancreatic insufficiency and more rarely diabetes mellitus.

Treatment

The principal objectives in treatment of acute pancreatitis are: (1) to restore circulating volume, (2) to prevent further release of pancreatic enzyme, (3) to stop secondary infection establishing, (4) to control pain; and (5) dietary management.

Intravenous fluids are essential in the initial stages of treatment to counter the fluid loss from vomiting, diarrhoea, reduced cardiac output and shock. If the circulation can be re-established then improved tissue perfusion will reduce the perpetuating damage occurring in the pancreas. If blood-gas analysis is available then check for signs of metabolic acidosis which is frequently present due to tissue ischaemia. Correction can be achieved by using sodium bicarbonate 5% solution intravenously in amounts dependent on the degree of acidosis. Alternatively, as most practices rarely have access to blood-gas analysis, lactated Ringer's solution may be used. Equally essential is the transfusion of whole blood, as this not only restores circulatory volume but provides essential alpha-2-macroglobulin. It is important to remember that normal liver function is required to convert lactate to bicarbonate. Plasma expander (Haemmaccel; Hoechst Animal Health) may also be used initially to correct circulating volume and improve tissue perfusion followed by isotonic saline or lactated Ringer's solution.

In the first 5 days of treatment it is essential to prevent the intake of any food or water, as this may further stimulate release of pancreatic secretion (Strombeck & Feldman 1983). Parenteral feeding may be used if the patients appetite returns early. Intake of food stimulates the release of gastrin and cholecystokinin which in turn stimulates the release of enzyme-rich pancreatic secretion. In addition, the presence of acid chyme in the duodenum releases secretin which stimulates the pancreas to produce an alkaline secretion low in enzymes, and the sight, smell and taste of food stimulates enzyme release from the pancreas via the vagus nerve. Even gastric distention due to water will result in reflex secretion from the pancreas via the vagus nerve. Removal of gastric secretion via a nasogastric tube was often advocated but removed the negative feedback mechanism for gastrin production. The use of H2 blockers will prevent acid secretion in the stomach far more effectively, when used in combination with food withdrawal, and results in total shutdown of pancreatic secretion.

Anticholinergic drugs such as atropine sulphate have been suggested to stop pancreatic secretion. However, this only works when the vagus nerve is actively stimulating the pancreas. In addition, atropine reduces intestinal motility and may predispose to bacterial overgrowth, with possible reflux of infection up the pancreatic duct. Glucagon is also a powerful suppressor of pancreatic secretion, and it also stimulates the myocardium increasing cardiac output and improving tissue perfusion. The dose should be 0.3 mg/kg intravenously. Such injections will reduce enzyme secretion and pain. Insulin given at 0.5 iu/kg intravenously will suppress the action of lipase, thereby preventing fat necrosis and pain.

Antibiotics should always be given in cases of acute pancreatitis to counter any primary or secondary bacterial infection. Such infections are likely to be caused by Gram-negative enteric bacteria which often have a high degree of resistance. Use penicillin with gentamicin, ampicillin, potentiated amoxycillin or chloramphenicol (Hall *et al.* 1988).

Corticosteroids should be used with extreme care. They can initiate acute pancreatitis and may exacerbate the clinical signs. Use these drugs only when the animal appears to be approaching a severe shocked state, as a single bolus intravenously. Prednisolone at 6 to 10 mg/kg may be used. Reducing the effects of pain will reduce the shock. Do not use morphine as this causes closure of the sphincter in the pancreatic duct, effectively causing obstruction.

When hypocalcaemia is present use 10% calcium borogluconate giving 10 to 40 ml intravenously but slowly, depending on size. If septic peritonitis develops initiate peritoneal lavage using 500 ml of a balanced electrolyte solution with added penicillin and gentamycin for a 15 kg dog carried out three times daily.

Even though the patient's appetite may return early, food should be withheld until the serum amylase and lipase levels have returned to normal. Relapses occur if food is introduced too early in the convalescent period. Use a high carbohydrate, low fat and protein diet initially. Gradually introduce to a normal diet depending on the response. The use of medium-chain triglycerides will not stimulate pancreatic secretion and will ensure adequate energy levels and fat soluble vitamins can be administered after the initial period. Boiled rice is considered an excellent carbohydrate source in the early stages of introducing diet.

Chronic pancreatitis

This may also be referred to as relapsing pancreatitis or subclinical interstitial pancreatitis. The same aetiological factors are implicated here as were described in acute pancreatitis. The difference lies in the fact that there are repeated episodes, together with subclinical inflammation. It is thought to be quite common in dogs but often misdiagnosed as acute gastritis (Brobst 1980). Cats are also thought to be commonly affected (Draffell 1975), it is often an incidental finding at post mortem (Williams 1988).

The acute flareups together with subclinical 'smouldering' inflammation will frequently lead to total loss of exocrine tissue being replaced by fibrous tissue. Clinically this results in exocrine pancreatic insufficiency (Brobst 1980).

Clinical diagnosis

The clinical signs are dependent on the stage of chronic pancreatitis and the degree of inflammation actively occurring (Hardy & Johnson 1980). This may be defined by the presence of either polymorphonucleocytes or lymphocytes, plasma cells and macrophages. Acute episodes with anorexia, depression, dehydration, vomiting and diarrhoea, exactly as in acute pancreatitis do occur. In between these episodes the patient may appear clinically normal but have subclinical disease. Unless the clinician is very alert, a diagnosis of acute gastritis is often given, but careful examination of the history may reveal previous episodes of 'acute gastritis' which should advise the clinician to re-evaluate the case.

During the acute episodes the diagnostic procedures described under acute pancreatitis apply. Radiographs may reveal some changes although they may not be as clear in chronic pancreatitis. Where the case is being evaluated, pancreatic biopsy should be considered after recovery from an acute episode to determine if there is a progressive chronic pancreatitis present, but the risk of postbiopsy leakage should not be overlooked. Occasionally the pancreas may appear macroscopically normal, so always collect a biopsy sample. Equally, chronic pancreatitis and adenocarcinoma of the pancreas may appear similar, so a biopsy is essential (Williams 1988).

Treatment

The patient should be treated in a similar manner to that described for acute pancreatitis. However in this case, follow-up examinations should be carried out to ensure there is no progression as subclinical disease. Treatment should be continued if such a situation exists.

Pancreatic neoplasia

Neoplasia which may involve the endocrine or the exocrine pancreas is not common in the dog and cat. Exocrine tumours are thought to be more common in the Poodle and Airedale Terrier breeds and certainly from middle age onwards. If it does ocur then usually this involves a highly malignant carcinoma of the acinar or duct cells. The tumours grow rapidly, initially show no clinical signs, and spread to the duodenum and liver initially and thereafter to the lungs. Histological examination of pancreatic tissue usually confirms a malignant character and reveals loss of functional exocrine tissue. There is normally no loss of endocrine function in these tumours.

Clinical diagnosis

The signs associated with adenocarcinoma of the pancreas are variable but are often sudden in onset and rapidly fatal. Occasionally the patient may only exhibit anorexia and weight-loss. The tumour is usually extensive before the animal shows obvious signs of ill health, often with metastasis to other tissues such as the liver and lungs and this results in a short postdiagnostic course.

Onset of vomiting, anorexia and weight-loss may be sudden. Abdominal pain may be seen and a large irregular mass in the cranial abdomen may be detected. Diarrhoea may occur with the production of bulky fatty faeces indicating exocrine failure. Indeed one clinical case report was presented with signs of exocrine pancreatic insufficiency rather than vomiting and anorexia (Bright 1985). Jaundice will frequently occur at some stage but only once the bile duct becomes obstructed (Perman & Stevens 1969).

Diagnosis is often based on clinical findings together with evidence of a radiodense mass on X-ray examination of the abdomen. If ascites is present then cytological examination may confirm the diagnosis as tumour cells may exfoliate. In many cases definitive diagnosis is reached following exploratory laparotomy where the extent of the tumour can also be assessed.

Treatment

Unfortunately in most cases by the time clinical signs are observed there is metastatic spread to other organs. This makes the prognosis extremely guarded. Even where the tumour is removed early the actual process of removal may stimulate any remaining cells to grow more vigorously. In such cases chemotherapy may be considered, together with replacement enzyme therapy and dietary management as for exocrine pancreatic insufficiency.

Exocrine pancreatic insufficiency (EPI)

The terms maldigestion, malabsorption and malassimilation have been used to refer to exocrine pancreatic insufficiency. This has led to considerable confusion as to whether failure of enzymic digestion has occurred or whether there is lack of absorption across the small intestinal mucosa. By definition, EPI is a maldigestive process although it is now accepted that EPI and small intestinal disease are considered together as malabsorption. EPI is considered to be the commonest cause of malabsorption in dogs, although it is very rare in cats (Williams 1988, Hoskins *et al.* 1983). Loss of exocrine tissue may be congenital, including juvenile atrophy and pancreatic hypoplasia or acquired following repeated episodes of pancreatitis. The former is most frequently observed in dogs, and postnatal atrophy is thought to occur in most cases. Although EPI may be hereditary in the German Shepherd, due to an

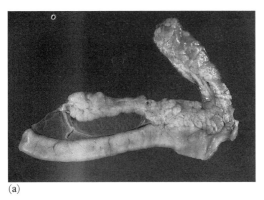 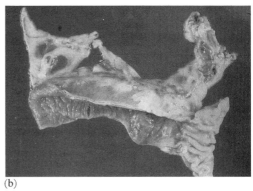

(a)   (b)

Fig. 8.3 Macroscopic appearance of (a) the normal canine pancreas with that of (b) a dog with exocrine pancreatic insufficiency.

autonomal recessive gene (Westermark 1980), in cats the few cases recorded are likely to be secondary to relapsing pancreatitis (Hoskins *et al.* 1983).

In cats there is no obvious breed or sex predisposition to EPI (Hoskins *et al.* 1983). However the condition is more commonly seen in large breeds of dog especially German Shepherds, Irish Setters and Rough Collies, and it is rare to observe the condition in the small breeds. There is no sex predisposition. Diagnosis of canine EPI is often made between 1 and 5 years of age, although cases may occur in the older age group secondary to pancreatitis.

As with other glands the pancreas has a large functional reserve and has good powers of regeneration, even following acute pancreatitis. Clinical signs only occur after 80 to 90% of the exocrine tissue is lost. Some extra-pancreatic digestion occurs in the stomach and small intestine and this may assist digestion in individual cases but ultimately marked weight loss develops in all cases.

The classical signs of EPI are very similar to small intestinal disease making differentiation between the two conditions very difficult on clinical grounds alone. The same breeds tend to be affected by either condition, providing another difficulty in recognition.

In spite of the major loss of exocrine tissue seen in EPI (Fig. 8.3) there is very rarely any sign of endocrine dysfunction in the congenital form. However those cases which arise following chronic pancreatitis may have signs of diabetes mellitus as well as EPI. The breed incidence is also different in this group, and may include dogs of the smaller breeds.

The diarrhoea associated with EPI is caused by two mechanisms: (1) the inability of the dog to utilize ingested food which remains in the intestine and causes an osmotic diarrhoea. Consequently the faeces are bulky because of the presence of undigested food and additional water; and (2) undigested fat is broken down by bacteria in the colon to produce hydroxy fatty acids which cause a secretory diarrhoea.

It is quite common for dogs with EPI to have bacterial overgrowth causing physical damage to the villous structure and impairing production of brush border enzymes of the small intestine. These changes reduce even further the ability to handle ingested food and add to the weight-loss. This may be described as secondary small intestinal disease associated with EPI.

Clinical diagnosis

Dogs with EPI develop normally in the first year of life with occasional bouts of diarrhoea. There then follows a period of time when in spite of a good appetite the dog begins to lose weight. As this develops, all the clinical signs associated with EPI become apparent.

Classically, dogs with EPI are presented with three major symptoms; weight-loss which can be up to 40% of body weight, ravenous appetite and diarrhoea. The dogs are almost invariably described as bright, alert and keen to exercise. The coat is dull and the skin scurfy and dry. The faeces are usually bulky, cow pat in form, and greasy in appearance. Borborygmi and flatus are common, as is coprophagia. Owners may report the presence of recognizable undigested food in the faeces. Vomiting is occasionally reported but is usually intermittent and variably associated with feeding. The authors have occasionally collected histories of marked polydipsia.

The differential diagnosis of weight-loss and polyphagia is large, and for this reason it is important to carry out a thorough investigation (see Chapter 7). Urine and faeces should be examined together with a blood profile. Routine haematology and serum chemistry often reveal little of significance in EPI. Cholesterol and triglyceride may be lower than normal. There should be no evidence of hypoproteinaemia and liver function should be normal. Changes in serum folate and B12 may indicate the presence of bacterial overgrowth, which is common in EPI. Xylose absorption is usually normal, although quantitative fat absorption is often poor (Simpson & Doxey 1983). Repeating this test with added lipase results in a marked increase in serum triglyceride levels.

Faecal analysis can be of great value as a screening procedure if carried out correctly. It is important the dog is on a standard diet of tinned meat and biscuit, and that at least two faecal samples are thoroughly examined. Each sample should be checked for bacterial pathogens, worm eggs, the presence of undigested food and trypsin. Where pathogenic bacteria or worm eggs are detected, treatment should be carried out and the dog reassessed at a later date. Microscopic examination of faeces involves making light faecal smears on microscope slides. The presence of starch is indicated by black granules following staining with Lugol's iodine, and fat is indicated by staining with Sudan IV (Fig. 8.4). Various methods have been employed to measure faecal trypsin. The authors use the gelatin tube test (Simpson & Doxey 1988) because it is simple and cheap to carry out and provides suitable results. To overcome any false results with the trypsin digest test, the results must be considered together with the results of the microscopic examination. Exocrine pancreatic insufficiency is likely where the trypsin digest titre is nil and there is evidence of undigested starch and fat (Simpson & Doxey 1988).

Having screened the dog for possible EPI, a definitive diagnosis can now be made by measuring a fasted TLI value. Normal dogs and those with small intestinal disease will have normal TLI values, in excess of 5 µg/l. Dogs with EPI have TLI values of less than 2.5 µg/l (Williams & Batt 1983). Previously the N-benzoyl-L-tyrosyl-p-aminobenzoic acid (BT-PABA) test was used to determine if EPI was present, but this has proved difficult to interpret in some cases as the absorption of PABA may be influenced by small intestinal disease as well as EPI (Batt & Mann 1981).

Very rarely, the TLI value and the pancreas may be normal in a dog showing signs of enzyme deficiency. This can occur due to congenital enterokinase deficiency, small intestinal disease causing a reduction in cholecystokinin and secretin secretion, or following individual enzyme deficiency states. Finally, in Zollinger−Ellison syndrome where excess gastrin leads to excess acid, there is inactivation of intestinal and pancreatic enzymes (Williams 1988).

Treatment

In our experience, failure in treating EPI is a consequence of too much

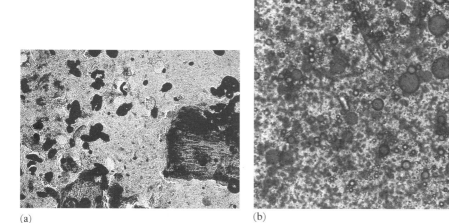

(a)   (b)

Fig. 8.4 The appearance of (a) starch granules, and (b) fat globules following staining of faeces from a dog with EPI.

attention being paid to the use of replacement enzyme therapy and too little attention to dietary management. Owners must be advised about the need for strict dietary control and the importance of not feeding tit-bits or altering the diet from day-to-day. Treatment is carried out in three stages: (1) to correct the diarrhoea and bacterial overgrowth, (2) to increase the diet intake to obtain maintenance and growth without inducing diarrhoea; and (3) to satisfy the dogs appetite. Any attempt to carry out the treatment in any other order than that described above will fail. For example it is impossible to expect a dog with EPI to gain weight by feeding large amounts of food while it still has diarrhoea and bacterial overgrowth.

Diet formulation is the most important initial step in treatment. Ideally a prescription diet such as Hills i/d or Waltham low fat diet should be used. Homemade diets should be avoided as they are rarely consistent from day-to-day. No tit-bits must be given, a constraint which is very difficult to achieve as the dogs are always very hungry and may steal food. Initially, feed the prescription diet at the minimum recommended by the manufacturer divided into two meals per day. Once the dog passes normal formed faeces the amount of food may be increased slowly. If required, a vitamin/mineral supplement may also be added to the prescription diet.

Pancreatic enzyme replacement should be added to the food either as a tablet, powder or granules (Pancrex V; Paines & Byrne). The tablets are enteric-coated while the powder has no protection against gastric acid. The granules have some degree of enteric coating and have been used most frequently by the authors. Give one teaspoonful of granules per 100 g food. There is no advantage in increasing the amount of enzyme as it is expensive and provides no improvement in response. Further protection of the enzyme granules may be provided by giving 4 mg/kg cimetidine (Tagamet; SmithKline Beecham Pharmaceuticals) orally about one-half hour before feeding. This reduces gastric acid production and will assist in protecting the enzyme supplement in food (Simpson 1988).

In addition to this treatment, the dog should also receive 20 to 40 mg/kg of tylosin (Tylan; Elanco Products) orally to treat the bacterial overgrowth. The combination of tylosin and dietary management will rapidly suppress bacterial growth and restore small intestinal function.

Once the dog starts to pass normal faeces, the amount fed each day can be increased, together with the amount of enzyme replacer, until the animal starts to gain weight. There is normally a maximum amount of food each individual dog will tolerate, even with enzyme replacer, before diarrhoea recurs. It is therefore better to find the maximum tolerated by the dog and allow weight gain to occur slowly than to try and obtain a quick response to treatment, which often fails. Once the dog regains its normal body weight, the appetite returns to normal, the dog will be more settled and the coat and skin condition improves. The author has noted female dogs which have failed to come into season start to cycle normally again.

Once the dog has returned to normal body weight, the amount of food and enzyme replacer may be reduced to that required simply to maintain weight. This reduces costs and maintains the improvement sought by the owner. Any sudden recurrence of diarrhoea usually follows access to extra food and should be treated by total withdrawal of food for 24 h.

References

Anderson N.V. (1973) Review of literature: Pancreas. *Journal of American Animal Hospital Association*, **9**; 89–100.

Batt R.M. & Mann L.C. (1981) Specificity of the BT-PABA test for the diagnosis of exocrine pancreatic insufficiency in the dog. *Veterinary Record*, **108**; 303–307.

Bright J. McI. (1985) Pancreatic adenocarcinoma in a dog with a maldigestion syndrome. *Journal of American Veterinary Medical Association*, **187**; 420–421.

Brobst D.F. (1980) Pancreatic function. In: *Clinical Biochemistry of Domestic Animals*. J.J. Kaneko (ed.), Academic Press, New York, 259–281.

Cornelius L.M. (1976) Laboratory diagnosis of acute pancreatitis and pancreatic adeno-carcinoma. *Veterinary Clinics of North America*, **6**; 671–685.

Creutzfeldt W. & Schmidt H. (1970) Aetiology and pathogenesis of pancreatitis. *Scandinavian Journal of Gastroenterology*, **5**; Supplement 6; 47–62.

Draffell, S.J. (1975) Some aspects of pancreatic disease in the cat. *Journal of Small Animal Pratice*, **16**; 365–374.

Drazner F.H. (1982) Clinical implications of disseminated intravascular coagulation. *Compendium on Continuing Education for the Practicing Veterinarian*, **4**; 974–982.

Drazner F.H. (1986) Diseases of the pancreas. In: *Canine and Feline Gastroenterology*. B.D. Jones (ed.), W.B. Saunders, Philadelphia, 295–344.

Hardy R.M. & Johnson G.F. (1980) The Pancreas. In: *Veterinary Gastroenterology*. N.V. Anderson (ed.), Lea & Febiger, Philadelphia, 621–650.

Hall J.A., Macy D.W. & Husted P.W. (1988) Acute canine pancreatitis. *Compendium on Continuing Education for the Practicing Veterinarian*, **10**; 403–416.

Hoskins J.D., Turk J.R. & Turk M.A. (1983) Feline pancreatic insufficiency. *Veterinary Medicine and Small Animal Clinics*, **77**; 1745–1748.

Neuman N.B. (1975) Acute pancreatic haemorrhage associated with iatrogenic hypercalcaemia in a dog. *Journal of American Veterinary Medical Association*, **166**; 381–383.

Owens J.M., Drazner F.H. & Gilberton S.R. (1975) Pancreatic disease in the cat. *Journal of American Animal Hospital Association*, **11**; 83–89.

Perman V. & Stevens J.B. (1969) Clinical evaluation of the acinar pancreas of the dog. *Journal of American Veterinary Medical Association*, **155**; 2053–2058.

Simpson J.W. (1988) Treatment of canine exocrine pancreatic insufficiency. *Veterinary Practice*, **20**; 5.

Simpson J.W. & Doxey D.L. (1988) Evaluation of faecal analysis as an aid to the detection of exocrine pancreatic insufficiency. *British Veterinary Journal*, **144**; 174–178.

Simpson J.W. & Doxey D.L. (1983) Quantitative assessment of fat absorption and its diagnostic value in exocrine pancreatic insufficiency. *Research in Veterinary Science*, **35**; 249–251.

Strombeck D.R., Faver T.F. & Kaneko J.J. (1981) Serum amylase and lipase activities in the diagnosis of pancreatitis in dogs. *American Journal of Veterinary Research*, **42**; 1966–1970.

Strombeck D.R. & Feldman B.F. (1983) Acute pancreatitis. In: *Current Veterinary Therapy VIII*, R.W. Kirk (ed.), W.B. Saunders, Philadelphia, 810–812.

Westermark E. (1980) The hereditary nature of canine pancreatic degenerative atrophy in the German Shepherd dog. *Acta Veterinaria Scandinavica*, **21**; 389–394.

Williams D.A. (1987) New tests of pancreatic and small intestinal function. *Compendium on Continuing Education for the Practicing Veterinarian*, **9**; 1167–1175.

Williams D.A. (1988) Exocrine pancreatic disease. In: *Proceedings of a course in Small Animal Gastroenterology and nutrition*. New Zealand Veterinary Association, 199–224.

Williams D.A. & Batt R.M. (1983) Diagnosis of canine exocrine pancreatic insufficiency by the assay of serum trypsin-like immunoreactivity. *Journal of Small Animal Practice*, **24**; 583–588.

9/Diseases of the Liver

Introduction

The liver is a vital body organ and is the largest gland in the body. It performs many functions which are essential for life and is the core organ for metabolic activity, providing a factory, storage depot, quality control unit and waste processing plant in one structure.

The organ has great functional capacity and many tissue insults can be tolerated without upsetting normal function or causing clinically manifest disease. This is largely attributable to the marked regenerative ability of hepatic tissue, principally through hepatocyte hyperplasia.

There is an important difference between a state of hepatic damage and liver failure. Liver damage does not necessarily result in clinically apparent disease. The use of the term liver failure, on the other hand, implies a serious dysfunction with clinical implications. It is the complexity and interdependence of liver function, together with the ability to withstand different levels of severity of insult, which makes clinical diagnosis of hepatic disease difficult. These problems arise for one or more of the following reasons;

1   Specific signs of early hepatic dysfunction or insult are difficult to detect and this means that an affected animal is often seriously ill at the time of first presentation for clinical examination. By the same token, liver lesions may be widespread in the organ or advanced by the time animals are clinically ill.

2   Hepatic disease presents a difficult differential diagnostic situation on many occasions. This is because the liver condition may be primary or secondary in origin and consequently clinical features may not necessarily indicate hepatic disease.

3   The diagnosis and assessment of liver disease relies heavily on the use of ancillary biochemical and enzyme assays concurrent with clinical assessment. However such assays by themselves do not always give an indication of the type of hepatic disease and its severity. Furthermore, no single test specifically defines a lesion.

Hepatic anatomy

The liver develops from a number of embryonic precursors. The bulk of the organ comprises cords of hepatocytes which are derived from mesenchyme.

The intrahepatic bile ducts form from differentiated elements of the hepatocytes whilst the extrahepatic bile ducts are derived from gut endoderm.

In both the adult dog and cat the liver lies immediately caudal to and partly in contact with the diaphragm. It is located well under the costal arch and topographically extends as far cranially as the level of the seventh rib. On the right side, the rib cage completely shields the organ laterally but on the left side the left lateral lobe extends slightly beyond the caudoventral border of the costal arch. This area is therefore available for palpation but is not easily detected in obese animals and muscular dogs.

The liver is a multi-lobed crescent-shaped organ which is convex cranially against the diaphragm. It weighs 127 to 1350 g in dogs whilst the feline liver ranges in weight from 70 to 80 g; there are exceptions at either end of the ranges. The organ is broadly divided into left and right lobes with smaller caudate, papillary and quadrate lobes (Fig. 9.1).

The gall bladder lies between the quadrate and right central lobe in both species. In the dog there is a common bile duct which extends from the gall bladder to the duodenum and is separate from the major pancreatic duct. In some dogs a smaller minor pancreatic duct may join the common bile duct at or just proximal to the papilla of Vater in the duodenal mucosa. The feline major pancreatic duct joins the single common bile duct prior to entry to the duodenum.

The liver is encapsulated in a thin elastic membrane (Glisson's capsule) giving it normally a smooth surface. The hepatic parenchyma consists of multitudinous cords of hepatocytes supported by a thin reticulin scaffolding

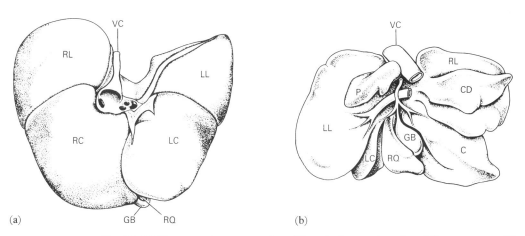

(a)   (b)

Fig. 9.1 (a) Diagrammatic representation of liver diaphragmatic surface. VC = vena cava, GB = gall bladder, RQ = right quadrate lobe, RC = right central lobe, RL = right lateral lobe, LC = left central lobe, LL = left lateral lobe. (b) Liver visceral surface. LL = left lateral lobe, LC = left central lobe, P = papillary lobe, RQ = quadrate lobe, GB = gall bladder, C = central lobe, CD = caudate lobe, RL = right lateral lobe.

which forms a network of vascular endothelial-lined channels (sinusoids) between hepatocyte cords. Scattered along the sinusoids are fixed macrophages, the Kupffer cells. There is a small space between the endothelial lining cells and the hepatocytes; this is occupied by thin collagen fibres and prelymph fluid. These spaces of Disse also harbour fat-storing Ito cells (Fig. 9.2). Running along the external cell walls of hepatocytes are the bile canniculi which join larger bile ducts and the latter eventually empty into the gall bladder via major bile ducts.

As befits its major metabolic functions, the liver has a well-developed vascular system. Arterial blood supply is via the hepatic artery from the aorta (30% of the total blood to the liver). The hepatic portal vein carries blood (70% of the total blood to the liver) from the stomach, small intestine and spleen to the liver. Smaller branches of these vessels are supported in the portal tracts alongside the bile ducts and eventually empty into the sinusoids (Fig. 9.2). Drainage is via the central veins in the centre of the hepatic lobules; these central veins drain into hepatic veins which empty into the caudal vena cava as it traverses the dorsal border of the liver. More focal areas of collagen support blood vessels and intrahepatic bile ducts and these constitute so-called portal tracts.

Concepts of liver microanatomy

The traditional view of the arrangement of hepatocellular parenchyma has been the hepatic lobule based on patterns of sinusoidal blood flow (Kiernan

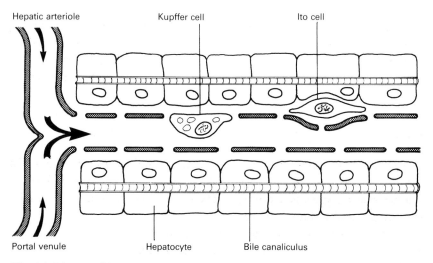

Fig. 9.2 Diagram of hepatic sinusoid microanatomy.

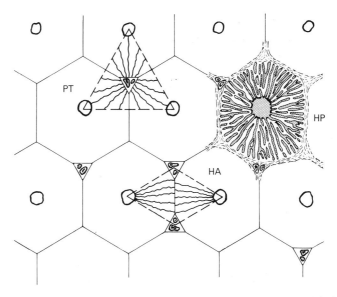

Fig. 9.3 Diagram illustrating concepts of hepatic microarchitecture. HP = hepatic lobule, PT = portal triad, HA = hepatic acinus.

1833). This consists of a hexagonal unit of hepatic cells formed from three-dimensional radiating hepatocyte cords and sinusoids draining into the central vein with hepatic portal venules, hepatic arterioles and bile ducts clustered at the edge of the lobule in the portal tracts.

An alternative model makes the portal triad the central feature based on the bile-secreting function of the liver. This model places the portal triad at the centre of the triangle with the central veins constituting the apices of the triangle.

A more recent concept has been that of the hepatic acinus based on the relative distribution of blood to hepatocytes, i.e. it is a vascular unit (Rappaport 1975). This is a less-easily visualized unit but has been used to explain the reactions observed in hepatotoxicity. These units are shown in Fig. 9.3.

Normal liver function

The liver plays an important role in a number of vital body functions. In addition to the major role of metabolic regulation, the liver is important in synthesizing enzymes and proteins. There are three main areas of activity with direct clinical implications:
1 Metabolic regulation in maintenance of homeostasis.
2 Processing of absorbed substances from the gut.
3 Bile metabolism and excretion.

Central metabolic regulation

A major role played by the liver is in carbohydrate regulation. In positive energy balance, excess glucose is processed and stored as glycogen in hepatocytes. In some situations, excess carbohydrates may be metabolized to fatty acids. In negative energy balance the glycogen stores are converted to glucose. In addition, in the latter situation the liver plays an important role in provision of glucose through gluconeogenesis.

Protein substances are deaminated in the liver. Excess amino acids may be converted to fatty acids. Excess amines or ammonia from these metabolic breakdown reactions are converted to urea prior to renal excretion.

Lipids are also metabolized and controlled in part by the liver. In carnivores the handling of fatty acid breakdown products is important since these species do not tolerate accumulations of ketone bodies.

An important liver function is in the synthesis of plasma proteins, particularly albumin and globulin. The liver is also responsible for maintaining adequate levels of proteins involved in blood coagulation (prothrombin and fibrinogen).

Vitamin synthesis occurs in the liver. Precursors of B vitamins are synthesized by hepatocytes together with precursors of active vitamin D (2,5-dihydroxycholecalciferol). There is evidence that vitamin A is also stored in the liver.

The liver plays a vital role in the biotransformation of excess hormones, drugs and many other toxic substances, by rendering them less lipid-soluble and therefore less able to enter cells. Cell debris, bacteria and their toxins may also be eliminated from the circulating blood by Kupffer cell activity.

The cat differs from the dog in liver metabolic activity in two important respects. Firstly, in the cat there is a relatively low level of glucuronyl transferase which makes the cat less able to metabolize and inactivate salicylate and acetaminaphen drugs. Secondly, the feline liver cannot synthesize arginine, an amino acid which is important in the conversion of ammonia to the excretory product urea.

Bile metabolism

The liver has a fundamental role in dealing with the products of haem breakdown through the mechanisms of bile formation and secretion. This process is summarized in Fig. 9.4. It depends on the uptake, conjugation and storage of bile pigments (bilirubin) by hepatocytes, followed by excretion as bile.

Bilirubin is produced from the haem fraction of haemoglobin in reticulo-endothelial cells, particularly in splenic red pulp. It is a fat-soluble substance which binds loosely to plasma albumin and is transported to the liver as

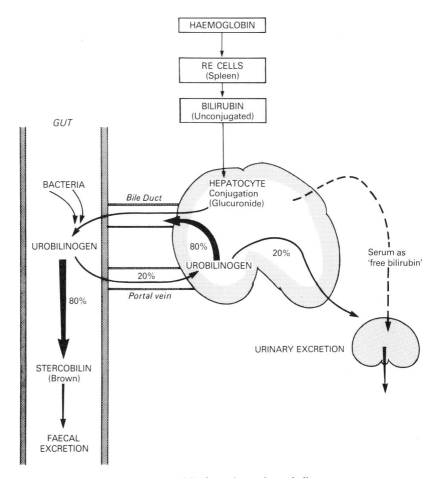

Fig. 9.4 Diagram to illustrate normal bile formation and metabolism.

free, or indirect bilirubin. In the hepatocyte, bilirubin is conjugated with glucuronic acid to form water-soluble glucuronide known as direct bilirubin. This direct bilirubin is secreted into the bile and stored in the gall bladder with bile salts, cholesterol, bicarbonate, chemical wastes and water prior to secretion into the duodenum.

In the small intestine most of the bilirubin glucuronide is converted enzymatically to urobilinogen and then oxidized by bacteria to urobilin (stercobilin), a brown fluid. Approximately 20% of the urobilinogen is resorbed from the intestine and re-excreted in bile. Some urobilinogen (20%) is excreted in the urine following vascular transport. Low levels of direct bilirubin are normally excreted in the canine urine but not in feline urine.

Bile salts are formed from cholesterol products. Primary bile salts (cholic and chenodeoxycholic acids) are conjugated with sodium and potassium salts of glycholic and taurocholic acids in the gall bladder. These bile salts are stored in the gall bladder until released under the influences of vagal activity and cholecystokinin. The latter is released from the duodenal mucosal cells when lipids are present in the intestine. Bile salts provide the correct environment for the emulsification and hence absorption of ingested fats.

Pathophysiology states

Clinical signs of liver disease often reflect a defect or inadequacy of one or more of the physiological functions described above and reference may be made to a temporary or permanent stoppage in one part of the factory rather than total closure. This leads to the concept of restricted impairments rather than total failure; the former can be minimized by clinical intervention and will often be amenable to therapy whilst the latter has serious prognostic implications. Depending on the relative importance of the factory unit involved, the impairment may be of more or less clinical significance.

Disturbance of bilirubin excretion

Disturbance of normal bilirubin excretion usually leads to excessive circulating levels of bilirubin and this is seen as jaundice, a yellow staining of the mucosae, skin and organs depending on severity. Three types of jaundice are recognized; prehepatic (haemolytic), hepatic and posthepatic (obstructive). Assay of the relative levels of free and conjugated bilirubin levels give a guide as to the pathogenesis of the jaundice but marked ratio changes are needed to be truly meaningful (see Chapter 10). Clinically jaundice is observed if the total serum bilirubin level exceeds 35 μmol/l. It has to be stated, however, that serum bilirubin levels alone are not sensitive indicators of hepatic damage.

Cholestasis

Retention of bile results in retention of cholesterol and bile salts in addition to bilirubin. This leads to interference in fat digestion in the small intestine. Bile acids may spill over into the circulation and serum bile acid assay provides the basis for an additional assessment of liver function (see Chapter 10). Cholestasis may be intrahepatic or extrahepatic, the latter associated with pancreatic disease or abnormalities of tissues in the proximity of the common bile duct. Cholestasis seems to be less common in the dog than in the cat (Hornbuckle & Allan 1980).

Inadequate ammonia metabolism (hepatic encephalopathy)

Failure to detoxify ammonia produced by bacterial activity in the intestine and deamination of amino acids leads to raised blood ammonia. The raised ammonia leads to neurological signs such as fits, blindness, abnormal behaviour and ataxia.

Depressed protein synthesis

A serious manifestation of depression in hepatic protein synthesis is the development of bleeding syndromes associated with deficiencies of prothrombin and fibrinogen. Clotting factors may be absent or reduced in amount. Inadequate albumin levels may result in fluid imbalances and generalized subcutaneous oedema and ascites. Other proteins (ceruloplasmin and macroglobulin) are involved in transport of metallic ions and iron transport may be deficient, leading to anaemia.

Disturbances in glucose metabolism

Serious fluctuations in glucose levels may occur; the most significant is hypoglycaemia leading to lethargy and serious neurological signs.

Drug and chemical metabolism

Liver disease may often lead to failure or depression of drug oxidation/reduction and glucuronide conjugation. This may lead to enhanced or persistent drug reactions and in part explains idiosyncratic reactions in liver disease (Wilke 1984).

Portal hypertension and ascites

Normal portal venous pressure is low; any condition which increases resistance to portal blood flow produces portal hypertension.

Prehepatic portal hypertension is rare in the dog and cat. It is rarely seen where there is extravascular pressure from adjacent abdominal space-occupying lesions such as tumours and abscesses or organ displacements. Portal vein thrombosis is very rare in dogs and cats.

Intrahepatic hypertension is not uncommon; it is usually associated with diffuse liver disease such as fibrosis.

Posthepatic hypertension is caused by impeding drainage in the post-hepatic caudal vena cava or hepatic veins. The most common cause in the dog is chronic congestive heart failure although this is less common in cats. Ascites may be associated with intrahepatic and posthepatic portal venous

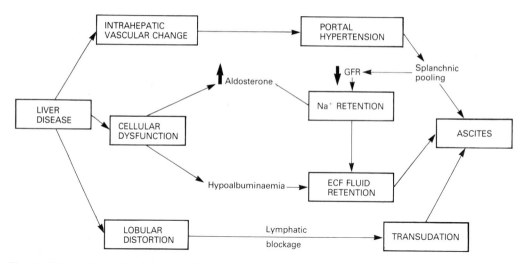

Fig. 9.5 Diagram illustrating formation of ascites as a result of liver disease. GFR = glomerular filtration rate, ECF = extra cellular fluid.

hypertension. However the development of ascites in liver failure is not solely related to a hypertensive mechanism; derangements of sodium and fluid balance and hypoalbuminaemia also play important roles (Fig. 9.5).

The spectrum of liver lesions

The range of clinical signs associated with liver malfunction is very wide and often the same symptoms may be caused by very different lesions. There is much that is not understood in the pathogenesis of liver lesions in the dog and cat but some broad categories of liver disease can be defined as follows.

Hepatic necrosis

This type of change may be acute or chronic, both in terms of pathological change and time course.

Acute necrosis refers to focal or more extensive destruction of liver tissues. Extreme and diffuse change produces irrevocable liver failure. Different patterns of acute necrosis have been identified: (1) zonal necrosis or centrilobular necrosis, which in terms of acinar units is periacinar in distribution; and (2) massive necrosis which implies a more serious and widespread change, with death of hepatocytes and disruption of stromal architecture. Acute forms of necrosis are most commonly associated with adverse drug reactions or toxic chemicals but severe viral or bacterial infection can cause such changes.

Chronic necrosis is more insidious, lower grade in nature and occurs over a more prolonged time. There is a progressive loss of viable hepatic tissue but attempted healing also occurs. This results in a distorted organ comprising areas of regenerative hyperplastic hepatocytes and irregular scar (fibrous) tissue. This type of chronic change is usually associated with prolonged or repeated exposure to low grade or insidious hepatotoxic agents.

Hepatitis

Inflammation of the liver may often be accompanied by necrotic change but unlike the necrosis above there is an acute or more chronic, sometimes persistent, inflammatory cell response. Where the condition is persistent or insidious then attempts at healing occur and fibrosis may coexist alongside more active inflammatory areas. Chronic hepatitis has been reported with increasing frequency in both dogs (Hardy 1986) and cats (Center 1986).

This type of disease is associated with infectious bacterial or viral agents but other agents (e.g. copper) may also be involved. Hepatitis is sometimes used as a blanket term where the true aetiology and pathogenesis of liver disease is uncertain.

Cholangitis/cholangiohepatitis

Inflammation of the biliary duct system (cholangitis) may also involve the hepatic parenchyma to varying degrees (cholangiohepatitis) as a result of involvement of peribiliary hepatocytes.

The inflammatory changes may be acute or chronic. The former are often thought to be associated with ascending infections from the gut in dogs (Hendricks et al. 1980) and may result in cholestasis and jaundice (Rogers & Cornelius 1985). A true chronic condition occurs in cats but the aetiology is not fully understood. An intestinal reflux or infection does not appear to be a major aetiological factor (Center 1986) although other authorities disagree (Hirsh & Doige 1983, Zawie & Garvey 1984).

Lipidosis

Excessive hepatocyte storage of triglyceride produces fatty change in the liver. The presence of small amounts of fat does not seem to depress liver function per se, particularly in dogs, although excessive accumulations result in reduction of sinusoidal blood and bile flow. This type of change is usually reversible although idiopathic lipidosis in cats is more serious (Cornelius & Jacobs 1989) and the fatty change seen in diabetes mellitus is indicative of severe ketone body accumulations.

Fatty infiltration occurs in obese animals and is characterized by storage of fat in Ito cells rather than hepatocytes. This change does not interfere with liver function.

Vascular anomalies

Vascular anomalies of the hepatic system are characterized by shunting blood away from the portal vein thereby reducing perfusion. These abnormal routes may be congenital in origin or acquired. The anomalies are most commonly seen in young dogs and are more unusual in cats. The usual congenital types have a connection between the portal vein and the caudal vena cava or the azygos vein. In the acquired conditions the shunts are often multiple, smaller, tortuous accessory veins draining to the spleen, kidney and colon.

Affected animals are often presented as stunted individuals with neurological symptoms resulting from hepatic encephalopathy.

Neoplasia

Primary hepatic tumours are uncommon in dogs and rare in cats (Center 1986). Benign hepatomas in dogs may be incidental necropsy findings with no reported clinical symptoms although large masses may lead to intra-abdominal compression. In the authors' experience malignant primary tumours are also uncommon, with the possible exception of cholangiocarcinoma in the cat.

In contrast, multifocal secondary neoplasia following lymphohaematogenous metastasis from malignant tumours elsewhere is common in both species. The liver is also frequently involved in lymphosarcoma or leukaemia.

Clinical signs of liver disease

Dogs and cats with liver abnormalities often present with either a wide variety of clinical symptoms or vague and non-specific signs. An initial presenting symptom may be misleading and liver disease may masquerade as malfunction of another body organ system. Hepatic encephalopathy is a classic example of this situation where the presenting symptoms are neurological.

Affected animals may have had disease progression for a number of days without the owner detecting changes.

Any dog or cat presenting with one or more symptoms of anorexia, vomiting, diarrhoea and/or weight-loss where there is no obvious explanation should be regarded as a potential liver abnormality case. More specific signs such as jaundice and ascites indicate the presence of serious or advanced liver abnormality.

Vomiting is commonly associated with acute necrosis and hepatitis and less commonly with chronic disease. The swelling of the liver with stretching of its capsule as a result of tissue destruction is thought to induce reflex vomiting through the vagus nerve. In addition, where there is massive necrosis, or in chronic states, toxicity also leads to vomiting.

Weight-loss is seen in chronic liver disease and this is probably related to the failure of the metabolic and synthesizing functions of the organ, particularly with regard to protein synthesis and carbohydrate metabolism. In addition, where bile formation and secretion are abnormal then fat digestion will be upset.

Changes in faecal character are commonly associated with liver malfunctions. These include changes in consistency and colour. Where there is blockage of the bile flow into the duodenum there is lack of bile pigment and stercobilin resulting in paler than normal faeces. If there is excessive bile secretion/excretion, then faecal colour may be more orange or darker. Diarrhoea is thought to be caused by marginal steatorrhoea following upset in fat absorption in the face of reduced bile secretion. Acholic faeces is a useful indicator of the presence of liver disease.

Hepatic encephalopathy is not uncommon in severe liver disease or accompanying vascular anomalies in young animals (Zawie & Garvey 1984). Grand mal fits, apparent blindness, behavioural changes, circling and ataxia

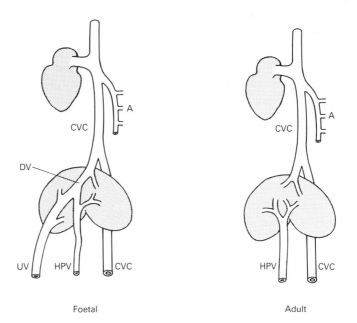

Foetal   Adult

Fig. 9.6(a) Diagrams of fetal and adult hepatic venous drainage. A = azygos vein, CVC = common and caudal vena cava, DV = ductus venosus, UV = umbilical vein, HPV = hepatic portal vein.

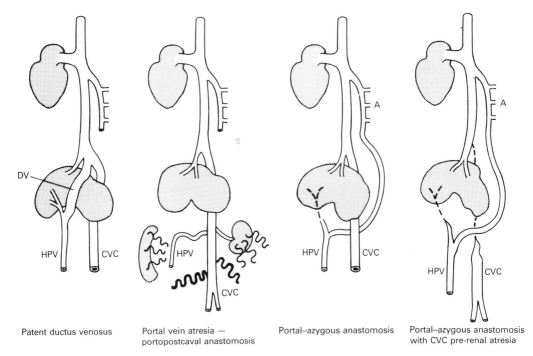

Patent ductus venosus | Portal vein atresia — portopostcaval anastomosis | Portal–azygous anastomosis | Portal–azygous anastomosis with CVC pre-renal atresia

Fig. 9.6(b) Diagrams of congenital and acquired portosystemic anastomoses. HPV = hepatic portal vein, DV = ductus venosus, CVC = common and caudal vena cava.

with compulsive walking may occur. These symptoms arise as a sequel to the high ammonia levels in the general circulation following shunting past the liver parenchyma (Fig. 9.6).

Upsets in normal urine production and character often accompany liver disease. Some of the reasons for these changes remain unclear but deranged urea and ammonia metabolism play key roles. The presence of glucosuria and ketonuria may be associated with some forms of liver damage but these phenomena are seen in other diseases, notably diabetes mellitus and hyper-adrenocorticism. The clinician should therefore by wary of overinterpreting such changes in terms of liver disease. Similarly, whilst the cat does not normally excrete conjugated bilirubin in urine, the dog does and so the detection of urinary bilirubin should be regarded in the light of this knowledge.

The presence of jaundice is always an indicator of serious disease of either prehepatic, hepatic or posthepatic origin (Rogers & Cornelius 1985, Meyer & Center 1986). Assessment of levels of total serum and urine bilirubin and particularly the ratio of conjugated to unconjugated are mandatory (Table 9.1).

An additional sign of serious liver impairment is the presence of ascites or more generalized oedema. However many other causes of ascites exist

Table 9.1 Plasma and urine bilirubin levels associated with jaundice

Type and cause of jaundice	Plasma bilirubin levels	Urine bilirubin levels
Haemolytic (prehepatic):		
Leptospirosis	90% Unconjugated	↑ Conjugated
(*L. icterohaemorrhagiae*)	10% Conjugated	↑ Urobilinogen
Autoimmune haemolytic anaemia	i.e. ↑ Unconjugated	
Incompatible blood transfusion		
Haemobartonellosis		
Piroplasmosis		
Copper poisoning		
Hepatic (failure of bilirubin conjugation):		
Leptospirosis	Very variable	↑ Conjugated
Cirrhosis	Biopsy more useful	↑ Urobilinogen
Neoplasia (includes myeloid leukaemia)		
Infectious canine hepatitis		
Toxic hepatitis		
Toxoplasmosis		
Acute necrotizing pancreatitis		
Posthepatic (impaired bile excretion):		
Extrahepatic biliary obstruction	10% Unconjugated	↑ Conjugated
Cholestasis (+ cholelithiasis)	90% Conjugated	No or reduced urobilinogen
Cholangitis	i.e. ↑ Conjugated	
Intestinal foreign body		
Biliary neoplasia		
Ruptured bile duct		

such as cardiac failure, renal failure and hypoproteinaemia associated with enteric disease, so it is important to eliminate these conditions. Because both the renal and hepatic organs are intimately associated with sodium and body water balance, disease in either organ may lead to secondary or coexistent abnormality in the other and it is often difficult to separate the two.

Animals with chronic liver disease frequently have haemorrhagic syndromes or diathesis. This is largely the result of low levels of prothrombin and fibrinogen and affected dogs and cats present with multiple petechial haemorrhages in visible mucosae, often with more extensive subcutaneous or organoid haemorrhage.

Abdominal pain is a variable manifestation of liver disease. In acute necrosis or hepatitis where there is increased intrahepatic pressure, then abdominal discomfort may be observed. This may be registered as unease, restlessness or tensing of the abdominal musculature but generally such pain is detected on palpation during clinical examination. More chronic liver disease rarely causes pain even on palpation unless the disease process causes raised intrahepatic pressure (e.g. large neoplasms).

Increased liver size as may occur in hepatitis or neoplasia (cf. chronic changes with fibrosis and atrophy) is often difficult to appreciate. Palpation is often misleading in obese animals and only dramatic increases in size can be detected with confidence by this method. Radiography is of considerable assistance in detecting and assessing hepatomegaly or changes in hepatic silhouette.

Canine and feline liver diseases

The following account deals with liver diseases under the headings of aetiologies where these are known together with individual species variations.

In the authors' experience acute liver disease is less common in cats than in dogs. The preponderance of chronic disease in both species may be closely related to the increase in the geriatric canine and feline populations, together with the development of greater diagnostic sophistication in modern small animal practice.

Mechanical conditions

Hepatic rupture or tissue disruption of variable degree can result from traumatic abdominal compression such as that associated with road traffic accidents or malicious wounding (kicks etc). Severe disruption leads to massive or insidious abdominal haemorrhage and haemorrhagic shock is frequently the presenting symptom accompanied by an appropriate history. Examination at laparotomy or necropsy reveals hepatic damage and bleeding points.

Diaphragmatic rupture of congenital or acquired origin may lead to sequestration of parts or all of the liver in the chest (Fig. 9.7). This usually compromises normal function and may lead to hepatic lobe torsion.

Obstruction of the common bile duct may be caused by compression from adjacent space-occupying lesions (abscesses, tumours, granulomatous formations) (Zawie & Garvey 1984, Hornbuckle & Allan 1980) or organ displacements. The bile duct may rupture if obstruction is complete particularly if the duct becomes involved in an inflammatory reaction or neoplasia. This results in jaundice and bile peritonitis (Hornbuckle & Allan 1980). In the cat this type of bile duct lesion is sometimes associated with pancreatitis (see below).

Vascular abnormalities

Vascular abnormalities usually involve portosystemic venous anastomosis where the liver is by-passed by abnormal channels of venous drainage from the hepatic portal vein to the caudal vena cava, azygos veins or more rarely the

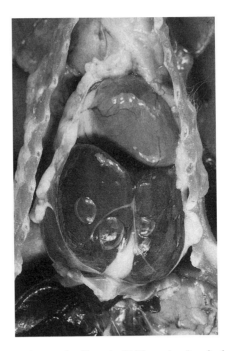

Fig. 9.7 Dissection of the thorax of a 12-week-old kitten showing the bulk of the liver compressing the heart following herniation through the diaphragm.

hepatic vein (Fig. 9.6). These routes are often congenital in origin. Acquired shunting in older animals is less common but may be associated with long-standing liver fibrosis leading to portal vein hypertension or prehepatic venous hypertension. In these cases tortuous vessels traverse the abdominal cavity from the portal vein to the colonic or renal vein systems.

The congenital condition is reported in cats at between 10 to 14 weeks of age (Blaxter 1987) and puppies are slightly older at 6 to 9 months of age. Canine cases are often more stunted than are feline, but the chief reasons for presentation are behavioural changes or neurological abnormality resulting from hepatic encephalopathy. The nervous signs may be correlated with feeding. Feline cases may be discovered following poor recovery from sedatives or anaesthetics for ovariohysterectomy.

Clinical examination should seek to eliminate specific neurological deficits or lesions. Radiography may reveal an atrophied or small liver. Contrast portal venography is helpful in identifying and tracing shunts (Blaxter 1987, Hardy 1989).

Clinical biochemistry may be variable; serum alanine aminotransferase and alkaline phosphatase may be raised or normal and serum proteins may be reduced. Bile acids are often slightly raised in cats and always raised in dogs. Bromsulphthalein clearance is usually normal. The most useful assay is blood ammonia; normal or raised fasting levels are seen, often correlated with severity of encephalopathy, but an ammonia tolerance test is always abnormal (Meyer *et al.* 1978). Ammonium biurate crystaluria develops inconsistently in cats (Center 1986) but is a common finding in dogs.

Livers of affected animals are small but macroscopically and histopathologically normal in cases of congenital origin or short duration (Fig. 9.8). Where the condition is of longer duration, the liver is more atrophied and may exhibit mild diffuse fibrosis, i.e. 'juvenile cirrhosis' (Vitums 1961, Van den Ingh & Rothuizen 1982). The acquired cases usually have more severe and overt degenerative fibrous changes.

Toxic hepatopathy

There is a vast potential range of toxic agents which cats and dogs may ingest with resultant hepatotoxicity. There is no breed, age or sex predisposition although younger animals, especially cats tend to be more prone. Clinical histories usually have a known access to a toxin such as a domestic

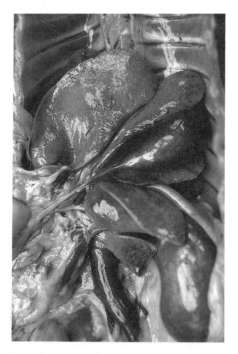

Fig. 9.8(a) Liver of a 7-month-old dog with a patent ductus venosus. Note the small liver volume and distended caudal vena cava.

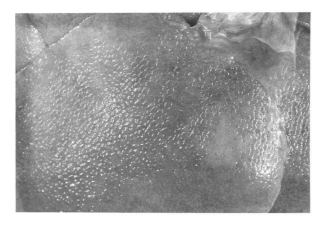

Fig. 9.8(b) Close-up view of the surface of a liver from a 4-month-old dog exhibiting juvenile cirrhosis. The liver was small, pale with a finely bosselated surface.

disinfectant, use of a rodenticide in premises or truly accidental or malicious administration.

The type of toxin may vary from a domestic detergent or disinfectant to a known toxin such as arsenic or an organochloride rodenticide. In addition, drug overdosage or an idiosyncratic reaction to an otherwise normally acceptable therapeutic substance may occur.

Signs of toxicity are usually dramatic and acute in onset with acute liver failure (Sherding 1985). Where the toxic agent is low grade or smaller amounts have been ingested, then toxic changes are more insidious. Toxicity in cats is more serious since they have a relatively poorer ability to conjugate noxious substances (due to lower glucuronide levels) than do dogs.

Clinical signs may vary depending on the nature of the toxin and some agents (rodenticides, slug baits) may induce predominantly neurological signs in addition to hepatic dysfunction especially in cats. A common presenting sign is acute onset jaundice with abdominal pain and depression. Vomiting is not often seen unless the substance is irritant, e.g. phosphorus. Where toxic agents are irritant or corrosive, affected animals may exhibit polydipsia. Low grade toxins cause increasing lethargy, anorexia and weight-loss with a borderline jaundice on examination.

Biochemical assays are often not very helpful. Dramatic elevations of serum alkaline phosphatase may be seen in acute widespread hepatic damage but the onset of toxicity may be peracute and death may supervene before assays can be performed.

Affected animals often have focal or massive hepatic necrosis, depending on the type of poison or drug damage. The affected organ may be diffusely swollen and friable or merely softened in some areas, depending on the

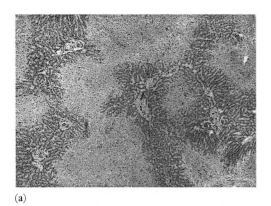
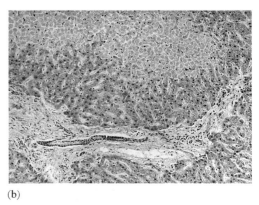

(a)   (b)

Fig. 9.9 Histopathological section of a liver from an adult dog showing large zones of necrosis.
Note there is 'ghost' tissue with no inflammatory response.

extent and nature of the insult. Histopathologically, changes are characterized
by hepatocellular necrosis, often zonal with haemorrhage (Fig. 9.9). Some
agents such as carbon tetrachloride induce zonal fatty change. Inflammation
does not occur in acute cases although more chronic cases may exhibit low
grade mononuclear inflammation, together with attempts at regeneration
and healing by fibrosis. Table 9.2 is a synopsis of some of the more common
hepatotoxins affecting dogs and cats in the UK. Cats are particularly sensitive
to phenacetin and salicylates (Eder 1964) as well as paracetamol (Davis
1985, Wilkinson 1984, Hardy 1989).

Infectious agents

The introduction of efficient vaccination programmes and use of antibiotics
in canine and feline practice has considerably reduced the incidence of what
were once serious infectious diseases. However, individual cases or group
outbreaks of the diseases may still occur especially in young animals.

Infectious canine hepatitis

This disease is caused by canine adenovirus type 1 which has a specific
tropism for vascular endothelium as well as hepatic parenchyma. It therefore
typically causes a haemorrhagic disease in severe acute infections in susceptible
dogs. Experimental work however has shown that chronic canine hepatitis
can also be induced (Gocke *et al.* 1967).

Affected animals usually present with non-specific anorexia, depression
and pyrexia. Vomiting and abdominal pain are common. Progress of the
disease is rapid and death often supervenes before jaundice develops. In
more chronic cases jaundice and haemoglobinuria are seen.

Table 9.2 Hepatotoxic agents* in the dog and cat

Compound	Dog or cat	Effects
Yellow phosphorus	Both	Fatty degeneration
Thallium	Both	Fatty degeneration
Arsenic	Mainly dog	Hepatitis
Salicylates	Mainly cat	Hepatitis
Carbon tetrachloride	Both	Centrilobular necrosis
Phenols (creosote, carbolic acid, tar)	Both	Centrilobular necrosis
Methoxyflurane	Both	Widespread necrosis
Halothane	Both	Widespread necrosis
Acetaminophen	Mainly cat	Widespread necrosis
Mebendazole	Mainly dog	Periacinar necrosis
Metophane	Mainly dog	Periacinar necrosis
Diethylcarbamazine	Mainly dog	Periacinar necrosis
Glucocorticoids*	Mainly dog	Focal necrosis
Metaldehyde	Both	Hyperaemia/haemorrhage
Warfarin (+ other coumarins)	Both	Haemorrhage
Lead	Mainly dog	Hepatocellular degeneration
Copper	Dog	Hepatocellular degeneration + storage
Phenobarbitone	Both	Cholestasis
Diphenylhydantoin	Both	Cholestasis
Phenytoin	Mainly dog	Cholestasis
Primidone	Mainly dog	Cholestasis

* i.e Long-term or high doses

Affected livers are turgid, swollen and friable with fibrin tags on the surface. The gall bladder wall may be oedematous. On gross section the liver parenchyma has liquefied necrotic zones with surviving yellow zones of fatty change. Histopathologically, there is usually centrilobular necrosis with fatty degeneration in surviving cells. Few if any inflammatory cells are present but characteristic intranuclear inclusions are usually seen (Fig. 9.10).

Other canine viruses

Herpesvirus infection causes focal necrosis in the liver of young puppies of 2 to 8 weeks of age. The condition is typified by weak, lethargic 'fading' puppies. At necropsy kidneys and livers have multiple petechial haemorrhages (Percy 1982). Viral inclusions can be demonstrated in hepatocytes but they are not abundant.

Jarrett and O'Neil (1985) described an acidophil cell hepatitis in adult dogs. They attributed areas of hepatocyte necrosis and fatty degeneration

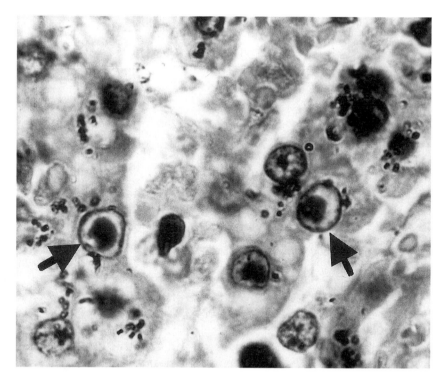

Fig. 9.10 Intranuclear inclusion bodies in hepatocytes from a dog characteristic of infectious canine hepatitis.

with minimal inflammation which progressed to chronic hepatitis and cirrhosis to a possible but unidentified infectious agent. This condition has not been reported to date elsewhere in the world.

Feline viral hepatitis

Feline infectious peritonitis caused by coronavirus infection is usually associated with chronic pleurisy and peritonitis (Wilkinson 1984), with liver involvement in some cases (August 1984). However, it may also be an unusual cause of acute multifocal hepatic necrosis in kittens younger than 3 months of age.

Coronavirus infection in older cats (2 to 10 years), especially oriental breeds, causes a more widespread syndrome characterized by vague clinical signs of lethargy, intermittent fever, anaemia and anorexia. The disease usually progresses with jaundice and ascites and respiratory involvement may result from pleural effusions.

Affected cats have marked hypergammaglobulinaemia and moderate elevations in liver enzymes. Ascitic fluid is rich in globulin. There may be a non-regenerative anaemia with leucocytosis with a lymphopenia. Serum assay for coronavirus antibody is usually positive (Pedersen 1983).

Lesions depend on the presence of the wet effusive or dry granulomatous form. The former is characterized by viscid proteinaceous fluid accumulations in pleural and abdominal cavities (Fig. 9.11) with fibrinous organ adhesions and peritonitis. The dry form is more common in chronic cases and is characterized by pyogranulomatous lesions in the liver. Pyogranulomata occur in other organs and chronic inflammatory reactions may be seen in the eye and meninges (Wilkinson 1984).

Some reports (Meyer & Center 1986, Center 1986) have suggested that feline calicivirus infection may cause hepatic necrosis.

Leptospirosis

Although both agents may cause liver damage, *Leptospira canicola* is thought to be more common than *L. icterohaemorrhagiae*.

Affected dogs present with an acute febrile disease with jaundice, vomiting, dehydration and bloody diarrhoea. Albuminuria is common. A coexistent nephritis may be present and polyuria with haemoglobinuria may result. Surviving dogs develop a chronic nephritis which ultimately leads to uraemia. One report (Bishop *et al.* 1979) has implicated leptospiral organisms in chronic hepatitis.

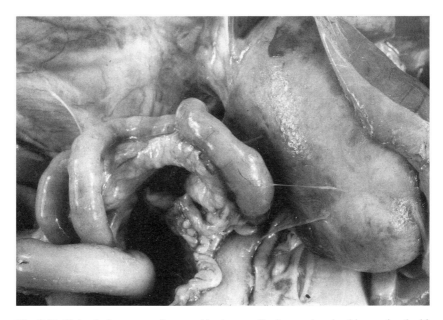

Fig. 9.11 Abdominal contents of a cat with viscous adhesions and peritonitis associated with feline infectious peritonitis.

Livers of dogs with acute leptospiral hepatitis may show little in the way of macroscopic change other than focal haemorrhages and softening. Histopathologically, hepatocytes shrink and dissociate resulting in liver cord fragmentation. Necrosis is not a feature. Leptospiral organisms may be demonstrated by silver staining techniques.

Other bacterial infections

Abscessation and focal necrosis may be encountered in young animals affected by septicaemia. The availability of broad spectrum antibiotics has rendered bacterial agents non-lethal in many infections although severe infections can be difficult to eradicate once established, and may be complicated by concurrent fungal growth in severe cases.

Puppies or kittens may be affected by septicaemia following umbilical infections or non-specific bacterial infections as sequelae to viral infections. Severe septicaemia cases present as whole body disease with pyrexia, depression, dehydration, vomiting and diarrhoea or respiratory symptoms, depending on the site of major or primary insult.

Acute infection may be caused in puppies and kittens by *Streptococcus*, *Staphylococcus*, *Proteus* and *Pseudomonas* spp. More chronic infections of serious consequence may establish in older animals, e.g. *Salmonella* spp. and *Nocardia* spp. At least one report has implicated clostridial infection arising from the small intestine in a dog (Smith 1980). In kittens, Tyzzer's disease caused by *Bacillus piliformis* has been recorded (Jones *et al.* 1985), although this is usually an infection of laboratory animals.

Generally, affected animals have focal solitary or multifocal hepatitis with periportal inflammation comprising polymorph and plasma cell infiltrations alongside focal necrosis. Abscess and granuloma formation are encountered, depending on the inciting agent.

Parasitic agents

In the UK hepatotropic parasites are relatively uncommon and potential non-specific parasites such as *Toxocara* and *Toxascaris* spp. are not a major problem, probably because of efficient anthelmintic preparations that are available.

Toxoplasmosis is potentially the most important parasitic infestation (Zawie & Garvey 1984, Center 1986). *T. gondii* has the cat as its definitive host with the target organ being the colon; a granulomatous colitis may occur in severely affected cats. Problems arise as a result of aberrant immature forms nidating in body organs such as the liver and muscles. Dogs become infected by ingestion of meat containing encysted forms or by feline faecal contamination (Beverley 1976, Frenkel 1985, Hall 1986).

Infestation may be asymptomatic but severe parasitic burdens result, with many tissue cysts containing immature organisms which may provoke low grade chronic inflammation. Affected livers show pale soft grey foci of necrosis with minimal inflammation. Organisms are difficult to demonstrate but serological dye tests or enzyme-linked immunosorbent assay (ELISA) methods are available for clinical diagnosis of significant titres.

Feline infectious anaemia is caused by *Haemobartonella felis* (Nash & Bobade 1986). This protozoan induces a haemolytic prehepatic jaundice but it may also affect liver parenchyma resulting in hepatocellular necrosis. Raised liver enzyme levels are present and affected cats have swollen livers. Protozoa can be demonstrated in red calls in haematological smears of peripheral blood.

Biliary system disorders

This is an important group of disorders which in some instances is poorly understood although well-recognized, particularly in the cat. In general, disorders of the biliary system are less common in the dog than in the cat (Center 1986, Hardy 1989). This may be related to the different anatomy of the bile duct system connection to the small intestine in the two species but this is not known for certain.

Cholestasis and cholelithiasis

Cholestasis is more common in cats than dogs but cholelithiasis is rare in both species (Walshaw 1985). Acute stasis may result from inspissated or sludged bile which induces obstructive jaundice. Cholestasis most commonly arises from occlusion pressure produced by adjacent abdominal masses such as tumours or abscesses. It may also arise as a distortion associated with granulation tissue or fibrous scarring. Acute cholestasis in the dog is also said to be related to ascending infection from severe enteritis or intestinal foreign body obstruction producing ascending cholangitis (Hendricks *et al.* 1980).

Affected animals are lethargic and anorexic with vague abdominal pain. Jaundice is variable, depending on the completeness of the obstruction. Ascites is not seen. A malabsorption of fat may be induced giving rise to steatorrhoea.

Biochemical tests reveal hyperbilirubinaemia, hypercholesterolaemia and moderately raised serum alkaline phosphatase and alanine aminotransferase levels. Bile acids may be raised if assayed post ingestion. Bile salt deposits may be seen in liver biopsies confirming stasis, although liver cells appear unaffected.

Radiography may reveal intra-abdominal masses but laparotomy is often

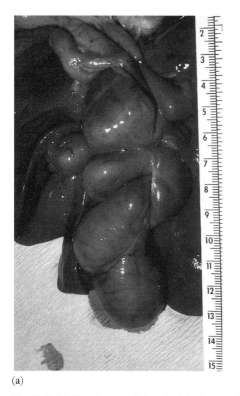

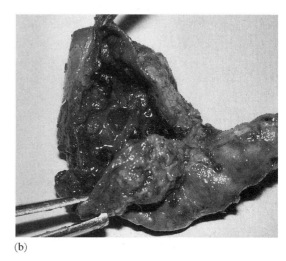

(a)   (b)

Fig. 9.12 (a) Grossly-distended major bile ducts and gall bladder in a canine liver. (b) Grossly-thickened gall bladder and bile ducts with cholelithiasis. The black foci are the choleliths.

needed to ascertain the cause of the bile duct obstruction since there is no specific diagnostic test for duct obstruction. Choleliths consist of cholesterol combined with sodium and potassium salts. Complete blockage may induce duct rupture and peritonitis (Mullowney & Tennant 1982).

Pathological findings include a grossly-distended gall bladder with possible inspissated bile, or rarely choleliths in the bile duct (Fig. 9.12). Adjacent neoplasia, abscesses and granulomas may be present, and in the case of the cat, pancreatitis may be associated.

Cholangitis and cholangiohepatitis

Pure inflammation of the biliary tree alone is not usually seen (Hardy 1989); the hepatocellular parenchyma is almost invariably involved. The disease is therefore usually referred to as the cholangiohepatitis complex. It is more common in cats than dogs in the authors' experience and the following account is largely based on the feline disease.

There is no sex predisposition. There does appear to be a difference in the type of disease pattern seen at different ages; some authorities consider that a non-suppurative process is more common in young cats, whereas a bacterial infection occurs or is suspected more frequently in the older age group.

A clinical syndrome of the waxing and waning type is observed with recurrent pyrexia, vomiting, lethargy and variable anorexia. Some abdominal pain is evident. Jaundice develops but ascites is only seen in advanced or long-standing cases. Typical cases show remissions and recurrences with increasing severity in latter episodes.

Assays show raised levels of conjugated bilirubin with elevated serum alanine aminotransferase, alkaline phosphatase and gamma glutamyl transferase. There are markedly raised globulin values in the presence of depressed albumin. Fasting bile acids are normal but are raised postfeeding in non-jaundiced cats. A mild non-regenerative anaemia with leucocytosis and neutrophilia is often seen. Coagulopathies may occur in advanced disease states where hepatocyte loss and scarring are severe.

Radiographs of the abdomen are rarely of diagnostic assistance. Liver biopsy is mandatory either following laparotomy or by needle sampling.

Pathological lesions vary and three types of change have been described although they may be progressions of the same disease spectrum. Macroscopic lesions vary from diffuse or focal minimal changes to severe distortion with fibrous scarring involving the whole organ. The three types of change are as follows:

1 A suppurative acute inflammatory change characterized by periportal inflammation and fibrosis with neutrophils. The biliary ducts are frequently plugged with neutrophils, giving rise to suppurative cholangitis (Hirsh & Doige 1983).

2 Chronic non-suppurative cholangiohepatitis may develop from 1 or arise 'de novo'. There is no age or sex predilection (Lucke & Davies 1984). There is more severe damage and macroscopically scarring, and distortion are more obvious. Histopathological changes are chiefly those of chronic inflammation (lymphocytes, plasma cells, macrophages and few polymorphs) with fibrosis, chiefly in portal areas. Biliary hyperplasia is common. There may be 'bridging' fibrosis between adjacent portal areas and adjacent hepatocellular hyperplasia. Advanced cases have distorted hyperplastic hepatic lobules and marked biliary duct hyperplasia, surrounded by extensive fibrosis and chronic inflammatory cells (Fig. 9.13).

3 A less-common state is sclerosing cholangitis (Edwards et al. 1983). There is exaggerated thickening of extrahepatic bile ducts by fibrous tissue with diffuse fibrosis in the hepatic parenchyma. The general appearance is suggestive of an 'end-stage' scenario. Some reports (Prasse et al. 1982, Rogers & Cornelius 1985) refer to this terminal condition as biliary cirrhosis, but in the authors' experience it does not resemble the canine condition often referred to as cirrhosis.

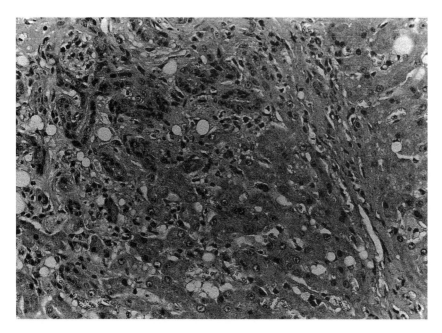

Fig. 9.13 Histopathological section of an advanced chronic cholangiohepatitis in a 7-year-old domestic short-haired cat.

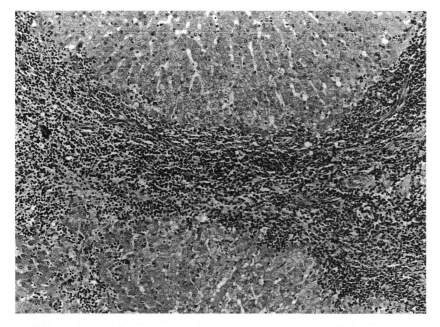

Fig. 9.14 Histopathological section of a liver from a 9-year-old domestic short-haired female neutered cat with lymphocytic cholangitis. Note the bridging zones of lymphocyte infiltration.

These changes may represent a progression of the same process or three different mechanisms. An ascending infection from the gut, possibly associated with cholestasis has been proposed for the suppurative condition (Rogers & Cornelius 1985). The changes in the second state have been interpreted by some workers as akin to human primary biliary cirrhosis which is thought to be the result of an immune-mediated process. Sclerosing cholangitis closely resembles a condition in man which is associated with chronic inflammatory bowel disease with a possible autoimmune basis. It is highly likely that the continual chronic reaction has an immune-mediated basis. In this connection the lymphocytic cholangitis described by Prasse et al. (1982) and Lucke & Davies (1984) may be evidence for cholangitis of immune origin. Affected livers are distorted as a result of extensive fibrosis with bile duct proliferation; intense lymphocyte infiltrations in portal tracts and bridging areas are seen (Fig. 9.14). The association with chronic pancreatitis in cats remains an unexplained but common phenomenon. In dogs experimental studies indicate that the right side of the liver is preferentially affected, probably resulting from the close proximity of the pancreas and distribution of portal blood flow to that side of the liver (Tuzhilin et al. 1975).

Hepatic neoplasia

Primary hepatic neoplasia in both dogs and cats is said to be uncommon (Moulton 1978). Whilst this is true for the dog, the authors' experience is that malignant hepatic neoplasia may be more common than previously supposed. Secondary or metastatic tumours affecting the liver in both species are common.

Primary hepatic neoplasia

Hepatomas, hepatocellular carcinomas, cholangiocarcinomas and haemangiosarcomas occur in both species with advancing age (greater than 6 years). Benign primary tumours are less common than malignant ones in the cat in our experience; cholangiocarcinoma is the commonest type in our series of cats (Fig. 9.15).

In dogs, hepatomas are often asymptomatic unless large and pressing upon adjacent abdominal viscera. Hepatomas may often be incidental necropsy findings (Fig. 9.16). Large tumours can usually be palpated or can be seen on a radiograph. Occasionally tumours produce insulin and this is manifest clinically as hypoglycaemia.

Large benign primary tumours may cause few symptoms until the disease is advanced; anorexia and weight-loss are common with ascites and jaundice developing late. There may be non-specific mild or variable elevation in liver enzymes. Mild elevation of serum bilirubin which increases with

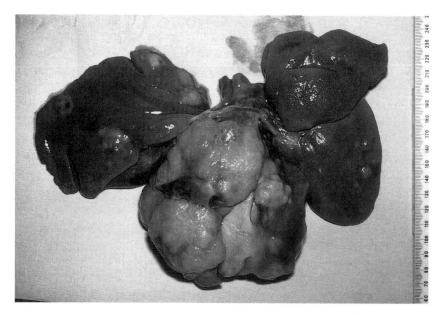

Fig. 9.15 Cholangiocarcinoma in a 12-year-old domestic short-haired cat. Note the association with the gall bladder, although the latter is not obviously neoplastic.

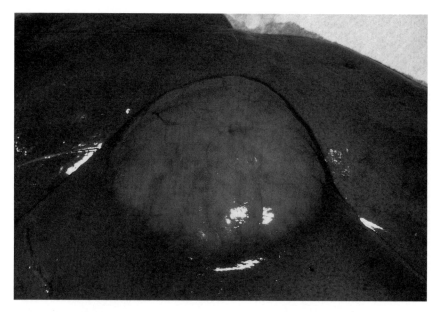

Fig. 9.16 A well defined solitary hepatic tumour in the liver of a 13-year-old dog. This was an incidental finding at necropsy.

advanced disease may occur (but levels are always lower than in cholangiohepatitis). Where biliary obstruction is present then total bilirubin rises dramatically, together with elevation of serum alanine aminotransferase and alkaline phosphatase. Malignant primary neoplasms cause more clinical symptoms as a result of abnormal functioning due to liver destruction. Levels of serum alanine aminotransferase and alkaline phosphatase are usually very high, together with marked elevation of total bilirubin. Serum globulin may be raised and albumin reduced. Reduced levels of clotting factors associated with hypoproteinaemia lead to haemorrhagic diathesis. Laparotomy and liver biopsy with histopathological examination give a definitive diagnosis.

Metastatic neoplasia

Metastatic hepatic neoplasia (Fig. 9.17) commonly arises following dissemination of cells from primary malignant tumours such as carcinomas (e.g. mammary) or sarcomas (e.g. haemangiosarcoma of the heart or spleen). Multiple foci establish following lymphohaematogenous spread of the tumour emboli which nidate in sinusoids. Normal function is compromised as multiple neoplasms superpopulate normal hepatic parenchyma.

Similar clinical symptoms to those described above are seen with greater severity and speed of onset. The bleeding syndromes and hypoproteinaemia

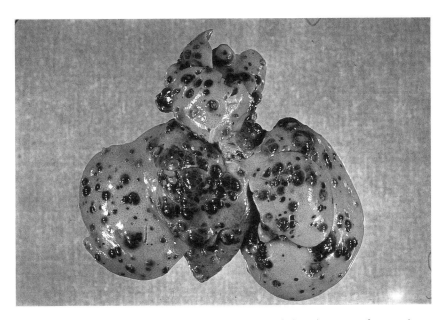

Fig. 9.17 Liver of a 6-year-old labrador bitch with metastatic hepatic tumours from a primary malignant haemangiosarcoma of the spleen.

are important components of the paraneoplastic syndrome in metastatic disease (Brown 1981).

Affected livers usually have multiple widespread metastatic tumour deposits. In the case of carcinomas, these are often white or cream, friable foci and more vascular in the case of haemangiosarcomas. Histopathological appearance is characteristic of a parent primary malignant tumour if this can be identified.

Diagnosis is confirmed by a combination of known history or diagnosis of a primary malignant tumour together with radiographic confirmation of liver masses or more general enlargement. Definitive diagnosis is usually made on laparotomy and/or liver biopsy, the latter depending on the accuracy of sampling if done by needle techniques.

Involvement of the liver also occurs in leukaemia or lymphosarcoma in both the dog and cat. In both species neoplastic cells superpopulate the liver leading to blockage of bile and blood flow, and eventually to hepatocellular degeneration. Normal function is compromised. Affected livers are pale, swollen and friable with widespread foci of tumour cells seen microscopically in sinusoids and portal tracts. Cats with any liver disease should always have their feline leukaemia virus (FeLV) status assessed.

In the cat, systemic mastocytosis or mast cell neoplasia affects the spleen and liver. The affected organs are enlarged and turgid with uniform but bulging parenchyma on gross section. Histopathologically, there is replacement of normal parenchyma by dense neoplastic mast cell populations. The histamine content of the mast cells induces gastric ulceration and this causes vomiting which is often the initial presenting symptom.

Cirrhosis

Cirrhosis is a term used in human medicine to describe a condition of fine diffuse fibrosis of the liver (Anthony *et al.* 1977). It is classically associated with alcohol abuse in man but also occurs in other diseases (MacSween *et al.* 1979). The canine and feline diseases of the liver which have in the past been referred to as cirrhosis are more correctly a combination of nodular regeneration and degenerative change accompanied by fibrosis. Some clinicians still prefer to view cirrhosis clinically as end-stage chronic liver disease regardless of cause (Hardy 1989).

In the veterinary literature various types of cirrhosis have also been described based on the pathogenesis or location of the fibrosis. Hence, portal cirrhosis refers to fibrous change centred on the portal triads, biliary cirrhosis results from chronic biliary obstruction (see cholangiohepatitis), and cardiac cirrhosis refers to centrilobular necrosis arising from chronic congestive heart failure with centrilobular hypoxia.

These types of change are more commonly recognized in dogs, and affected animals usually present with depression, jaundice and ascites. Gastric

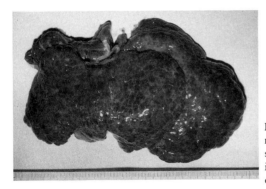

(a)

Fig. 9.18 (a) A cirrhotic liver from a 14-year-old male neutered Yorkshire Terrier. (b) Histopathological section from the same liver showing lobule distortion, irregular hepatocytes and fibrosis with sparse numbers of chronic inflammatory cells.

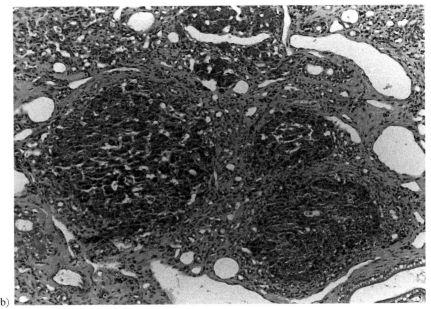

(b)

ulceration is said to be a feature of these cases (Ng *et al.* 1981). Livers are often distorted and reduced in size and thus radiography may not be of assistance in diagnosis. Liver biopsy is useful for establishing the presence of fibrosis and chronic inflammatory changes (Simpson & Else 1987).

Biochemical assays show high serum alkaline phosphatase but alanine aminotransferase may be normal or only moderately raised, Bromsulphthalein (BSP) clearance rate is reduced.

At laparotomy or necropsy, livers of affected animals are discoloured, contracted, distorted and nodular (Fig. 9.18) as a result of a combination of fibrosis, and attempted nodular hepatocyte regeneration. Bile ducts are usually thickened and distorted, thereby generally contributing to the irregularity. Histopathological examination reveals replacement by fibrous tissue with hepatocellular hyperplasia, low grade chronic inflammation and bile duct hyperplasia.

Chronic active hepatitis

This is a descriptive term borrowed from human medicine where it refers to an autoimmune disease characterized by so-called 'piece-meal' necrosis of hepatocytes at the limiting plate of the acinus (Whitcomb 1979). Some authors have described similar hepatic changes in dogs in recent years and referred to them as chronic active hepatitis (CAH) (Strombeck & Gribble 1978). To date however, nobody has demonstrated a convincing autoimmune mechanism in canine livers to account for the changes. Some reports in the veterinary literature (Hardy 1989) have included copper-associated hepatitis (see below) in the CAH complex and Franklin & Saunders (1988) have noted the association specifically in Doberman Pinschers.

Clinical symptoms are often vague and inconsistent with intermittent depression, variable jaundice and possible encephalopathy. Ascites may also develop eventually. There is no age predisposition but there is some evidence of a higher incidence in females. There has been a preponderance of reports of the Doberman breed being involved (Johnson *et al.* 1982, Crawford *et al.* 1985) but the autoimmune component does not appear to be involved.

Liver function is abnormal with raised serum alanine aminotransferase and alkaline phosphatase and reduced BSP clearance. Plasma proteins are markedly raised with globulin levels particularly involved. Antinuclear antibody reaction is used to establish the immune nature of the disease (Hardy

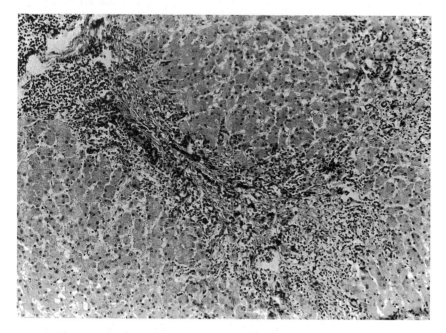

Fig. 9.19 Histopathological section of liver from a 10-year-old Doberman bitch with liver failure. Note the bridging cellular infiltration and disruption.

1986). Cholestasis may occur. Liver biopsy is mandatory for diagnosis.

Affected livers may be relatively unaffected macroscopically but distortion with diffuse pallor or pale foci has been reported (Strombeck & Gribble 1978, Doige & Lester 1981). Periportal ('piecemeal') necrosis with bridging between adjacent portal tracts is seen histologically. Portal areas have infiltrations by a range of inflammatory cells (neutrophils, lymphocytes, plasma cells and macrophages) and fibrosis is present in these sites (Fig. 9.19). Bile duct proliferation also occurs.

A related condition, lobular dissecting hepatitis has been reported in a small series of dogs (Bennett et al. 1983) which were depressed and ascitic. Liver enzymes were normal or only slightly raised, whilst serum albumin was low. Blood ammonia levels were raised and BSP clearance was reduced. At necropsy the livers were swollen or shrunken with distended portal veins. Histopathological examination showed disruption of the normal reticulin-supporting framework and 'piecemeal' necrosis similar to CAH but with milder cellular infiltrations; the portal areas were not affected (cf. CAH). Although the condition bears some resemblance to CAH, the aetiology of both conditions remains obscure and it is not certain whether they are related.

Storage diseases

The hepatocellular parenchyma is capable of acting as a site for storage or sequestration of abnormal metabolic products or wastes. Such accumulations may compromise normal liver function.

Copper-associated hepatitis

This condition was first described in Bedlington Terriers (Hardy et al. 1975, Kelly et al. 1984) and has subsequently been recorded in Dobermans (Johnson et al. 1982, Crawford et al. 1985), West Highland White Terriers (Thornburg et al. 1986a) and some other breeds of dog (Thornburg 1984).

Affected dogs show no age or sex predilection. They may be asymptomatic or be affected by progressive liver failure with ill thrift, nervous signs, jaundice (variable) and eventually ascites.

Biochemical tests reveal slightly raised bilirubin levels, elevated serum alkaline phosphatase but alanine aminotransferase may be normal. Liver copper levels are diagnostic with increases of five to 50 times normal levels (normal less than 300 μg/g dry weight; up to 10 000 μg/g recorded in affected dogs) (Lucke & Herrtage 1987). Liver biopsies show copper deposits particularly if rhodamine or rubeanic acid stains are used.

Livers are pale and fibrous with finely nodular surfaces in advanced disease. Golden brown granules are seen histologically in hepatocytes particularly in centrilobular locations. The granules are mixtures of copper and iron but lipofuscin may also be present. There may be random fatty change with sparse periportal infiltrations by neutrophil polymorphs together with piecemeal necrosis. Portal fibrosis may be seen. Overall the pattern of changes resembles CAH.

The significance of the copper accumulations remains in doubt; copper deposits may be primary events or secondary to bile stasis.

Lysosomal storage disease

Lysosomal storage diseases are specific congenital abnormalities or deletion of enzymes involved in metabolic pathways. The majority manifest as storage metabolites or excess substances in neurones, and hence present as primary neurological cases. Some variants do involve visceral organs and here the liver may become affected, e.g. Gm_1-gangliosidosis in Beagles, glucocerebrosidosis in Sydney Silky Terriers. A glycogen storage disease involving a deficiency of the enzyme amylo-1,6-glucosidase has been reported in German Shepherd dogs by Rafiquzzaman et al. (1976). Abnormal storage products are formed in hepatocytes and Kupffer cells as well as neurones. They are not common diseases.

Miscellaneous diseases

Amyloidosis

This may occur rarely in dogs as part of a primary idiopathic multisystem disease with involvement of kidneys and intestines as well as liver. Jaundice and ascites are late manifestations in advanced disease but renal failure and intestinal malabsorption are major symptoms. Liver enzymes and serum globulin are elevated. Liver and colon biopsies are useful in detecting amyloid and the arteritis which accompanies the amyloid deposits. Affected livers are enlarged, firm and pale; amyloid deposits can be demonstrated by special stains and immunofluorescence.

Secondary amyloidosis may be seen more often where it is a sequel to a chronic inflammatory process with antigen–antibody reaction (Hardy 1989). Pancreatic primary amyloidosis occurs in cats but liver involvement is not common.

Hepatic lipidosis

Fatty infiltration in obese animals is usually an incidental finding at necropsy. The affected cells are parasinusoidal Ito cells. The condition is usually of no clinical significance.

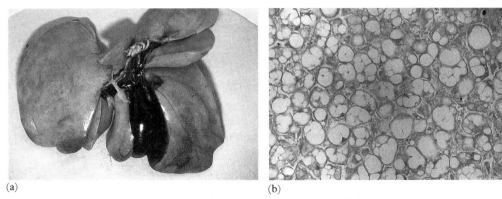

(a)   (b)

Fig. 9.20 (a) The liver of a 13-year-old domestic short-haired obese queen cat. There is extensive pallor characteristic of lipidosis. The liver was friable and greasy on gross examination. (b) Histopathological section from the same liver; the hepatocytes have extreme fatty degeneration.

Fatty change in hepatocytes is associated with a metabolic upset such as that accompanying diabetes mellitus and hyperadrenocorticism in dogs. It is fairly common (Cornelius & Jacobs 1989) and potentially reversible, but if widespread it is accompanied by liver failure. Affected organs are pale cream if severely affected, greasy and friable. Fatty vacuoles distend hepatocytes. If cholestasis develops then serum liver enzymes may rise but the more dramatic clinical features are those associated with the primary diseases of diabetes mellitus or hyperadrenocorticism.

In cats a primary idiopathic lipidosis occurs and this is a serious condition. It is said to occur more frequently in obese animals but there is no age or sex predisposition. It is associated with prolonged anorexia (Thornburg *et al.* 1986b). There is severe weight-loss and dehydration with ensuing neurological depression terminating as coma. Some cats exhibit polyuria and polydipsia.

Serum assays reveal normal alanine aminotransferase and bile acids but alkaline phosphatase is markedly elevated. Blood glucose and cholesterol levels are raised together with hyperbilirubinaemia. Serum proteins are normal.

Affected livers are enlarged with rounded borders and are pale, greasy and friable. There is no necrosis or inflammation histologically but virtually all hepatocytes are distended with fatty vacuoles (Fig. 9.20).

The aetiology of the condition is unknown; relative arginine deficiency in cats may lead to high ammonia levels, hence the nervous signs (Hardy 1989). Other suggested aetiological factors include low protein intake, ornithine deficiency (Rogers & Cornelius 1985), bacterial toxin, endocrine abnormality involving insulin and/or glucagon (Zawie & Garvey 1984) and reduced apoprotein synthesis in the liver leading to increased hepatocyte triglyceride storage.

Steroid hepatopathy

This condition has been recorded in dogs undergoing long-term steroid administration (Rogers & Ruebner 1977) but may also occur in hyper-adrenocorticism (Hardy 1989). Clinically dogs are presented in liver failure with elevated serum alanine aminotransferase (SALT) and serum alkaline phosphatase (SAP) levels and increased BSP retention. This rise in SAP is nearly always greater than that of SALT. Affected livers are enlarged and pale; the latter is not the result of fatty change but storage of excess glycogen and water (Fittschen & Bellamy 1984). This condition resolves with removal of steroid therapy.

Congenital hepatic cysts

Single or multiple congenital hepatic cysts may occur in dogs and cats (Van den Ingh & Rothuizen 1985, Black 1983). They probably arise as abnor-malities of the intra- or extra-hepatic biliary system and are often asymp-tomatic. The cysts may however become large (Fig. 9.21) and act as a space-occupying lesion requiring surgical removal or drainage.

Hyperthyroidism in cats

At least two authors (Petersen 1984, Blaxter 1987) have noted the association of feline hyperthyroidism with raised liver enzyme and bilirubin levels. It is

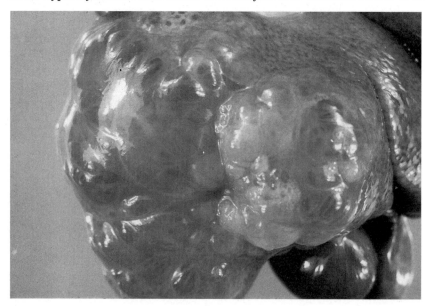

Fig. 9.21 Part of the liver of a 2-year-old domestic short-haired neutered female cat showing multiple but confluent cysts.

not certain whether this is a primary or secondary event but checking of thyroxine levels and liver biopsy should be carried out in these cases.

Treatment of hepatic disease

It is often difficult to make a specific recommendation on treatment because of our lack of knowledge of the pathogenesis of liver disease and the reluctance of some clients to permit liver biopsy, thereby allowing a definitive diagnosis to be made. In many cases, therefore, treatment is empirical, directed towards correcting the immediate metabolic aberrations of fluid imbalance and encephalopathy while supporting nutritional requirements and attempting to control inflammatory or degenerative changes.

Treatment can be divided into more immediate requirements to deal with potentially life-threatening situations such as fluid balance, encephalopathy and infection. Treatment should support the patient on a long-term basis through dietary requirements and attempt to suppress fibrosis and scarring.

Fluid balance

Patients with chronic liver failure and ascites tend to retain sodium and water, lose potassium and develop hypoalbuminaemia. Metabolic acidosis or alkalosis and hypoglycaemia are also features of liver disease (Magne & Chiapella 1986). Hypokalaemia, metabolic alkalosis and hypoglycaemia potentiate the effects of encephalopathy (Center 1986).

These situations must be corrected at an early stage to ensure a good response by the patient. The accurate detection of acidosis or alkalosis requires the use of blood-gas analysis, and great care is required when only clinical judgement is used to make this assessment. The latter is usually inaccurate and corrective measures are likely to make matters worse rather than improve the patient's condition. In most situations the acid−base balance can be readily corrected without blood-gas analysis by dealing with the hypokalaemia and dehydration, leading to better tissue perfusion especially to the kidneys.

In acidosis lactated Ringer's solution should be given while in alkalosis, isotonic dextrose saline with a potassium supplement should be employed. Great care is needed in the use of solutions containing high levels of sodium, which is often retained in chronic liver disease (Magne & Chiapella 1986).

Ascites of hepatic origin may be due to retention of sodium and water, hypoalbuminaemia or portal hypertension. Correction of the ascites is not an emergency procedure unless the volume is so great that it interferes with normal respiratory function through pressure on the diaphragm. Reduction of ascites may be achieved using diuretics, low salt diets and in some cases abdominal paracentesis.

Diuretics such as frusemide, which is commonly employed for rapid fluid removal, must be used with care as it tends to cause further losses of potassium. Spironolactone (Aldactone; Searle Pharmaceuticals) at 1 to 2 mg/kg twice daily and the thiazide diuretics (Vetidrex; Ciba-Geigy Agrochemicals) at 2 mg/kg daily are both potassium sparing and can be safely used long term.

Abdominal paracentesis should not be used routinely to correct ascites. This is because the procedure depletes the protein levels even further, increases the risk of peritonitis and may cause hypovolaemic shock. Fluid removed in this manner often collects again within a few days unless the underlying problems have been corrected so the benefit is only short-lived. The only real indication for paracentesis of the abdomen is where there is marked respiratory embarrassment.

Intravenous plasma expanders such as Haemaccel (Hoechst Animal Health) may be of value in some cases where ascites is present. This works by expanding the circulating volume, improving renal perfusion and allowing increased urine production to assist the elimination of retained fluid.

Correction of encephalopathy

Encephalopathy of varying severity is not uncommon in the dog but is rare in the cat. Problems arise from failure of the liver to metabolize intestinal ammonia to urea, so that ammonia remains in the circulation and in the central nervous system leading to reduced levels of excitatory neurotransmitters and increased levels of inhibitory neurotransmitters. Absorbed mercaptens and volatile fatty acids produced by bacteria in the intestine are also implicated in the development of encephalopathy (Strombeck 1980).

Where hepatic coma has occurred, immediate treatment to reduce the circulating ammonia levels should be carried out. This involves withholding all food, evacuation of the colon with enemas, infusing neomycin and lactulose as a retention enema and starting intravenous fluid therapy to correct hypokalaemia, hypoglycaemia and metabolic alkalosis. The infusion of branched-chain amino acids intravenously has also met with some success (Laflamme 1988).

Where encephalopathy is not life threatening, treatment should aim at reducing the formation and absorption of ammonia from the intestine. This can be achieved by making the environment for urease-producing bacteria less favourable by reducing the pH within the intestine and by speeding the transit of faecal material through the colon without inducing frank diarrhoea. The low pH converts ammonia to ammonium salt which is less-easily absorbed (Drazner 1983). This can be achieved by giving lactulose (Lactulose

Solution BP; Duphar Laboratories) a semi-synthetic disaccharide orally at 1 to 2 ml/kg three times daily although the dosage employed should be adjusted to the response by the patient and the faecal character. In cats the dose of lactulose should be 1 ml bid orally (Center 1986).

Bacterial growth may be suppressed by giving antibiotics. Neomycin has been indicated for this purpose at 20 mg/kg bid, but it has also been implicated in causing bacterial resistance and in toxicity especially in cats. Metronidazole (Flagyl; RMB Animal Health) has also proved useful in the control of encephalopathy used at 7.5 mg/kg tid (Morgan & Read 1982). Probiotics have also been advocated in the control of encephalopathy, but the authors have found them of little value. The oral administration of lactulose together with neomycin in the initial stages of encephalopathy has been suggested and, once effective control has been achieved, the neomycin may be stopped while lactulose is maintained. Ten to 20 ml of a 1% neomycin solution with 5 to 10 ml of lactulose may be given per rectum (Twedt 1981). Povidone plus iodine 10% solution has also been suggested given at 5 to 10 ml infused into the colon to reduce bacterial growth.

The conversion of ammonia to urea can be improved by ensuring the blood sugar level is maintained and the effects of encephalopathy can be reduced further by correction of hypokalaemia, azotaemia and alkalosis. In addition, every effort should be made to reduce protein catabolism which increases ammonia production and demand on the liver for its conversion to urea. Arginine is also required in the urea cycle and may be given in acute encephalopathy. The use of all sedatives, tranquillizers and anaesthetic agents should be avoided as they further depress the central nervous system. Methionine and lipotrophic drugs should also be avoided as they increase mercapten formation. Haemorrhage into the gastrointestinal tract through ulceration should also be controlled using cimetidine at 4 mg/kg bid orally, as this provides a rich protein source for bacterial fermentation and ammonia production (Magne & Chiapella 1986).

In some cases of encephalopathy there is a requirement to correct a vascular anomaly such as a portosystemic shunt. In such cases the patient should be treated medically prior to surgery to reduce the anaesthetic risk.

Dietary management

Dietary protein of high biological value is essential to support surviving and regenerating hepatocytes. Excess protein leads to protein catabolism and exacerbation of encephalopathy. It is important to feed small meals frequently during the day to ensure maximum hepatic function and to reduce the amount of protein reaching the colon for bacterial fermentation. The use of a balanced proprietary prescription diet with a reduced protein content (e.g. Hills k/d diet) would be suitable.

The energy source should be highly digestible carbohydrate to prevent fat and protein being metabolized, thereby resulting in further ammonia production. Again a proprietary prescription diet meets this requirement. Choline and methionine-containing foods are contraindicated as they produce mercaptens.

Other diets which may be used include milk and cottage cheese both of which contain good balances of amino acids, being low in aromatic amino acids. Vegetable protein is less suitable than animal protein, but if animal protein is used the level must be carefully controlled. Boiled rice is the most suitable source of readily digestible carbohydrate. Fat should be present in small amounts and never more than 6% of the total diet.

Cats are frequently anorexic and may not take diets prepared for hepatic disease. In this situation it is better to encourage cats to eat rather than to be in a negative nitrogen balance. Proprietary prescription (Hills c/d) diet may provide the best alternative in these cases.

Vitamin deficiency may occur, especially in the respect of the B vitamins. If a prescription diet is employed this should not be a problem. However thiamine deficiency may mimic encephalopathy so a good vitamin supplement should be provided in all cases. If cholestasis is present then vitamin K should be included in the therapeutic regime. Where salt and water retention is a problem the diet should be low in salt. In such cases a balance must be made between providing a low protein and a low salt diet.

Antibiotics

The reticuloendothelial function of the liver is usually reduced in hepatic disease so that filtration of bacteria from portal blood is impaired (Strombeck 1980) and septacaemia is more likely to occur. Antibiotic cover should be provided with ampicillin, amoxycillin and cephalosporins or aminoglycoside. Chloramphenicol, tetracyclines, sulphonamides and erythromycin should be avoided especially in cats as they are normally metabolized by the liver (Center 1986).

Anabolic steroids

The use of anabolic steroids is controversial. Nandrolone (Nandrolin; Intervet UK) will increase erythropoietin production thus stimulating stem cells in the bone marrow. It will also stimulate appetite but as it may be hepatotoxic and lead to sodium and water retention, it is contraindicated in liver disease.

Diazepam (Valium; Roche Products) acts centrally to stimulate the appetite in the cat which often becomes anorexic with liver disease. Diazepam and more especially oxazepam may be used at 0.2 mg/kg orally, resulting in a response within 1 hour as well as producing mild sedation (Center 1986).

Steroids

Corticosteroids may be employed to reduce inflammation and fibrosis in chronic liver disease. They are normally metabolized by the liver and must be used with caution. Thus the dose should be reduced as the half-life will increase in liver disease. If they are used in viral conditions they result in increased viral replication and higher mortality (Strombeck 1980). They should not be used where there is ascites or encephalopathy as they are catabolic, immunosuppressive and fluid-retaining.

However, they may be very usefully employed in chronic active hepatitis and lymphocytic cholangitis to reduce the inflammatory reaction and development of fibrosis. Where there is infiltration by plasma cells and lymphocytes which leads to loss of hepatocytes, prednisolone reduces this infiltration and thus conserves hepatocytes. In addition it has been shown to reduce the development of fibrosis tissue scarring following severe hepatocyte destruction.

Prednisone is converted to prednisolone in the liver so only the latter should be used in liver disease. Corticosteroid has been shown significantly to improve the long-term outcome of chronic liver disease (Strombeck *et al*. 1988). Azathioprine (Imuran; Calmic Medical Division) has also been indicated in the treatment of chronic liver disease. Both prednisolone and azathioprine should be used at 1 mg/kg daily or twice daily.

Colchicine and zinc gluconate have been used for their antifibrotic action in human liver disease. They reduce microtubule formation, increase collagenase activity and reduce collagen formation. They may however cause haemorrhagic gastroenteritis, pyrexia, alopecia, hypocalcaemia and bone marrow suppression. They are experimental drugs and have not been evaluated in dogs and cats. Penicillamine (Distamine; Dista Products) may be more effective than prednisolone in preventing fibrosis by interfering with collagen deposition and maturation (Chen *et al*. 1979).

In cats prednisolone is very useful in the treatment of lymphocytic cholangitis. It improves appetite and bile flow. A daily dosage of 2 mg/kg should be used initially, tapering to alternate day therapy once a satisfactory response has been obtained.

Copper chelation

Copper accumulation may be important in some forms of liver disease. D-penicillamine (Distamine; Dista Products) at 10 to 15 mg/kg bid chelates serum copper and excretes the chelated product in the urine, so reducing copper accumulation in the liver. The drug may cause side effects of vomiting and diarrhoea (Magne & Chiapella 1986).

Concurrent disease

Coagulopathy

In chronic hepatic disease, disseminated intravascular coagulation (DIC) and clotting factor deficiencies may develop. These are manifest as bleeding syndromes. Management and treatment of these cases can be difficult; the main aim is to reduce fibrinolysis and restore levels of clotting factors. Administration of heparin at 100 units/kg tid is recommended as it blocks the clotting mechanism, but it must be given with whole blood in order to replace clotting factors or fatal haemorrhage occurs (Strombeck 1980). Cimetidine (Tagamet; SmithKline Beecham Pharmaceuticals) should be given at 2 to 4 mg/kg bid to help control gastrointestinal ulceration and bleeding. In combination with these drugs a good source of dietary protein is required. The prognosis in cases of hepatic disease with DIC is very poor, especially where there is haemorrhage into the intestine, since it is very difficult to control.

Renal disease

Hepatic disease especially in older animals may be exacerbated by the presence of renal disease with fluid imbalance. Renal disease also contributes to the presence of ascites through retention of sodium and water. Diuretics such as frusemide, which causes potassium loss, are also metabolized by the liver and so they are contraindicated. Thiazide diuretics and spironolactone should be employed as previously described.

Prerenal uraemia should be treated by careful use of intravenous fluids to restore renal perfusion. Even if the intravenous fluids increase the amount of ascitic fluid, it is nonetheless essential to give fluids in order to establish renal perfusion. Once this has been achieved then the ascites can be corrected with diuretics or a hypertonic solution of dextrose or mannitol.

As the treatments for hepatic and renal disease are not always compatible and because of the seriousness of the combined dysfunction, cases with involvement of both systems should carry a very guarded prognosis (Strombeck 1980).

References

Anthony P.P., Ishak K.G., Nayak N.C., Poulsen H.E., Scheurer P.J. & Sobin L.H. (1977) The morphology of cirrhosis. Definition, nomenclature and classification. *WHO Bulletin*, **55**; 521–540.

August J.R. (1984) Feline infectious peritonitis. An immune-mediated coronaviral vasculitis. *Veterinary Clinics of North America*, **14**; 971–984.

Bennett A.M., Davies J.D., Gaskell C.J. & Lucke V.M. (1983) Lobular dissecting hepatitis in the dog. *Veterinary Pathology*, **20**; 179–188.

Beverley J.K.A. (1976) Toxoplasmosis in animals. *Veterinary Record*, **99**; 123−127.

Bishop L., Strandling J.D. & Adams R.J. (1979) Chronic active hepatitis in dogs associated with Leptospires. *American Journal of Veterinary Research*, **40**; 839−844.

Black A.P. (1983) A solitary congenital hepatic cyst in a cat. *Australian Veterinary Practice*, **13**; 166−168.

Blaxter A. (1987) Diagnosis and management of hepatic disorders in the cat. *In Practice*, **9**; 178−185.

Brown N.O. (1981) Paraneoplastic syndromes of humans, dogs and cats. *Journal of American Animal Hospital Association*, **17**; 911−916.

Center S.A. (1986) Feline liver disorders and their management. *Compendium on Continuing Education for the Practicing Veterinarian*, **8**; 889−901.

Chen T.S., Zaki G.F. & Levy C.M. (1979) Studies of nucleic acid and collagen synthesis; current status in assessing liver repair *Medical Clinics of North America*, **63**; 583−591.

Cornelius L.M. & Jacobs G. (1989) Feline hepatic lipidosis. In: *Current Veterinary Therapy* Vol. X, R.W. Kirk (ed.), W.B. Saunders, Philadelphia, 869−873.

Crawford M.A., Schall W.D. & Jensen R.K. (1985) Hepatopathy in 24 Doberman Pinschers. *Journal of American Veterinary Medical Association*, **187**; 1343−1350.

Davis M.R. (1985) Paracetamol poisoning in a cat. *Veterinary Record*, **116**; 223.

Doige C.E. & Lester, S. (1981) Chronic active hepatitis in dogs; a review of fourteen cases. *Journal of American Animal Hospital Association*, **17**; 725−730.

Drazner F.H. (1983) Hepatic encephalopathy in the dog. In: *Current Veterinary Therapy* Vol. VIII, R.W. Kirk (ed.), W.B. Saunders, Philadelphia, 829−834.

Eder H. (1964) Chronic toxicity studies on phenacetin n-acetyl-p-amino penol (NAPA) and acetylsalicylic acid on cats. *Acta Pharmacologie Toxicologie*, **21**; 197−204.

Edwards D.F. McCracken M.D. & Richardson D.C. (1983) Sclerosing cholangitis in a cat. *Journal of American Veterinary Medical Association*, **182**; 710−712.

Fittschen C. & Bellamy J.E.C. (1984) Prenisone induced morphologic and chemical changes in the liver of dogs. *Veterinary Pathology*, **21**; 399−406.

Franklin J.E. & Saunders G.K. (1988) Chronic active hepatitis in Doberman Pinschers. *Compendium on Continuing Education for the Practicing Veterinarian*, **10**; 1247−1254.

Frenkel J.K. (1985) Toxoplasmosis. *Pediatric Clinics of North America*, **32**; 917−982.

Gocke D.J., Presig R. & Morris T.D. (1967) Experimental viral hepatitis in the dog; production of persistent disease in partially immune animals. *Journal of Clinical Investigation*, **46**; 1506−1517.

Hall S.M. (1986) Toxoplasmosis. *Journal of Small Animal Practice*, **27**; 705−715.

Hardy R.M. (1986) Chronic hepatitis in dogs: a syndrome. *Compendium on Continuing Education for the Practicing Veterinarian*, **8**; 904−913.

Hardy R.M. (1989) Diseases of the liver and their treatment. In: *Textbook of Veterinary Internal Medicine, Diseases of the dog and cat*, Vol. 2, Ettinger, S.J. (ed.), W.B. Saunders, Philadelphia.

Hardy R.M. Stevens J.B. & Stove C.M. (1975) Chronic progressive hepatitis in Bedlington Terriers associated with elevated liver copper concentrations. *Minnesota Veterinarian*, **15**; 13−24.

Hendricks J.D., DiMagno E.P., Go V.L.W. (1980) Reflux of duodenal contents into the pancreatic duct of dogs. *Journal of Laboratory and Clinical Medicine*, **96**; 912−921.

Hirsh V.M. & Doige C.E. (1983) Suppurative cholangitis in cats. *Journal of American Veterinary Medical Association*, **182**; 1223−1226.

Hornbuckle W.E. & Allan G.S. (1980) Feline liver disease. In: *Current Veterinary Therapy* Vol. VII, R.W. Kirk (ed.), W.B. Saunders, Philadelphia, 891−895.

Jarrett W.F.H. & O'Neil B.W. (1985) A new transmissible agent causing acute hepatitis, chronic hepatitis and cirrhosis in dogs. *Veterinary Record*, **116**; 629−635.

Johnson G.K. Zawie D.A. & Gilbertson S.R. (1982) Chronic active hepatitis in Doberman Pinschers. *Journal of American Veterinary Medical Association*, **180**; 1438−1442.

Jones B.R., Johnstone A.C. & Hancock W.S. (1985) Tyzzer's disease in kittens with familial primary hyperlipoproteinaemia. *Journal of Small Animal Practice*, **26**; 411−419.

Kelly D.F., Haywood S. & Bennett A.M. (1984) Copper toxicosis in Bedlington Terriers in the United Kingdom. *Journal of Small Animal Practice*, **25**; 293–298.

Kiernan F. (1833) The anatomy and physiology of the liver. *Philosophical Transactions of the Royal Society of London*, Series B, **123**; 711–770.

Laflamme D.P. (1988) Dietary management of canine hepatic encephalopathy. *Compendium on Continuing Education for the Practicing Veterinarian*, **10**; 1258–1262.

Lucke V.M. & Davies J.D. (1984) Progressive lymphocytic cholangitis in the cat. *Journal of Small Animal Practice*, **25**; 249–260.

Lucke V.M. & Herrtage M.E. (1987) Copper associated liver disease in the dog. In: *The Veterinary Annual*, G.S.C. Grunsell, F.W.G. Hill & M.E. Raw (eds). Scientechnica, Bristol, 264–269.

MacSween R.N.M., Anthony P.P. & Scheuer P.J. (1979) *Pathology of the Liver*. Churchill Livingstone, Edinburgh.

Magne, M.L. & Chiapella, A.M. (1986) Medical management of canine chronic hepatitis. *Compendium on Continuing Education for the Practicing Veterinarian*, **8**; 915–921.

Meyer D.J. & Center S.A. (1986) Approach to the diagnosis of liver disorders in dogs and cats. *Compendium on Continuing Education for the Practicing Veterinarian*, **8**; 880–888.

Meyer D.J., Strombeck D.R. & Stone E.A. (1978) Ammonium tolerance test in clinically normal dogs and dogs with portosystemic shunts. *Journal of American Veterinary Medical Association*, **173**; 377–379.

Morgan M.H. & Read A.E. (1982) Treatment of hepatic encephalopathy with metronidazole. *Gut*, **23**; 1–7.

Moulton J.E. (1978) Tumours of the pancreas, liver, gall bladder and mesothelium. In: *Tumours in Domestic Animals*, J.E. Moulton (ed.). University of California Press, Berkeley, 276–282.

Mullowney P.C. & Tennant B.C. (1982) Choledocholelithiasis in the dog: a review and report of a case with rupture of the common bile duct. *Journal of Small Animal Practice*, **23**; 631–638.

Nash A.S. & Bobade P.A. (1986) Haemobartonella felis infection in cats from the Glasgow area. *Veterinary Record*, **119**; 373–375.

Ng B.K., Noor F. & Omar A.R.S. (1981) Hepatic cirrhosis with duodenal ulcers in a dog. *Australian Veterinary Practitioner*, **11**; 14–17.

Pedersen N.C. (1983) Feline infectious peritonitis and feline enteric coronavirus infections. *Feline Medicine*, **13**; 5–20.

Percy D.H. (1982) Type 2 Herpes simplex infection, animal model. *Armed Forces Institute for Pathology, Comparative Pathology Bulletin*, **14**; 2–4.

Petersen M.E. (1984) Feline hyperthyroidism. *Veterinary Clinics of North America*, **14**; 809–826.

Prasse K.W., Mahaffey E.A., DeNovo R. & Cornelius L. (1982) Chronic lymphocytic cholangitis in three cats. *Veterinary Pathology*, **19**; 99–108.

Rafiquzzaman M., Svenkeind P., Straude A. & Hauge J.G. (1976) Glycogenosis in the dog. *Acta Veterinaria Scandinavia*, **17**; 196–209.

Rappaport A.M. (1975) Anatomic considerations. In: *Disease of the Liver*, L. Schiff (ed.). W.B. Saunder, Philadelphia.

Rogers K.S. & Cornelius L.M. (1985) Feline icterus. *Compendium on Continuing Education for the Practicing Veterinarian*, **7**; 391–399.

Rogers W.A. & Ruebner B.H. (1977) A retrospective study of probable glucocorticoid induced hepatopathy in dogs. *Journal of American Veterinary Medical Association*, **170**; 603–606.

Sherding R.G. (1985) Acute hepatic failure. *Veterinary Clinics of North America*, **15**; 119–132.

Simpson J.W. & Else R.W. (1987) Diagnostic value of tissue biopsy in gastrointestinal and liver disease. *Veterinary Record*, **120**; 230–233.

Smith L.T. (1980) Hepatitis due to *Clostridium perfringens* in a dog. *Veterinary Medicine: Small Animal Clinician*, **75**; 1380–1383.

Strombeck D.R. (1980) Management of canine chronic active hepatitis. In: *Current Veterinary Therapy* Vol. VII, R.W. Kirk (ed.). W.B. Saunders, Philadelphia, 885–891.

Strombeck D.R. & Gribble D.G. (1978) Chronic active hepatitis in the dog. *Journal of American Veterinary Medical Association*, **173**; 380–386.

Strombeck D.R., Miller L.M. & Harrold D. (1988) Effects of corticosteroid treatment on survival time in dogs with chronic hepatitis: 151 cases (1977–85). *Journal of American Veterinary Medical Association*, **193**; 1109–1113.

Thornburg L.P., Polley D. & Dimmitt R. (1984) The diagnosis and treatment of copper toxicosis in dogs. *Canine Practice*, **11**; 36–39.

Thornburg L.P. Simpson S. & Digilio K. (1986a) Fatty liver syndrome in cats. *Journal of American Animal Hospital Association*, **18**; 397–400.

Thornburg L.P., Shaw D., Dolan M., Raisbeck M., Crawford S., Dennis G.L. & Olwin D.B. (1986b) Hereditary copper toxicosis in West Highland White Terriers. *Veterinary Pathology*, **23**; 148–154.

Tuzhilin S.A. Podolsky A.E. & Drieling D.A. (1975) Hepatic lesions in pancreatitis: clinico-experimental data. *American Journal of Gastroenterology*, **64**; 108–114.

Twedt D.C. (1981) Jaundice: hepatic coma and hepatic encephalopathy. *Veterinary Clinics of North America*, **11**; 121–146.

Van den Ingh, T.S.G.A.M. & Rothuizen, J. (1982) Hepatoportal fibrosis in three young dogs. *Veterinary Record*, **110**; 575–577.

Van den Ingh, T.S.G.A.M. & Rothuizen, J. (1985) Congenital cystic disease of the liver in seven dogs. *Journal of Comparative Pathology*, **95**; 405–414.

Vitums A. (1961) Porosystemic communications in animals with hepatic cirrhosis and malignant lymphoma. *Journal of American Veterinary Medical Association*, **138**; 31–34.

Walshaw R. (1985) Liver and biliary system. In: *Textbook of Small Animal Surgery*, D.H. Slatter (ed.). W.B. Saunders, Philadelphia, 798–827.

Whitcomb F.F. (1979) Chronic active liver disease. Definition, diagnosis and management. *Medical Clinics of North America*, **63**; 413–422.

Wilke, J.R. (1984) Idiosyncrasies of drug metabolism in cats. *Veterinary Clinics of North America*. **14**; 1345–1354.

Wilkinson G.T. (1984) *Diseases of Cats and their Management*. Blackwell Scientific, Oxford.

Zawie D.A. & Garvey M.S. (1984) Feline hepatic disease. In: Symposium on Advances in Feline Medicine II. *Veterinary Clinics of North America*, **14**; 1201–1231.

10/Laboratory Methods and Biopsy Collection

This chapter contains information on the various diagnostic procedures described throughout the book (Table 10.1). The methods for carrying out the diagnostic tests are described, together with information on the interpretation of results.

The values may vary from those observed in other laboratories and they should not be directly compared. The general degree of change from normal will be maintained in most cases but the actual values must be considered in the light of the normal values for each laboratory.

Routine faecal analysis

Where a dog or cat is presented with chronic diarrhoea, faecal analysis

Table 10.1 Diagnostic procedures described in this chapter

Faecal analysis	Trypsin digest test
	Microscopic examination for undigested food
	Worm egg count
	Bacteriological examination
Dynamic tests	Xylose absorption test
	Quantitative fat absorption test
	BT-PABA test
	Ammonium tolerance test
	BSP retention test
Biopsy techniques	Oesophageal and gastric biopsy
	Colonic biopsy
	Small intestinal biopsy
	Percutaneous liver biopsy
	Abdominal paracentesis
Haematology	Routine haematology
Biochemistry	Serum proteins
	Serum sodium and potassium
	Trypsin-like immunoreactivity test
	Serum folate and vitamin B12 assay
	Liver enzymes and function tests
Radiography	Motility studies
	Obstructions
	Mucosal changes
	Assessment of liver
	Ascites and peritonitis

should be used as an initial screening procedure to assist the clinician in determining the type of problem that may be present.

Routine faecal analysis should include a trypsin digest test, microscopic examination of faeces for undigested food, worm egg count and bacteriological examination. It is important that the examination is complete and this means at least two faecal samples should be examined if meaningful information is to be obtained. For example, a single trypsin digest test is totally meaningless but together with the microscopic examination of faeces for undigested food it will provide useful information and in combination with results from additional tests may provide a definitive diagnosis.

Trypsin digest test

In normal dogs and cats the faeces contain some trypsin activity, although the amount may vary considerably. By incubating faeces with a suitable protein substrate (e.g. gelatin) it is possible to assess the level of trypsin activity. The gelatin tube test is simple and easy to perform and gives a good indication of trypsin activity. At least two faecal trypsin estimations should be carried out and the results interpreted in conjunction with the microscopic examination of faeces for undigested food.

The method of carrying out the gelatin tube test is shown in Table 10.2. The trypsin titre may vary considerably and it is not uncommon to have nil titres in normal dogs. Dogs with exocrine pancreatic insufficiency (EPI) always have titres of less than 1/10. If the titre is less than 1/10 *and* there is

Table 10.2 Method of carrying out the gelatin tube test

Preparation of faecal suspension
1 Weigh out 1 g of faeces
2 Sieve faeces into a bowl with 9 ml of 5% sodium bicarbonate
3 Final dilution is 1/10 ready for double dilution

Dilution of faecal suspension

	1	2	3	4*
Add 7.5% gelatin solution	2 ml	2 ml	2 ml	2 ml
Add 1/10 faecal suspension	1 ml	0.5 ml	0.25 ml	—
Add sodium bicarbonate	—	0.5 ml	0.75 ml	1 ml

Mix tubes thoroughly

Incubation and interpretation
1 Incubate tubes at 37°C for 60 min
2 Refrigerate tubes at 4°C for 20 min
3 Examine tubes for digestion
   Control tube should always be solid
   Tubes which remain liquid indicate digestion has occurred

* Tube no.

undigested starch and fat present in the faeces this strongly suggests the presence of EPI. In such cases a trypsin-like immunoreactivity (TLI) test should be carried out in order to obtain a definitive diagnosis.

Microscopic examination of faeces

This simple technique is valuable in detecting the presence of undigested fat and starch in faecal samples. In the past, some importance has been attached to the detection of undigested muscle fibres but this has now been shown to be of limited value (Simpson & Doxey 1988). It is important that the animal is placed on a properly-balanced diet containing both carbohydrate and fats, if the microscopic examination is to be of any value. Sudden changes in diet, to facilitate this test, may lead to the presence of undigested starch and fat in the faeces, which is not associated with maldigestion but entirely due to the sudden dietary change.

The faeces sample is prepared as follows; a thin film of fresh faeces should be smeared onto three microscope slides. Before the smears dry, Lugol's iodine (for the detection of starch) should be applied to one slide, Sudan IV (for the detection of fat) to another slide. The third slide may be prepared to examine faeces for split fats or fatty acids. In the latter case a faecal smear is flooded with Sudan IV and a few drops of acetic acid, heated until it just boils and then allowed to cool for 5 min. In all cases following staining for 5 min the excess stain should be decanted, the underside of the slide dried and the slide viewed under a ×4 objective lens.

Normally no evidence of undigested fat or starch should be present on the slide. Faeces from dogs with EPI show large numbers of fat globules (see Fig. 8.4(b)) and starch granules (see Fig. 8.4(a)). Ten random fields should be examined under the microscope and if more than 200 fat globules and starch granules per field are detected this should be considered significant. Where split fats take up the stain this means that fatty acids are present, suggesting adequate digestion but poor absorption.

The results of this test should be interpreted together with results of a trypsin digest test in order to determine if EPI is likely to be present. If the results suggest the presence of exocrine pancreatic insufficiency, the TLI test should then be carried out. Where steatorrhoea occurs in the presence of normal trypsin titres, this may suggest the presence of bacterial overgrowth. In such cases bacteria may deconjugate bile acids or produce hydroxy fatty acids leading to malabsorption of fat. Infection with *Giardia* spp. may also cause steatorrhoea without affecting the trypsin titre or digestion of starch.

Worm egg count

A worm egg count should always be carried out as part of the routine faecal examination. In general a quantitative concentration technique is the most useful. It is important to carry out a worm egg count on at least two different faecal samples, as eggs can be excreted intermittently.

The most commonly-used method is the McMaster technique. With this method, 3 g of fresh faeces are thoroughly mixed with 42 ml of water and poured through a 100 mesh sieve into a bowl. The filtrate is placed in two centrifuge tubes and centrifuged for 3 min. The supernatant is discarded and the deposit resuspended in saturated salt solution and thoroughly mixed. A Pasteur pipette is used to collect the resuspended deposit from each tube and is used to fill each chamber of the McMaster slide. The slide is then examined microscopically under the ×4 objective lens and all parasitic eggs within each chamber are counted (Fig. 10.1). This number is multiplied by 50 to give the number of eggs per gram of faeces.

Bacteriological examination

The last component of the routine faecal examination is a bacteriological examination. It is always advisable to collect faecal samples rather than faecal swabs which may not be representative of rectal contents or may dry out, destroying bacteria and giving false negative results. At least two faecal samples should be examined as bacteria may be excreted intermittently, especially *Salmonella* spp. and *Campylobacter* spp. Interpretation of the significance of coliforms in faeces is difficult and may require serial sampling. In addition, faecal culture does not reflect the balance of bacterial flora in

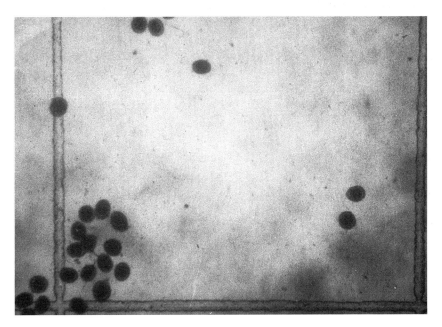

Fig. 10.1 Examination of faeces for *Toxocara canis* eggs using the McMaster counting chamber.

the small intestine and relative proliferation of different populations is better assessed using serum folate and vitamin B12 estimations.

Dynamic tests

Xylose absorption test

The xylose absorption test is one of the simplest assays to test the efficiency of small intestinal absorption. Its use in the dog was first described by Hill *et al.* (1970). D-xylose is a pentose monosaccharide which is not normally found in the diet or circulation. No digestion of xylose is required prior to passive and active absorption across the small intestinal mucosa. Xylose enters the portal blood and then the general circulation where it can easily be measured indicating the degree of absorption that has taken place.

Following an overnight fast, the dog or cat is given 0.5 g/kg liveweight of xylose (Analar; BDH) mixed with 150 g of a standard dog or cat food. This presentation has two advantages; the animal will eat the food without need for stressful dosing, and secondly it allows an assessment of xylose absorption in the presence of other dietary components. One millilitre blood samples in fluoride (glucose) bottles are collected prior to feeding and at hourly intervals for 4 h after feeding.

Normal animals have a nil or very low resting value which will increase to at least 3 mmol/l at 2 to 3 h post feeding, before falling again by 4 h (see Fig. 7.4). In small intestinal disease (malabsorption) values are reduced and the degree of reduction tends to reflect the degree of dysfunction present. Not all animals with malabsorption however will yield reduced xylose values as this depends on the type of malabsorption present and the extent to which the small intestine is involved. Disadvantages of the test include the possibility of delayed gastric emptying, bacterial utilization of xylose, and the fact that results reflect only the absorption of one dietary component, compared with the normal situation where a complete meal is fed and absorbed.

In spite of these limitations, the xylose absorption test is still a useful test of small intestinal function. If the test is used together with the fat absorption test, serum folate and B12 assay for small intestinal function, the clinician will be able to determine whether small intestinal disease is present.

Quantitative fat absorption test

The diet normally contains fat consisting of long-chain triglyceride (LCT) which must be broken down by the action of lipase and bile salts before absorption can occur. Following absorption the fat is removed from the small intestine by way of the lymphatic system to enter the general circulation.

Measurement of serum triglyceride will indicate the amount of fat that has been digested and absorbed. Medium- and short-chain triglycerides (MCT and SCT) are absorbed intact across the small intestine and enter the portal blood where they are removed by the liver. Thus measurement of serum triglyceride levels are of no value when these fats are fed.

The fat absorption test may be used to detect a deficiency in lipase, bile salts or small intestinal malabsorption. By measuring the serum triglyceride levels, the test allows an accurate assessment of fat absorption to be made by comparison with normal values.

The dog or cat should be starved overnight and fed 3 ml/kg liveweight of vegetable oil (i.e. LCT), to a maximum dose of 90 ml. Clotted blood samples are collected before feeding the fat and at hourly intervals thereafter for 4 h. Samples are analysed for serum triglyceride levels.

The mean normal resting triglyceride value is 0.5 mmol/l and after feeding vegetable oil the value should triple by 3 h, with a mean of 1.6 mmol/l (see Fig. 7.5).

If the serum triglyceride values have not increased, then the test should be repeated with added lipase (Pancrex granules; Paines & Byrne) at one teaspoonful per 20 ml of vegetable oil. If the values increase on this occasion then exocrine pancreatic insufficiency is the likely cause. If no elevation occurs repeat the test with added bile salts (Panteric; Upjohn) at one tablet per 20 ml of vegetable oil. Elevation on this occasion suggests bile salt deficiency. No elevation suggests small intestinal malabsorption. Other tests should now be carried out to confirm the diagnosis of small intestinal malabsorption including xylose absorption, serum folate and vitamin B12 assay and ultimately biopsy of the small intestine.

BT-PABA test

Exocrine pancreatic insufficiency (EPI) may be detected by feeding the synthetic substrate N-benzoyl-L-tyrosyl-p-aminobenzoic acid (BT-PABA) which is specifically split by chymotrypsin from the exocrine pancreas. The free p-aminobenzoic acid (PABA) can then be absorbed and measured in blood samples or urine (Batt and Mann 1981).

After an overnight fast BT-PABA (Sigma Chemicals) is fed at 35 μmol/kg liveweight as an aqueous solution (16.5 mg/10 ml/kg). Heparinized blood samples are collected at rest and every 30 min for 3 h.

Normal dogs show a steady increase in value of PABA in the plasma up to a peak at 90 min with a value exceeding 30 μmol/l. Dogs with EPI will have values of less than 5 μmol/l at 90 min (Fig. 10.2).

Unfortunately the test can yield misleading results, as a consequence of reduced gastric emptying, hydrolysis of BT-PABA by bacterial proteases or where there is small intestinal malabsorption. All these factors may signifi-

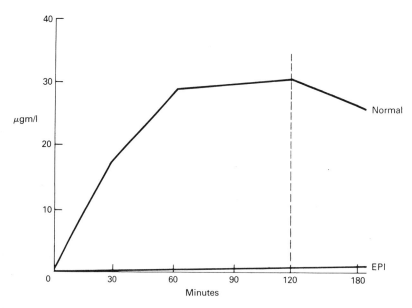

Fig. 10.2 BT-PABA curve observed in normal dogs and those with exocrine pancreatic insufficiency.

cantly alter the absorption of the PABA and make interpretation difficult. For this reason it has been superseded by a more reliable test, the trypsin-like immunoreactivity (TLI) test (see later).

Ammonia tolerance test

Ammonia absorbed from the intestine is rapidly removed from the portal blood by the liver, converted to urea and excreted in the kidneys. If the ammonia is not removed from the portal circulation, high levels persist in the circulation causing marked central nervous symptoms. The ammonia tolerance test is therefore important in assessing the ability of the liver to clear ammonia from the portal blood (Meyer and Center 1986).

Following an overnight fast, 100 mg/kg of ammonium chloride in warm water is given orally. A heparinized blood sample is collected before feeding and 30 min later. It is important to ensure blood samples are stored in ice and assayed as rapidly as possible after collection, as ammonia is volatile and the value falls rapidly after collection. Values in excess of 70 μmol/l are abnormal, and values of more than 200 μmol/l suggest either the presence of a congenital portosystemic shunt or cirrhosis of the liver, causing blood to by-pass the liver into the vena cava (Drazner 1983). A concurrent low blood urea level (less than 2 mmol/l) will often complement the high ammonia level.

Bromsulphthalein retention test

Another method of assessing liver function is the bromsulphthalein (BSP) retention test. The exogenous dye, which the normal liver will rapidly remove, is injected intravenously. The liver conjugates BSP and excretes it in the bile (Bush 1980). Where more than 55% of liver function is lost, BSP retention occurs.

Interference with the test may occur if bilirubin levels are elevated or albumin levels are reduced and in the presence of ascites. The test is less reliable in cats than in dogs. The BSP half-life $(T_{\frac{1}{2}})$ is used in large animals but cannot be used in dogs because BSP is excreted in two phases in the latter species. There is an initial fast phase of excretion followed by a slow phase and this pattern interferes with interpretation of BSP $T_{\frac{1}{2}}$ estimation.

Following an overnight fast, the dog or cat is given an intravenous injection of BSP at 5 mg/kg liveweight. A heparinized blood sample is collected before the dye is injected and after a further 15 min in cats and 30 min in dogs. In normal dogs less than 5% of the BSP is retained in the circulation at 30 min, while values of more than 10% are considered abnormal. In cats less than 10% of the BSP should be retained at 15 min, and values higher than this are considered abnormal. The BSP retention test has to some extent been superseded by the measurement of bile acids and by the ammonia tolerance test.

Biopsy collection

Fibre-optic endoscopy

The use of fibre-optic endoscopy has revolutionized diagnosis in gastro-enterology. It is now possible to carry out a detailed examination of the pharynx, oesophagus, stomach and colon without recourse to invasive surgery. This has resulted in more effective diagnosis, faster recovery for the patients and has met with great enthusiasm from the owners. It also allows complete assessment of therapy because follow-up endoscopy subjects the patient to very little stress, particularly where laparotomy could not be routinely considered.

The main disadvantages of endoscopy include: (1) the risk of causing major haemorrhage on biopsy collection, although this has not been a problem recognized by the authors, (2) the inability to detect pathological changes which lie outwith the mucosa; and (3) difficulties in examining areas such as the small intestine with the inherent problem of representative sampling. However in skilled hands it offers the clinician a powerful diag-nostic tool which permits biopsy collection and diagnosis of conditions without recourse to invasive surgery (e.g. in atrophic gastritis, hypertrophic gastritis, gastric ulceration and neoplasia).

Endoscopes are available in varying diameters from 7.5 mm to 12 mm. The former are very useful in small dogs and cats while the latter should be used in larger breeds of dog. The larger the diameter the greater the number of fibres and hence the amount of light available and hence image quality. The endoscope tips may be 'side viewing' or 'end viewing' and are designed for different purposes. The 'end viewing' endoscope is used routinely as it allows the operator to examine the tissues immediately in front of the endoscope as it passes along the gastrointestinal tract (Fig. 10.3). Biopsy forceps come in various sizes and shapes. Basically they comprise two cups which close to capture and retrieve a biopsy sample. The cups may be fenestrated to reduce crushing damage to the biopsy sample when the forceps close, and some have a central needle which assists in stabilizing the forceps while collecting a biopsy sample from a selected site (Fig. 10.4).

Oesophageal/gastric examination

1   Fast the patient for 24 h prior to endoscopy. This is especially important where there may be problems with gastric retention and atony, where food or fluid in the stomach make endoscopic examination impossible. If required, confirm the stomach is empty with a lateral radiograph before general anaesthesia is given.

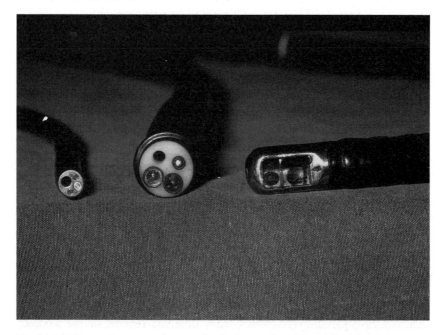

Fig. 10.3 Different diameters and types of end piece used on fibre-optic endoscopes.

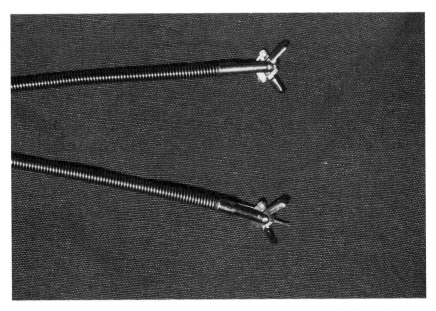

Fig. 10.4 Different types of biopsy forceps used for biopsy collection with fibre-optic endoscopes.

2 Following premedication, induce general anaesthesia, intubate to prevent any risk of gastric regurgitation and tie the endotracheal tube to the mandible and not the maxilla. Maintain with gaseous anaesthetics.

3 Place patient in left lateral recumbency.

4 Always use a mouth gag to prevent damage occurring to the endoscope.

5 Lubricate the tip of the endoscope and slowly advance into the pharynx. It is usually necessary to inflate the oesophagus with air to visualize the tissues and prevent 'red out' which is the term used when nothing is in focus and there is a uniform red colour observed down the endoscope. Examine the oesophagus as the endoscope is advanced and collect biopsy samples of any abnormal tissues detected. Oesophageal tissue is not easy to biopsy as it is very tough. In this respect biopsy forceps with a central needle are most useful in assisting sampling in this site.

6 The cardia of the stomach may or may not be patent. Usually some resistance is felt as the endoscope is advanced into the stomach. Inflate the stomach with only a small amount of air as the pylorus and duodenum are more easily examined if the stomach is not overdistended. This is because the tip of the endoscope is more easily directed under these conditions.

7 Examine all regions of the stomach carefully and systematically. Collect biopsy samples from any abnormal tissue detected. Where no abnormality is detected multiple biopsy samples from different regions of the stomach should always be collected.

8 Biopsy samples should be carefully removed from the forceps and mounted mucosal surface uppermost on thin cardboard before being labelled and placed in 10% formol saline.

9 Following endoscopy the stomach should be deflated using a stomach tube to ensure very little free gas remains.

10 Seepage of blood is common from a biopsy site. If more extensive haemorrhage does occur instill 1 : 10 000 adrenaline solution with iced water through the biopsy channel using an endoscopic catheter (Portex). If this fails to stop the haemorrhage, laparotomy may have to be carried out to control the bleeding.

Colonic examination

1 Starve the dog or cat for 24 h before the procedure.

2 Give a warm water enema first thing in the morning and repeat the procedure 1 h later.

3 Repeat the enemas until the colon contains no further faecal material.

4 Avoid soap and other irritant enemas as they cause inflammatory changes to the colonic mucosa which makes interpretation of changes observed at endoscopy very difficult.

5 Sedate the patient using acepromazine (ACP; C-Vet) 0.05 mg/kg and buprenorphine (Temgesic; Reckitt & Colman) 0.01 mg/kg given intramuscularly. This has been found to be very satisfactory for colonoscopy, eliminating the need for a general anaesthetic and giving a very fast recovery time.

6 Place patient in left lateral recumbency.

7 Lubricate the tip of the endoscope and insert through the anus.

8 Examine the colon carefully as the endoscope is advanced and collect biopsy samples of any abnormal tissue.

9 Try to examine the entire colon if possible. The ascending colon is the most difficult region to examine, while the transverse and descending colon should be accessible on all occasions.

10 If no obvious abnormality is detected, multiple biopsy samples should be collected from all regions of the colon.

11 Biopsy samples should be carefully mounted on cardboard and stored in 10% formol saline until examined.

12 No special post procedural care is required with these patients other than to observe for signs of haemorrhage.

Small intestinal biopsy

It is difficult to collect biopsy samples from the small intestine using fibreoptic endoscopy. The normal route for collection of samples from this site is following laparotomy. For this reason the clinician should first obtain satisfactory evidence that small intestinal disease is present, from dynamic tests and measurement of serum folate and vitamin B12 levels.

Where the patient has a protein-losing enteropathy (PLE), the need for biopsy collection is just as valid but the risk of laparotomy to the patient is much greater. Animals with PLE are poor anaesthetic risks, and they have reduced powers of healing and are immunodeficient.

Whenever a laparotomy is carried out to collect small intestinal biopsy samples, the whole length of the small intestine should be carefully examined and a biopsy sample collected wherever an abnormality is detected. It is not unusual for no gross abnormality to be detected, and under these conditions biopsy samples should always be collected from the duodenum, jejunum and ileum together with a representative portion of mesenteric lymph node. Many small intestinal conditions give rise to microscopic rather than macroscopic changes, so that lack of gross changes should not discourage biopsy collection.

The authors have found the use of a 4 mm skin biopsy punch (Stiefel Laboratories UK) very useful in collecting full thickness biopsy samples without damaging the mucosa. The resultant wound is cleaner and more easily closed. Biopsy samples should be mounted on cardboard and fixed in 10% formol saline prior to histopathological examination. Alternatively, samples may be snap frozen for histochemical assay or frozen sections, biochemical or immunological assay.

Liver biopsy

Although the clinical symptoms and results of serum biochemistry may indicate hepatic malfunction, the only method of obtaining a definitive diagnosis in suspected liver disease is by liver biopsy. Normally clinicians would carry out a laparotomy to obtain a suitable tissue wedge biopsy but increased and unacceptable risk may attend severely debilitated or old animals. The alternative technique for obtaining a liver biopsy using a percutaneous needle may be preferred in such cases but there is still some risk involved. Although general anaesthesia is not usually required with this latter method, there are some disadvantages such as a danger of rupturing the gall bladder, or causing an unobserved intra-abdominal haemorrhage. Furthermore, it may not be possible to sample smaller focal lesions by this technique.

The authors routinely use the following percutaneous biopsy procedure for collection of liver samples, using a Menghini or Tru-cut needle. Once a tentative diagnosis of liver disease has been made two additional tests are carried out: (1) a radiograph of the abdomen is taken to access the size and

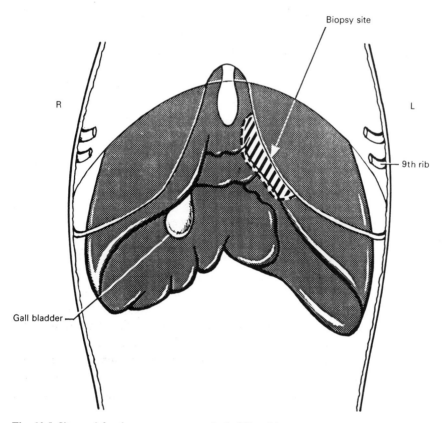

Fig. 10.5 Site used for the percutaneous method of liver biopsy.

position of the liver; this will also indicate the presence of a focal lesion. A large liver mass is usually easier to biopsy, while a small liver mass can make the procedure much more difficult; and (2) a prothrombin time is always determined in order to ensure there is no major bleeding tendency.

About 1 h before a sedative is given, the patient should receive 1 ml/kg body weight of vegetable oil, which will encourage the gall bladder to contract, making it much smaller during the biopsy procedure. The dog or cat is then given a sedative such as acepromazine (ACP; C-Vet) at 0.05 mg/kg with buprenorphine (Temgesic; Reckitt & Colman) at 0.01 mg/kg intramuscularly. After placing the patient in dorsal recumbency the area caudal to the ziphisternum and to its left is shaved and surgically prepared (Fig. 10.5). Local anaesthetic is infiltrated into the triangular area bounded by the costal arch, ziphisternum and linea alba. The skin is incised with a scalpel blade to permit the biopsy needle (Tru-cut; Travenol) to enter the muscle layer and pass through into the abdominal cavity. The needle should be directed in a dorsal, lateral and slightly cranial direction. This will reduce any risk of puncturing the gall bladder. Once the needle enters the peritoneal cavity it will feel 'loose' and if advanced further will 'firm' again as it enters the liver at which point a biopsy may be collected (Simpson & Else 1987).

Biopsy samples should be carefully removed from the needle onto card-board and fixed in 10% formol saline prior to histopathological examination. Portions of needle biopsies can also be used for bacteriological culture or immunological examination (Else 1989).

Abdominal paracentesis

Paracentesis of ascitic fluid can be of considerable diagnostic value. The technique is easily carried out by clipping the hair on the ventral abdomen from the xiphisternum to a point caudal to the umbilicus, and the area should be thoroughly cleaned with surgical spirit. Local anaesthetic may be infiltrated into a point midway between the xiphisternum and the umbilicus before inserting a sterile 20 gauge needle on a 20 ml syringe directly into the abdomen. Depending on the amount of fluid thought to be present, the patient may be held in lateral recumbency or kept in the standing position. Fluid collected should be stored in plain glass tubes and in heparin and sent for cytological examination and assessment of composition. Fluid accumu-lations in the abdomen may be true transudates through to exudates, and the cellular content may vary from negligible to inflammatory or neoplastic (Table 10.3).

Haematology and clinical chemistry

Routine haematology

Changes in the red cell indices are infrequently encountered in gastrointesti-nal disease. Haemoconcentration may occur where the animal becomes dehydrated following vomiting and/or diarrhoea. Bleeding from gastrointesti-

Table 10.3 Differentiation of ascitic fluid accumulations

Parameter	True transudate	Modified transudate	Exudate	Chyle	Urine
S.G.	<1.015	<1.015	>1.015	<1.015	>1.015
Colour	Clear	Pink	Turbid	Milky	Yellow
Clotting	—	—	Yes	—	—
Cells	—	Some	Many	—	Some
Protein	<30 g/l	30 g/l	>30 g/l	<30 g/l	>30 g/l
Bacteria	—	—	Yes	—	Yes
Urea	Low	Low	Low	Low	High

nal ulceration may lead to anaemia if the loss has been extensive and prolonged, but this is not common in small animals compared with man.

Persistent eosinophilia in association with gastrointestinal symptoms may suggest the presence of an eosinophilic gastroenteritis which should be investigated further. Where there is eosinophilia and lymphocytosis this may suggest the presence of hypoadrenocorticism, and further tests should be carried out to confirm this diagnosis (see below). Lymphocytosis may occur alone in advanced cases of enteric lymphosarcoma, but this is a rare finding and should not be used as the sole criterion for diagnosis of that condition. Neutrophilia is rare in gastrointestinal disorders although it occurs in association with secondary infection of tumours, peritonitis, acute pancreatitis, suppurative cholangitis and granulomatous enteritis. Leucopenia is more likely to be observed where viral gastroenteritis is present, with total white cells counts falling to less than 1×10^9/litre in the authors' experience.

Serum proteins

Hypoproteinaemia is a feature of some advanced forms of small intestinal disease such as lymphangiectasia, eosinophilic enteritis and lymphosarcoma. These cases are often referred to as protein-losing enteropathies because there is a major loss of serum protein into the lumen of the intestine. Both albumin and globulin tend to be lost in these cases, resulting in a substantial fall in total protein and values less than 30 g/l.

It is important to rule out other causes of hypoproteinaemia which may be associated with gastrointestinal symptoms. Liver failure and renal disease are the most important differentials. In both these conditions the hypoproteinaemia is predominently due to a reduction in albumin and not globulin. A careful check of hepatic and renal function (see below) will ensure these organs are functioning correctly and are not the cause of the hypoproteinaemia. This allows the clinician to concentrate attention on the type of intestinal disease which may be present.

Hyperglobulinaemia is an important and useful feature of two feline conditions; feline infectious peritonitis and lymphocytic cholangitis. In both these conditions globulin values may exceed 50 g/l and are often more than 70 g/l. In such situations further definitive tests should be carried out to confirm which condition is present, including serology and liver biopsy.

Sodium and potassium ratio

Where the clinical symptoms exhibited by the dog suggest the possibility of hypoadrenocorticism, measurement of serum sodium and potassium levels should be carried out. In the normal dog the ratio of sodium to potassium should be greater than 27:1; in Addison's disease the ratio may be less than 25:1 and often more than 20:1. Where the ratio is abnormal an adreno-corticotrophic hormone (ACTH) response test should be carried out which will reveal a low resting cortisol value and a poor response to ACTH in Addison's disease.

Trypsin-like immunoreactivity test (TLI)

The normal exocrine pancreas is thought to 'leak' small amounts of trypsino-gen into the general circulation where they can be measured by a radio-immunoassay. Measurement of the level of trypsinogen is considered to be a simple but specific test of exocrine pancreatic function (EPI) (Williams and Batt 1983). There is no oral dosing or problems with delayed stomach emptying or small intestinal malabsorption with this test, compared with the BT-PABA test. The most important procedural point is to ensure that the clotted blood sample is collected from a fasted dog. TLI values are not available for the cat, in which EPI is a very rare condition. The TLI test may also have value in detecting acute pancreatitis, when elevated levels of trypsinogen are present in serum, but no studies have been published to date on dogs.

The TLI value in normal fasted canine serum is more than 5 µg/l. Values less than 2 µg/l are considered diagnostic of EPI, whilst values which lie in the range 2 to 5 µg/l, are suggestive of EPI. In these cases the dog should be retested in 4 weeks' time, when the value is often found to be in the abnormal range.

Serum folate and vitamin B12

Folate is a water-soluble vitamin which is plentiful in the diet, where it takes the form of folate polyglutamate. Before absorption can occur folate polyglutamate must be split by the brush border enzyme folate deconjugase to folate monoglutamate. Absorption occurs only in the jejunum on specific carriers and because drugs such as sulphasalazine and phenytoin may interfere with absorption they should not be given when serum folate estimations are being carried out.

Vitamin B12 (cobalamin) is another water-soluble vitamin which is plentiful in the diet. Pepsin and acid in the stomach free vitamin B12 from dietary protein, while the acid pH favours the combination of vitamin B12 to R proteins present in saliva and gastric juice. In the duodenum proteases split the R proteins, freeing vitamin B12 which combines with intrinsic factor produced by the pancreas. The vitamin combined with intrinsic factor is then absorbed on specific carriers in the ileum (Williams 1987). Absorption cannot occur at any other site. Conditions such as atrophic gastritis, EPI, bacterial overgrowth and malabsorption may all cause reduced serum vitamin B12 levels (Batt & Morgan 1982).

The normal values for serum folate are 3.5 to 8.5 µg/l and those for vitamin B12 are 215 to 500 µg/l. Where there is proximal small intestinal disease the serum folate level falls while B12 level is maintained. Where the small intestinal disease occurs in the ileum, folate levels are maintained but B12 levels are reduced. If small intestinal disease affects the jejunum and ileum then both folate and B12 will be reduced. A high serum folate and low B12 level may suggest bacterial overgrowth, as proliferating bacteria often produce folate and bind B12. In bacterial overgrowth the xylose absorption curve is also depressed due to bacterial utilization of xylose and because of small intestinal damage caused by bacterial proliferation (Simpson 1982).

Assessment of liver disease

Because of the multifunctional nature of the liver and its great functional reserve capacity there is no single test which can be used to make a definitive diagnosis of hepatic disease. For this reason a 'liver profile' should be obtained where liver disease is suspected. This profile should include the assessment of liver enzyme levels and liver function tests as shown in Table 10.4.

Serum alanine aminotransferase (SALT)

In the dog and cat SALT is a liver-specific enzyme and elevations in this enzyme indicate active hepatocyte damage or increased membrane permeability. This occurs because the enzyme lies free within the cytoplasm of hepatocytes and is easily lost when the cell is damaged. Normal values depend on the laboratory used but range from 15 to 60 iu/l. In cases of acute hepatitis, values may increase to several thousand international units per litre. Values may be within the normal range in advanced chronic liver disease where no further active cell damage is occurring, it is therefore not a liver function test. Measurement of SALT is useful in indicating the level or degree of liver damage but it does not indicate what type of damage has occurred or what pathological changes are present.

Serum aspartate aminotransferase (SAST)

This enzyme is not liver-specific, and is found in several body tissues, including the liver and muscle. Elevations in SAST tend to follow those of SALT, so there is no real advantage in measuring this enzyme. Normal values range from 15 to 65 iu/l.

Table 10.4 Assessment of liver cell damage and function

Liver enzyme assay	SALT, SAST, SAP, GGT and bilirubin levels
Liver function tests	Plasma ammonia, serum albumin, BSP retention, bile acids.

Gamma glutamyl transferase (GGT)

The enzyme is found within hepatocytes associated with the cell membrane and is found in highest concentrations in cells located near bile caniculi. Although this enzyme is found in several other tissues, serum levels appear to reflect release of enzyme from hepatic cells. GGT is not a good indicator of hepatocellular damage but elevations are most frequently observed in cholestasis and usually in parallel with the elevation in serum alkaline phosphatase (SAP) levels. However GGT increases more slowly than SAP and tends to remain elevated for longer periods of time. Normal values for serum GGT range from 2 to 8 iu/l.

Serum alkaline phosphatase (SAP)

Alkaline phosphatase is bound to the microsomes of hepatocytes and is not free within the cytoplasm (cf. SALT). Values do not therefore increase when hepatocyte damage occurs or cell membrane permeability increases. Values do increase where there is cholestasis, as this causes increased production of the enzyme. SAP in conjunction with elevated bilirubin levels, may help to confirm cholestasis and determine the type of jaundice present (see later).

Increased values of SAP also occur in conditions unrelated to liver disease. In young animals where bone growth is occurring and in older animals with bone disorders SAP may be elevated. Metabolic conditions such as hyperparathyroidism may also elevate the SAP value. There are four isoenzymes known, one originating from the intestine, one from bone and two from the liver. The liver isoenzymes differ in their activities. One is elevated as a consequence of corticosteroid administration or in hyperadreno-corticism. The other is increased in cholestasis.

In the cat the SAP content of the liver is lower than the dog and it has a shorter half-life, being rapidly excreted in the urine. Therefore care is needed in interpreting normal SAP levels in cats, as this does not preclude the presence of cholestasis. In these cases bilirubin and GGT levels may be of more value.

Normal values of SAP range from 20 to 100 iu/l while values of more than 1000 iu/l may occur in cholestasis and metabolic disorders described above.

Serum bilirubin

Serum bilirubin is not a sensitive indicator of hepatocyte destruction, as jaundice may occur in a haemolytic crisis as well as in acute hepatitis, chronic liver failure and biliary obstruction. It therefore also reflects a state of cholestasis or excessive red cell destruction. Total serum bilirubin does not normally exceed 7 μmol/l and is composed of unconjugated and conjugated bilirubin. Clinical jaundice is observed when values are greater than 35 μmol/l. An assessment of the proportions of unconjugated to conjugated bilirubin in the jaundiced animal may help to determine the cause (Table 10.5).

Measurement of total bilirubin and the percentages of unconjugated to conjugated should be carried out. Where 90% of serum bilirubin is unconjugated and only 10% conjugated bilirubin, this suggests a haemolytic jaundice. Where the percentages are reversed this suggests an obstructive jaundice. Intermediate ratios are usually indicative of intrahepatic jaundice.

Serum bile acids

The measurement of serum bile acids in dogs and cats is rapidly replacing the BSP retention test as the routine test for assessing liver function, because the bile acids act as an endogenous dye which should normally be efficiently cleared from the circulation by the liver (Meyer & Center 1986). Following the ingestion of a large meal, bile salts are secreted into the duodenum to assist in the digestion and absorption of fat. Once this process has been completed and products of fat digestion have been absorbed across the small intestine, the bile salts themselves are resorbed in the ileum. They enter the portal vein and are normally removed by the liver for recycling. This is often termed the enterohepatic recirculation of bile salts which may occur several times during a large meal. If there is liver failure

Table 10.5 The differential diagnosis of jaundice

Parameter	Haemolytic jaundice	Hepatocellular jaundice	Biliary jaundice
Faecal colour	Dark	Normal	White
Bilirubin			
Conjugated	10%	50%	90%
Unconjugated	90%	50%	10%
Urine bilirubin	Present	Present	Present
Urobilinogen	Increased	Present	None
SAP	Normal	Normal/raised	Raised
SALT	Normal	Raised	Normal/raised
Albumin	Normal	Lowered	Normal

or a portosystemic shunt present, most of the bile salts remain in the circulation, giving elevated levels. Because there is no exogenous dye to inject and only one blood sample to be collected it has obvious attractions. Normal values lie within the range of 0 to 8 μmol/l. Values in excess of 30 μmol/l are considered significant (Simpson & Keay unpublished data). The greatest increases have been observed in cirrhosis or portosystemic shunts where values of 200 to 300 μmol/l have been observed. In other liver conditions the elevations are more variable. It is important that blood is collected from the fasted dog or cat as values may be elevated following feeding.

Plasma ammonia

Ammonia is normally absorbed from the intestine in the dog or cat. It enters the portal blood and is effectively cleared by the liver. Within the liver, ammonia is converted to urea and excreted in the kidneys. Where the portal blood by-passes the liver in conditions such as cirrhosis and porto-systemic shunts, the circulating ammonia level remains high. The normal value is usually less than 70 μmol/l, while values of more than 300 μmol/l occur in the conditions mentioned above. A compensatory fall in blood urea is often observed with values of less than 2 mmol/l. In some less-advanced forms of liver disease an ammonium tolerance test may be required in order to confirm liver dysfunction (see dynamic tests).

Radiography

Radiographic examination of the gastrointestinal tract may be of considerable assistance to the clinician in reaching a diagnosis. However the procedures adopted depend on the site and type of condition thought to be involved. In addition some conditions require sophisticated equipment in order to obtain diagnostic information, such as fluoroscopy, which may not be available to the practitioner. The clinician may require plain radiographs, contrast radiography, fluoroscopy or angiography in order to reach a diagnosis. Interpretation of radiographs can be very difficult as there is considerable normal variation which can be misinterpreted, giving a misleading diagnosis. In order to obtain the most diagnostic information from radiographs of the gastrointestinal tract their use will be considered under the following headings:

Motility disorders

Obstructions: foreign bodies, tumours, intussusceptions

Mucosal changes to small and large intestine

Liver size, position and angiography

Detection of ascites, peritonitis, abdominal masses

Motility disorders are usually associated with the swallowing process and therefore involve pharynx, oesophagus or stomach. In all these cases plain radiographs are often of little value, although occasionally they may reveal an underlying cause such as a tumour, or foreign body. Plain radiographs should always be taken in the first instance. The greatest diagnostic information however comes from contrast studies, using barium sulphate (Micropaque; Nicholas Laboratories), 2 ml/kg liveweight is given by mouth and radiographs are collected over the next 30 min depending on the progress of the barium. Fluoroscopic examination of the actual swallowing process enables oesophageal and gastric motility to be observed and provides the most accurate information. If possible such fluoroscopic examination should be recorded on video tape and examined in detail at a later date. These latter types of examination and recordings rely on costly and sophisticated equipment.

In general, barium should empty completely from the pharynx, pass along the oesophagus in one or two peristaltic contractions and enter the stomach. Very occasionally small amounts of barium will be retained in the distal cervical or thoracic oesophagus. The bulk of the barium should reach the stomach quickly and lie within the fundus. Antral contractions should occur at regular intervals moving towards the closed pylorus, forcing barium back into the body of the stomach. When liquid barium is given this should start to leave the stomach quickly, and certainly within 30 min of ingestion. The jejunum should be filling within 40 min and barium should have reached the ileocaecocolic junction within 2 h. The stomach should be empty by 3 to 5 h, with all the barium in the large intestine. Food empties from the stomach in a specific order; liquids always empty faster than solids, carbohydrates faster than fats and undigestible foods last of all.

Where liquid barium studies fail to reveal an abnormality which is thought to exist in the upper digestive tract, barium mixed in dog or cat food should be given. Sufficient barium to give some contrast to the food without masking its flavour should be added. This technique is excellent for high-lighting partial obstructions such as vascular ring anomalies, extra oesophageal masses, and problems in normal gastric motility.

Obstructions are often caused by bones or other radiodense objects which are readily detected on plain radiographs. Two views should always be taken to determine the exact location of the obstruction. With non-radiodense obstructions and intussusceptions a dilated loop of bowel is usually observed, being at least three times the diameter of normal bowel. The affected bowel loop often contains gas and 'gravel' both of which lie cranial to the obstruction. A barium meal is contraindicated in these cases, because perforation of the bowel may allow barium to escape into the abdomen where it cannot be resorbed. An iodine based product (Gastrografin; Schering Chemicals), which is resorbed from the peritoneum can however be safely used as a contrast medium in these situations.

Mucosal changes in the intestine can show up using a barium meal. Plain radiographs should be obtained before giving the barium, in order to determine the best exposure settings and to eliminate any obvious lesions. When a barium meal is given, 2 to 5 ml/kg liveweight of barium (Micropaque; Nicholas Laboratories) should be administered. If too much is given overlying loops of bowel will give a 'white out' effect with loss of definition. Too small a volume of barium will result in poor bowel filling and difficulty in interpretation.

Barium meals are expensive, time consuming and difficult to interpret as there is considerable normal morphological variation. The changes to the mucosa in malabsorption and colitis are very subtle and are rarely detected using simple, one dose barium studies. These cases require two different radiographic views every 30 min to 1 h. Even if an abnormality is detected, a biopsy is necessary to obtain a definitive diagnosis. The authors rarely use barium meals in the investigation of small and large intestinal disease unless some gross abnormality motility disorder or obstruction is thought to be

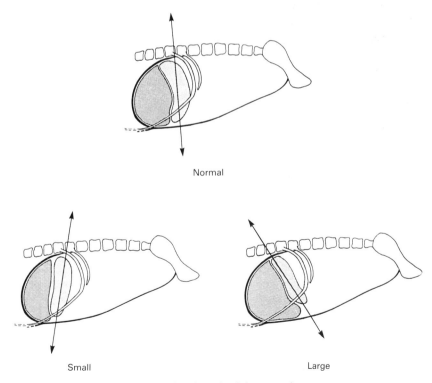

Normal

Small   Large

Fig. 10.6 Assessment of liver size using the axis of the stomach.

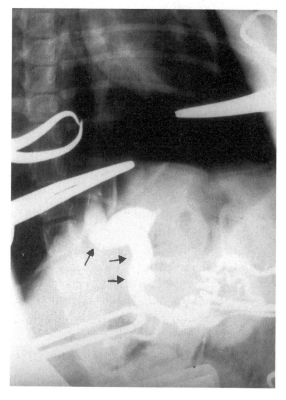

Fig. 10.7 Portal angiography showing (arrowed) the large blood vessel carrying blood past the liver.

present. Biochemical and dynamic tests together with biopsy collection and endoscopic examination are used to greater effect.

Radiographic assessment of the size and shape of the liver is important in determining the best site for liver biopsy. The longitudinal axis of the stomach may be used to assess changes in liver size (Fig. 10.6). Increases in liver size may be observed in hepatitis, Cushing's disease and neoplasia, while reduced liver size may be observed in advanced cirrhosis and porto-systemic shunts. Angiography is useful in providing a definitive diagnosis of a portosystemic shunt by delineating the aberrant blood vessel which shunts portal blood away from the liver and directly into the vena cava. Once located in this way the vessel can be ligated surgically.

Portoangiography is carried out under general anaesthesia to allow a laparotomy to be performed together with easy access to good X-ray facilities. A mesenteric blood vessel is cannulated and a radiodense dye (Conray 420; RMB Animal Health) injected. Lateral radiographs are taken over the next

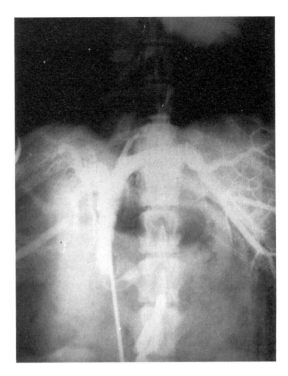

Fig. 10.8 Portal angiography following surgical correction of the portosystemic shunt, showing blood now entering into the substance of the liver.

10 min and should highlight the large blood vessel bypassing the liver (Fig. 10.7). Once located the vessel may be partially ligated and the dye injected again when the more normal tree-like branching of blood vessels in the liver should be observed (Fig. 10.8).

Ascites and peritonitis may be suspected on clinical examination and confirmed by radiological examination. Plain radiographs will reveal a loss of contrast or a 'ground glass' appearance within the abdomen, which may in the case of peritonitis be focal or general, and in the case of ascites appears generalized. Ascites may be better recognized by taking a standing lateral radiograph which will reveal an obvious fluid line, whereas in peritonitis the uniform ground glass appearance will persist.

References

Batt R.M. & Mann L.C. (1981) Specificity of the BT-PABA test for the diagnosis of exocrine pancreatic insufficiency in the dog. *Veterinary Record*, **108**; 303–307.

Batt R.M. & Morgan J.O. (1982) Role of serum folate and vitamin B12 concentrations in the differentiation of small intestinal abnormalities in the dog. *Research in Veterinary Science*, **32**; 17–22.

Bush B.M. (1980) The laboratory evaluation of canine hepatic disease. *The Veterinary Annual*. C.S.G. Grunsell F.W.G. Hill & M.E. Raw (eds). Scientechnica, Bristol, 57–65.

Drazner F.H. (1983) Hepatic encephalopathy in the dog. In: *Current Veterinary Therapy VIII*. R.W. Kirk (ed.), W.B. Saunders, Philadelphia, 829–834.

Else R.W. (1989) Biopsy — Special techniques and tissues. *In Practice*, **11**; 27–34.

Hill F.W.G., Kidder D.E. & Frew J. (1970) A xylose absorption test for the dog. *Veterinary Record*, **87**; 250–255.

Meyer D.J. & Center S.A. (1986) Approach to the diagnosis of liver disorders in dogs and cats. *Compendium on Continuing Education for the Practicing Veterinarian*, **8**; 880–888.

Simpson J.W. (1982) Bacterial overgrowth causing intestinal malabsorption in a dog. *Veterinary Record*, **110**; 335–336.

Simpson J.W. & Doxey D.L. (1988) Evaluation of faecal analysis as an aid to the detection of exocrine pancreatic insufficiency. *British Veterinary Journal*, **144**; 174–178.

Simpson J.W. & Else R.W. (1987) Diagnostic value of tissue biopsy in gastrointestinal and liver disease. *Veterinary Record*, **120**; 230–233.

Williams D.A. & Batt R.M. (1983) Diagnosis of canine exocrine pancreatic insufficiency by the assay of serum trypsin-like immunoreactivity. *Journal of Small Animal Practice*, **24**; 583–588.

Williams D.A. (1987) New tests of pancreatic and small intestinal function. *Compendium on Continuing Education for the Practicing Veterinarian*, **9**; 1167–1174.

Index